Health Reference Series

Fourth Edition

Adolescent Health

SOURCEBOOK

Basic Consumer Health Information about Adolescent Growth and Development, Puberty, Sexuality, Reproductive Health, and Physical, Emotional, Social, and Mental Health Concerns of Teens and Their Parents, Including Facts about Nutrition, Physical Activity, Weight Management, Acne, Allergies, Cancer, Diabetes, Growth Disorders, Juvenile Arthritis, Infections, Substance Abuse, and More

Along with Information about Adolescent Safety Concerns, Youth Violence, a Glossary of Related Terms, and a Directory of Resources

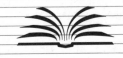

OMNIGRAPHICS

615 Griswold, Ste. 901, Detroit, MI 48226

Bibliographic Note
Because this page cannot legibly accommodate all the copyright notices, the Bibliographic
Note portion of the Preface constitutes an extension of the copyright notice.

* * *

OMNIGRAPHICS
Siva Ganesh Maharaja, *Managing Editor*
***

Copyright © 2018 Omnigraphics

ISBN 978-0-7808-1611-4
E-ISBN 978-0-7808-1612-1

Library of Congress Cataloging-in-Publication Data

Names: Omnigraphics, Inc., issuing body.

Title: Adolescent health sourcebook: basic consumer health information about
adolescent growth and development, puberty, sexuality, reproductive health,
and physical, emotional, social, and mental health concerns of teens and their
parents, including facts about nutrition, physical activity, weight management,
acne, allergies, cancer, diabetes, growth disorders, juvenile arthritis, infections,
substance abuse, and more; along with information about adolescent safety
concerns, youth violence, a glossary of related terms, and a directory of resources.

Description: Fourth edition. | Detroit, MI: Omnigraphics, [2018] | Series: Health
reference series | Includes bibliographical references and index.

Identifiers: LCCN 2017048576 (print) | LCCN 2017049634 (ebook) | ISBN
9780780816121 (eBook) | ISBN 9780780816114 (hardcover: alk. paper)

Subjects: LCSH: Teenagers--Health and hygiene. | Adolescent psychology. |
Consumer education. | Adolescence.

Classification: LCC RJ140 (ebook) | LCC RJ140.A335 2018 (print) | DDC
616.89/140835--dc23

LC record available at https://lccn.loc.gov/2017048576

Table of Contents

Preface xv

Part I: An Overview of Adolescent Health

Chapter 1 — Statistics on Adolescent Health in the
United States 3

Chapter 2 — Understanding Adolescent Health 15

Chapter 3 — Physical and Emotional Changes in
Teens 21

Chapter 4 — Understanding Adolescent Brain
Development 25

Chapter 5 — Key Indicators of Adolescent
Well-Being... 33

Chapter 6 — For Parents: Talking to Teens about
Health Issues 59

    Section 6.1 — Positive Parenting 60

    Section 6.2 — Communicating with Your
        Child 63

    Section 6.3 — Talking about Substance
        Abuse 67

    Section 6.4 — Talking about Healthy
        Relationships 72

    Section 6.5 — Talking about Sex....................... 75

Section 6.6 — Monitoring Your Teen's
Activities 80

Chapter 7 — For Teens: Talking to Your Parents
or Guardians 83

Part II: Staying Healthy during Adolescence

Chapter 8 — Medical Care and Your Teen............................... 89

Section 8.1 — What to Expect at the
Doctor's Office
(Ages 11 to 14)............................. 90

Section 8.2 — What to Expect at the
Doctor's Office
(Ages 15 to 17)............................. 95

Section 8.3 — Vaccines Teens Need 100

Chapter 9 — Nutrition Recommendations for Teens............... 103

Chapter 10 — Healthy Food Choices for Teens 109

Chapter 11 — Calcium, Vitamin D, and Teens.......................... 113

Section 11.1 — Facts about Calcium 114

Section 11.2 — Facts about Vitamin D 121

Chapter 12 — Teens and Caffeine Use.. 127

Section 12.1 — Energy Drinks........................... 128

Section 12.2 — Caffeine and Its Effects on
the Body 130

Chapter 13 — Physical Activity and Teens................................ 133

Section 13.1 — Physical Activity Facts............. 134

Section 13.2 — Importance of Physical
Activity 136

Section 13.3 — Physical Activity Guidelines
for Children and Adolescents... 138

Chapter 14 — Weight Management in Teens 143

Section 14.1 — Understanding Your Teen's
Body Mass Index
Measurement 144

Section 14.2—Helping Your Overweight
            Child 148

Section 14.3—Tips to Help Teens to Lose
            Weight 153

Chapter 15—Body Image in Youth 157

Section 15.1—For Teens: Developing
            Body Image and Self-Esteem ... 158

Section 15.2—Why Do Teens Get Cosmetic
            Surgery? 162

Chapter 16—Sleep and Adolescents 165

Section 16.1—Sleep Deprivation among
            Teens 166

Section 16.2—Sleep-Smart Tips for Teens 169

Part III: Puberty, Sexuality, and Reproductive Health

Chapter 17—Overview of Reproductive and Sexual
            Health Trends in Teens 175

Chapter 18—Male Reproductive System and Puberty 181

Chapter 19—Male Reproductive Concerns 187

Section 19.1—Erectile Dysfunction 188

Section 19.2—Disorders of the Scrotum
            and Testicles 197

Section 19.3—Testicular Cancer and Self-
            Examination............................. 200

Section 19.4—Gynecomastia (Male Breast
            Development) 206

Chapter 20—Female Reproductive System and
            Puberty 211

Chapter 21—Menstruation and the Menstrual Cycle 219

Chapter 22—Female Reproductive Health Concerns 227

Section 22.1—Why See a Gynecologist? 228

Section 22.2—Premenstrual
            Syndrome (PMS)...................... 231

vii

Section 22.3—Menstrual Irregularities 237

Section 22.4—Vaginal Yeast Infections 240

Section 22.5—Vaginal Discharge Concerns 245

Chapter 23—Precocious and Delayed Puberty........................ 251

Section 23.1—Precocious Puberty 252

Section 23.2—Delayed Puberty 257

Chapter 24—Teaching Teens about Sexual Activity 261

Section 24.1—Making Healthy Sexual
Decisions 262

Section 24.2—Facts on Sex Education in the
United States 266

Chapter 25—Sexually Transmitted Diseases (STDs)
and Their Prevention... 273

Section 25.1—Frequently Asked
Questions about STDs and
STIs 274

Section 25.2—Human Immunodeficiency
Virus (HIV) Testing among
Adolescents............................... 279

Section 25.3—Vaccine to Prevent Human
Papillomavirus.......................... 281

Section 25.4—Practicing Safer Sex 287

Chapter 26—Understanding Abstinence................................. 293

Chapter 27—Birth Control Methods (Contraception) 297

Chapter 28—Teen Pregnancy 313

Section 28.1—Statistics on Teen Pregnancy
in the United States 314

Section 28.2—Could I Get Pregnant If...?....... 316

Section 28.3—Prenatal Care for Pregnant
Teens 318

Section 28.4—Teen Parents... You're Not
Alone!....................................... 320

Chapter 29—Lesbian, Gay, Bisexual, and
Transgender Youth... 323

Part IV: Common Health Concerns of Teens and Their Parents

Chapter 30—Dealing with Chronic Health Problems 329

Chapter 31—Acne 333

Chapter 32—Allergies in Adolescents 339

Chapter 33—Asthma and Teens 343

Chapter 34—Cancer in Childhood and Adolescence................. 347

Chapter 35—Diabetes in Children and Teens 355

Chapter 36—Growing Concerns.. 359

    Section 36.1—Growing Pains........................ 360

    Section 36.2—Common Growth
                Disorders 363

Chapter 37—Juvenile Arthritis 365

Chapter 38—Infections Often Spread in Schools..................... 369

    Section 38.1—Preventing Influenza in
                Schools.................................... 370

    Section 38.2—Meningococcal Infection on
                Campus.................................... 375

    Section 38.3—Staphylococcal Infections
                in Teens.................................. 380

    Section 38.4—Mononucleosis........................ 386

Chapter 39—Malocclusion.. 389

Chapter 40—Scoliosis 393

Part V: Emotional, Social, and Mental Health Concerns in Adolescents

Chapter 41—Adolescent Stress... 399

Chapter 42—School Pressures 403

    Section 42.1—Test Anxiety............................ 404

    Section 42.2—Cheating................................. 409

    Section 42.3—Helping Your Child Feel
                Connected to School................. 412

Chapter 43—Adolescent Social Development and
    Concerns 417

    Section 43.1—Encouraging Healthy
                 Relationships: Tips to Help
                 Your Child 418

    Section 43.2—Peer Pressure 421

    Section 43.3—Parental Monitoring 425

Chapter 44—Facts about Mental Health Disorders in
    Adolescents 431

Chapter 45—Treating Mental Health Disorders in
    Teens 435

Chapter 46—Depression 441

    Section 46.1—Depression in Teens 442

    Section 46.2—Antidepressants and
                 Teens 446

Chapter 47—Other Common Mental Health
    Disorders Affecting Adolescents 451

    Section 47.1—Anxiety Disorders 452

    Section 47.2—Attention Deficit
                 Hyperactivity Disorder
                 (ADHD) 457

    Section 47.3—Behavior or Conduct
                 Problems 464

    Section 47.4—Bipolar Disorder in
                 Children and Teens 467

    Section 47.5—Borderline Personality
                 Disorder 472

    Section 47.6—Eating Disorders 478

    Section 47.7—Obsessive-Compulsive
                 Disorder (OCD) 482

    Section 47.8—Schizophrenia 486

    Section 47.9—Tics and Tourette
                 Syndrome in Youth 490

Chapter 48—Understanding Self-Harm 493

Chapter 49—Teen Suicide... 497

Part VI: Substance Abuse and Adolescents

Chapter 50—Addiction and the Adolescent Brain.................... 503

Chapter 51—Preventing and Treating Substance
    Abuse... 509

Chapter 52—Smoking and Nicotine Use among
    Adolescents... 515

    Section 52.1—Nicotine Addiction 516

    Section 52.2—Smokeless Tobacco.................... 520

    Section 52.3—Hookah (Water Pipe)
        Smoking....................................... 523

    Section 52.4—Smoking and How to Quit........ 526

Chapter 53—Alcohol Use among Adolescents......................... 531

    Section 53.1—Underage Drinking.................. 532

    Section 53.2—Talk to Your Child about
        Alcohol....................................... 534

Chapter 54—Marijuana Use among Adolescents 539

Chapter 55—Prescription Medicine Abuse 547

Chapter 56—Inhalants... 563

Chapter 57—Helping Your Teen Who Has a
    Problem with Drugs... 569

Part VII: Adolescent Safety Concerns

Chapter 58—Youth Risk Behavior Surveillance
    System (YRBSS) 579

Chapter 59—Driving Safety for Teens 583

    Section 59.1—Facts about Teen Drivers......... 584

    Section 59.2—Teen Driving Risks 587

    Section 59.3—Role of Parents in Guiding
        Teens for Safe Driving.............. 591

Chapter 60—Internet Safety 597

    Section 60.1—Electronic Aggression 598

    Section 60.2—Sextortion................................ 600

    Section 60.3—Social Networking Sites:
                  Safety Tips for Teens................ 603

Chapter 61—Skin Safety Concerns 609

    Section 61.1—Cosmetics 610

    Section 61.2—Safe Hair Removal................... 614

    Section 61.3—The Risks of Tanning............... 616

    Section 61.4—Tattoos and Teens.................... 622

    Section 61.5—Tinea Infections: Ringworm,
                  Athlete's Foot, and Jock Itch.... 625

Chapter 62—Work Safety for Teens 633

Chapter 63—Other Teen Safety Concerns 639

    Section 63.1—Concussion 640

    Section 63.2—Noise and Hearing Damage 643

    Section 63.3—Repetitive Stress Injuries in
                  Teens 648

Part VIII: Violence against Adolescents

Chapter 64—Youth Violence: A Public Health
               Problem 655

    Section 64.1—Understanding Youth
                  Violence 656

    Section 64.2—Statistics on Youth Violence 658

    Section 64.3—Youth Violence Risk and
                  Protective Factors..................... 661

Chapter 65—Bullying and Other Types of
               Aggressive Behavior 665

    Section 65.1—Understanding Bullying........... 666

    Section 65.2—Facts and Statistics on
                  Bullying..................................... 671

    Section 65.3—Stalking.................................... 673

    Section 65.4—Hazing 677

Chapter 66—Dating Violence and Abusive
Relationships 679

Chapter 67—Sexual Assault 683

Chapter 68—Youth Gangs and Violence 693

Chapter 69—Coping with Violence and Trauma 701

Part IX: Additional Help and Information

Chapter 70—Glossary of Terms about Adolescent
Health.. 711

Chapter 71—Directory of Adolescent Health
Organizations for Parents and Teens.................. 717

Index... 731

Preface

About This Book

Adolescents (ages 10 to 17) and young adults (ages 18 to 25) make up 22% of the United States population. During adolescence, as teenagers transition into adulthood, they experience significant physical, mental, and emotional changes. The choices they make during this period can have profound ramifications on their health and well-being. Teens who get involved in unhealthy or risky behaviors—such as substance abuse, unprotected sexual activity, or dangerous driving— may find themselves at risk for long-term, even lifelong health consequences. In addition, because social connections are so critical during the adolescent years, the demands of friendships, peer pressure, and other relationship stresses can complicate healthy decision-making processes.

Adolescent Health Sourcebook, Fourth Edition offers parents and teens basic information about growth and development during adolescence and related safety issues. It discusses the importance of routine medical care, adequate nutrition, physical activity, and sleep. It offers facts about reproductive development and the health consequences of sexual decisions. It also describes many of the most common health problems that affect adolescents, including acne, allergies, asthma, diabetes, and infections. Emotional, social, and mental health concerns—including depression, anxiety disorders, self-injury, suicide, and addictions—are also discussed. The book concludes with a glossary of related terms and a directory of resources for additional help and information.

How to Use This Book

This book is divided into parts and chapters. Parts focus on broad areas of interest. Chapters are devoted to single topics within a part.

Part I: An Overview of Adolescent Health discusses the physical, mental, and emotional components of adolescent well-being, and emerging issues related to them. Facts about brain development during the teen years, the role of risk taking during the transition to adulthood, and also includes the challenges of parent-teen communication.

Part II: Staying Healthy during Adolescence explores strategies teens can take to promote good health. These include getting recommended physical activities, vaccinations, eating right, exercising, limiting caffeine use, managing weight, and avoiding sleep deprivation.

Part III: Puberty, Sexuality, and Reproductive Health provides detailed information about gender-related concerns. For males, these issues include testicular self-exams, disorders of the testes, and gynecomastia (male breast development). For females, topics include menstruation and the menstrual cycle, and vaginal yeast infections. This part also offers information about sexually transmitted diseases, sexual abstinence, birth control, and teen pregnancy.

Part IV: Common Health Concerns of Teens and Their Parents discusses chronic health conditions that may affect adolescents. These include acne, allergies, asthma, cancer, diabetes, growth disorders, juvenile arthritis, and infectious diseases spread in schools.

Part V: Emotional, Social, and Mental Health Concerns in Adolescents identifies stresses, pressures, and disorders that interfere with a teen's ability to function at home, work, and school, including depression, anxiety disorders, attention deficit hyperactivity disorder, bipolar disorder, eating disorders, self-injury, obsessive-compulsive disorder, schizophrenia, tics, and Tourette syndrome. Information about the risk factors, warning signs of adolescent suicide, and need for parental monitoring is also included.

Part VI: Substance Abuse and Adolescents provides information about why teens are susceptible to addiction and discusses risk factors and treatment strategies for the most commonly abused substances, including nicotine, alcohol, marijuana, prescription medications, and inhalants.

Part VII: Adolescent Safety Concerns offers advice on preventing adolescent injuries and accidents. Teens and parents will find information on reducing the risk of motor vehicle accidents, avoiding online sexual solicitation and electronic aggression, and averting problems with body piercings, tattoos, and other skin issues. Tips on staying safe at work and preventing sports injuries are also included.

Part VIII: Violence against Adolescents identifies factors that protect teens against violence, such as family support, academic achievement, and community infrastructure. Adolescent aggression, which may take the form of bullying, hazing, choking games, dating violence, abusive violence, sexual assault, and gang-related activity, is discussed.

Part IX: Additional Help and Information provides a glossary of important terms related to adolescence. A directory of organizations that provide health information to teens and their parents and a list of hotlines and referral services specifically for teens in trouble are also included.

Bibliographic Note

This volume contains documents and excerpts from publications issued by the following government agencies: Centers for Disease Control and Prevention (CDC); Child Welfare Information Gateway; The Cool Spot; *Eunice Kennedy Shriver* National Institute of Child Health and Human Development (NICHD); Federal Bureau of Investigation (FBI); Federal Interagency Forum on Child and Family Statistics; Genetic and Rare Diseases Information Center (GARD); National Cancer Institute (NCI); National Center for Complementary and Integrative Health (NCCIH); National Heart, Lung, and Blood Institute (NHLBI); National Highway Traffic Safety Administration (NHTSA); National Institute of Arthritis and Musculoskeletal and Skin Diseases (NIAMS); National Institute of Diabetes and Digestive and Kidney Diseases (NIDDK); National Institute of Justice (NIJ); National Institute of Mental Health (NIMH); National Institute on Alcohol Abuse and Alcoholism (NIAAA); National Institute on Deafness and Other Communication Disorders (NIDCD); National Institute on Drug Abuse (NIDA) for Teens; National Institutes of Health (NIH); National Women's Health Information Center (NWHIC); *NIH News in Health*; Office of Dietary Supplements (ODS); Office of Disease Prevention and Health

Promotion (ODPHP); Office of the Surgeon General (OGS); Office on Women's Health (OWH); U.S. Department of Agriculture (USDA); U.S. Department of Health and Human Services (HHS); U.S. Department of Justice (DOJ); U.S. Department of Veterans Affairs (VA); U.S. Food and Drug Administration (FDA); United States Computer Emergency Readiness Team (US-CERT); and Youth.gov.

It may also contain original material produced by Omnigraphics and reviewed by medical consultants.

About the Health Reference Series

The *Health Reference Series* is designed to provide basic medical information for patients, families, caregivers, and the general public. Each volume takes a particular topic and provides comprehensive coverage. This is especially important for people who may be dealing with a newly diagnosed disease or a chronic disorder in themselves or in a family member. People looking for preventive guidance, information about disease warning signs, medical statistics, and risk factors for health problems will also find answers to their questions in the *Health Reference Series*. The *Series*, however, is not intended to serve as a tool for diagnosing illness, in prescribing treatments, or as a substitute for the physician/patient relationship. All people concerned about medical symptoms or the possibility of disease are encouraged to seek professional care from an appropriate healthcare provider.

A Note about Spelling and Style

Health Reference Series editors use *Stedman's Medical Dictionary* as an authority for questions related to the spelling of medical terms and the *Chicago Manual of Style* for questions related to grammatical structures, punctuation, and other editorial concerns. Consistent adherence is not always possible, however, because the individual volumes within the *Series* include many documents from a wide variety of different producers, and the editor's primary goal is to present material from each source as accurately as is possible. This sometimes means that information in different chapters or sections may follow other guidelines and alternate spelling authorities. For example, occasionally a copyright holder may require that eponymous terms be shown in possessive forms (Crohn's disease vs. Crohn disease) or that British spelling norms be retained (leukaemia vs. leukemia).

Medical Review

Omnigraphics contracts with a team of qualified, senior medical professionals who serve as medical consultants for the *Health Reference Series*. As necessary, medical consultants review reprinted and originally written material for currency and accuracy. Citations including the phrase, "Reviewed (month, year)" indicate material reviewed by this team. Medical consultation services are provided to the *Health Reference Series* editors by:

Dr. Vijayalakshmi, MBBS, DGO, MD
Dr. Senthil Selvan, MBBS, DCH, MD
Dr. K. Sivanandham, MBBS, DCH, MS (Research), PhD

Our Advisory Board

We would like to thank the following board members for providing initial guidance on the development of this series:

- Dr. Lynda Baker, Associate Professor of Library and Information Science, Wayne State University, Detroit, MI
- Nancy Bulgarelli, William Beaumont Hospital Library, Royal Oak, MI
- Karen Imarisio, Bloomfield Township Public Library, Bloomfield Township, MI
- Karen Morgan, Mardigian Library, University of Michigan-Dearborn, Dearborn, MI
- Rosemary Orlando, St. Clair Shores Public Library, St. Clair Shores, MI

Health Reference Series *Update Policy*

The inaugural book in the *Health Reference Series* was the first edition of *Cancer Sourcebook* published in 1989. Since then, the *Series* has been enthusiastically received by librarians and in the medical community. In order to maintain the standard of providing high-quality health information for the layperson the editorial staff at Omnigraphics felt it was necessary to implement a policy of updating volumes when warranted.

Medical researchers have been making tremendous strides, and it is the purpose of the *Health Reference Series* to stay current with the most recent advances. Each decision to update a volume is made on an individual basis. Some of the considerations include how much new information is available and the feedback we receive from people who use the books. If there is a topic you would like to see added to the update list, or an area of medical concern you feel has not been adequately addressed, please write to:

Managing Editor
Health Reference Series
Omnigraphics
615 Griswold, Ste. 901
Detroit, MI 48226

Part One

An Overview of Adolescent Health

Chapter 1

Statistics on Adolescent Health in the United States

More than 12 percent of people in the United States—almost 42 million—are between the ages of 10 and 19. These adolescents are increasingly diverse and reflect the changing racial/ethnic, socioeconomic, and geographic structure of the U.S. population.

As young people develop their identities and habits, these diverse characteristics are connected to their health outcomes and access to services. If adults who work with youth understand the demographic characteristics and diversity of adolescents, they can do a better job of planning and delivering health services to this population.

Number of Adolescents

Adolescents make up 13.2 percent of the population. As the U.S. population ages, adolescents will represent a smaller proportion of the total. By 2050, estimates show that adolescents will make up 11.2 percent of the population. While adolescents are predicted to represent a smaller portion of the total population, estimates show that the number of adolescents in the population will continue to grow, reaching almost 45 million in 2050.

This chapter includes text excerpted from "The Changing Face of America's Adolescents," U.S. Department of Health and Human Services (HHS), November 1, 2016.

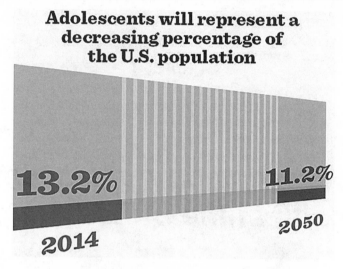

**Adolescents will represent a
decreasing percentage of
the U.S. population**

13.2%   11.2%

2014   2050

Figure 1.1. *Adolescent Population in the United States*

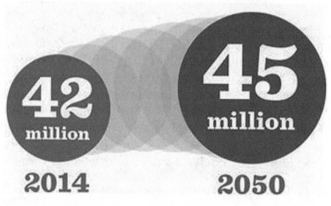

42 million   45 million

2014   2050

Figure 1.2. *Adolescent Population Projection*

(Source: 2014 Current Population Survey Estimate and the 2012 National Population Projections Middle Series.)

Age and Gender

There are important developmental, physical, and behavioral differences between younger (10–14) and older (15–19) adolescents. For instance, older youth are more likely to engage in unsafe behaviors—including drug use and risky sexual activity—than are younger teens.

There are also differences between male and female adolescents in risky health behaviors. For example, male adolescents are more likely to

4

use tobacco, alcohol, and other drugs while female adolescents are more likely to be physically inactive and to engage in unhealthy eating behaviors (such as intentionally vomiting and skipping meals), which often leads to eating disorders to control their weight and body composition.

Differences by age and gender also show up in how adolescents use health services. For example, as they get older, male adolescents are less likely to see a doctor than female adolescents. Professional guidelines recommend that providers spend some time alone with adolescent patients during health visits. This one-on-one time helps build a relationship with a health professional, encourages adolescents to share health information, and improves adolescents' ability to manage their healthcare.

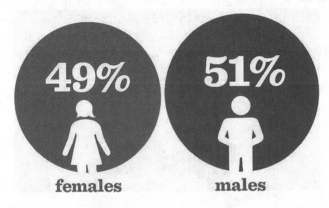

Figure 1.3. *Adolescents by Gender*

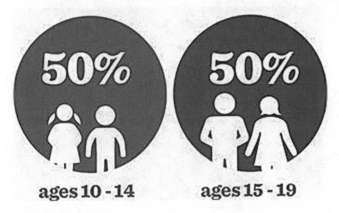

Figure 1.4. *Adolescents by Age*

(Source: Table 3 of Current Population Survey. Projections of the population by sex and selected age groups for the United States: 2015 to 2060.)

Race and Ethnicity

Differences by race/ethnicity in access to healthcare, health-related behaviors, and health outcomes are widely known. Members of racial and ethnic minority groups, in general, have less access to healthcare, experience more serious health conditions, and have higher mortality rates than whites. In part, these disparities reflect higher poverty rates among racial and ethnic minorities, which are also linked to poorer health. Health professionals can improve the delivery of services to minority youth by incorporating culturally informed practices.

The proportion of adolescents who are racial and ethnic minorities is expected to rise in the future. More than half of U.S. adolescents (54%) were white in 2014, but by 2050 that proportion is projected to drop to 40 percent as Hispanic and multiracial teens, in particular, come to represent a larger share of the population. Health equity among the diverse adolescent population will be difficult to achieve if racial and ethnic disparities are not addressed.

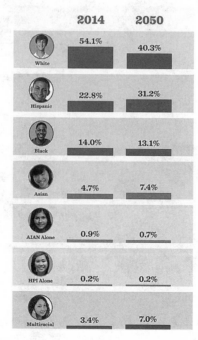

Figure 1.5. *Race and Ethnicity of America's Adolescents*

(Source: Current Population Survey: Projected Population by Single Year of Age, Sex, Race, and Hispanic Origin for the United States: 2014 to 2060.)

Hispanics/Latinos can be of any race. As listed all race categories, except for Hispanic and multiracial, exclude Hispanics/Latinos. AIAN stands for American Indian Alaska Native. HPI stands for Hawaiian or Other Pacific Islander.

Socioeconomic Status

Poverty is a reality for many adolescents in the United States. In 2014, almost one in five adolescents (18%) were living in families with incomes below the federal poverty line (defined as an income of $23,850 or less for a family of four with two children in 2014). Poverty rates were especially high for children growing up in a single-parent family.

Growing up in poverty can have negative health implications for adolescents. Compared to adolescents in higher income families, adolescents in lower income families have worse academic outcomes. These adolescents are also more likely to suffer from behavioral or emotional problems and engage in unhealthy behaviors, such as smoking and early initiation of sexual activity.

In general, low-income adolescents have also been more likely to be uninsured. However, the Patient Protection and Affordable Care Act (ACA) of 2010 has expanded health insurance coverage in recent years. As a result, more than nine in 10 adolescents ages 10 to 19 (91%) now have health insurance. Still, almost two million adolescents between the ages of 12 and 17 lacked health insurance in 2014.

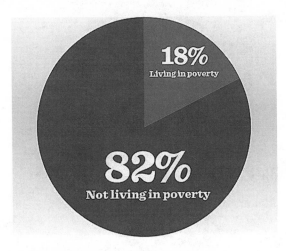

Figure 1.6. *Poverty Status*

Not including youth in foster care or those under the age of 15 living with nonrelatives

Geographic Location

Where adolescents live affects the number and types of services that they can access and their health behaviors. Most adolescents in the United States live in or just outside an urban area. Adolescents in urban areas, particularly those who live in poverty, may be exposed to higher levels of certain environmental toxins, violent crime, and may live in neighborhoods with limited options to purchase healthy food. However, urban children are more likely than rural children to have access to community or recreation centers and parks or playgrounds.

More than six million adolescents live in a rural area. Rural adolescents are more likely to be poor than adolescents in urban areas. They also face barriers to accessing health services due to a shortage of providers and transportation challenges. Moreover, mental health services are notably limited in rural areas. Youth in rural areas, compared to youth in urban areas, are more likely to be overweight or obese, to spend more time watching television or videos, and to live with someone who smokes. Nevertheless, rural children (particularly those in small rural areas) are more likely than other children to share a meal with their family every day of the week and attend religious services at least weekly—both of which are linked to more positive health outcomes.

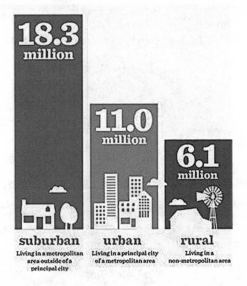

Figure 1.7. *Where Adolescents Live*

Note: Nearly six million adolescents (6,013,724) live in a "not identified" Census area. (Source: U.S. Census Bureau. (2014). Current Population Survey, Annual Social and Economic Supplement, 2014.)

A Picture of Adolescent Health

The adolescent years are critical for teens' current and future health. Good health enables adolescents to learn and grow. While adolescents are generally healthy, mental health, substance abuse, obesity, and risky sexual behaviors are common problems adolescents come across. These health issues can have long-term effects; however, they are often avoided by having supportive relationships and healthy communities. Here's how America's teens measure up.

Physical Health and Nutrition

Physical Activity

In 2013, male high school students (57%) were much more likely than female high school students (37%) to report getting the recommended 60 minutes of physical activity on five or more days in the past week. Overall, just under half of all high school students (47%) said they were physically active in a biennial national survey. Regular and continued physical activity promotes overall health and helps people achieve or maintain a healthy weight.

Note: The Youth Risk Behavior Surveillance System (YRBS) defines this measure as: "Physically active at least 60 minutes per day on 5 or more days in the past seven days; doing any kind of physical activity that increased their heart rate and made them breathe hard some of the time."

Obesity

In 2011–12, about one in five adolescents ages 12 to 19 (21%) were categorized as obese. About the same percentage of female adolescents (21%) and male adolescents (20%) were obese. When added together the number of overweight or obese adolescents was more than one in three (35 percent). Being overweight can increase the risk of health problems, such as cardiovascular disease, Type 2 diabetes, high cholesterol, and asthma.

Note: The National Health and Nutrition Examination Survey (NHANES) includes a physical examination where weight and height are measured, which was used to calculate body mass index (BMI). NHANES defines obese as: "In children and adolescents aged 2 to 19 years, obesity was defined as a BMI at or above the 95th percentile of the Centers for Disease Control and Prevention (CDC) sex-specific BMI-for-age growth charts from 2000."

Chronic Conditions

Almost one in three adolescents ages 12–17 (31%) had at least one chronic health condition in 2011–12, with 13 percent of adolescents having two or more conditions. Chronic health conditions can interfere with many activities. Teens with chronic conditions can benefit from having information about their condition, including ways to manage symptoms appropriately.

Asthma—the single most common chronic condition among adolescents—affected more than one in five high school students (21%) in 2013. It is a leading cause of hospitalization among children under age 15, which can lead to school absences. Males and females are equally likely to have asthma.

Note: The National Survey of Children's Health defines this measure as: "Chronic conditions surveyed include learning disability; Attention Deficit Disorder (ADD) or Attention Deficit Hyperactivity Disorder (ADHD); depression; anxiety problems; behavioral or conduct problems; autism or other autism spectrum disorder; developmental delay; speech problems; asthma; diabetes; Tourette Syndrome; epilepsy or seizure disorder; hearing problems; vision problems; bone or joint problems; and brain injury or concussion. For each condition, parent respondents were asked whether they have ever been told by a healthcare professional that the adolescent has the condition, and whether the adolescent currently has the condition."

Mental Health

Depression

A surprisingly high number of students report depression during adolescence. Female high school students (39%) were almost twice as likely as male high school students (21%) to report depressive symptoms. In 2013, three in 10 high school students (30%) reported symptoms of depression in the past year. Of students diagnosed with a major depressive episode, more than six in 10 did not receive treatment. Untreated depression can lead to serious health risks, including suicide. However, effective treatments exist and intervening promptly, before symptoms get more serious, could help.

Note: The YRBS measure of feeling sad or hopeless asks whether students felt so sad or hopeless almost every day for 2 or more weeks in a row that they stopped doing some usual activities. Persistent sadness can be a symptom or precursor of clinical depression, though this is not enough for a clinical diagnosis.

Attention Deficit Hyperactivity Disorder

In 2013, one in nine adolescents ages 12–17 (11%) experienced attention deficit hyperactivity disorder (ADHD). Adolescent males were more than twice as likely to be diagnosed with ADHD as adolescent females (16% versus 7%). Untreated ADHD can interfere with family and peer relationships, lead to unintended injury, and negatively affect academic performance.

Note: The National Health Interview Survey (NHIS) defines this measure as: "Has a doctor or health professional ever told you that [child's name] had attention deficit hyperactivity disorder (ADHD) or attention deficit disorder (ADD)?"

Reproductive Health

Sexual Activity

Teens who delay first sex are more likely to use contraception and have fewer sexual partners, lowering their risk of teen pregnancy and sexually transmitted diseases. In 2013, almost half of high school students (47%) reported they had sexual intercourse (46% of females and 48% of males).

Note: The YRBS defines this measure as "ever had sexual intercourse."

Substance Abuse

Tobacco Use

Tobacco use is one of the leading causes of preventable death and disease. Most smokers begin smoking in adolescence.

In 2013, about one in 13 adolescents ages 12–17 (8%) reported having used one or more tobacco products, including cigarettes, chewing tobacco, snuff, cigars, and pipe tobacco during the past month. In 2014, almost one in 15 high school seniors (7%) identified as being a daily smoker, and almost one in seven (14%) had smoked at least once in the previous month. In 2014, more teenagers smoked electronic cigarettes (or e-cigarettes) than smoked tobacco cigarettes.

Drinking Alcohol

In 2013, more than one in three high school students (35%) reported drinking alcohol in the past month (34% for males and 35% for females). Binge drinking is the most common form of alcohol abuse among adolescents, although any consumption may be harmful.

Note: YRBS defines this measure as: "Had at least one drink of alcohol on at least one day 30 days prior to taking the survey."

Substance-Free Status

In 2013, the majority of 8th to 12th grade students reported that they were substance free (they didn't use tobacco, alcohol, or illicit drugs in the past month). Students in the 8th grade (86%) were more likely to be substance free than 10th grade students (66%) and 12th grade students (52%). Use of tobacco, alcohol, and drugs is associated with numerous adverse health outcomes.

Educational Attainment

Good health promotes education and education promotes good health. Healthy students are generally better learners than their peers who lack healthy behaviors. In addition, youth who perform better in school and complete more education are healthier over the course of their adult lives. They engage in fewer risky behaviors such as smoking and binge drinking and participate in healthier behaviors such as exercise, which helps them to live longer. Some of the long-term relationship between education and health is due to the potential for increased employment and earnings that more education can provide.

Math Proficiency

In 2013 in the United States, only about one in three 8th grade students (35%) were at the proficient or advanced level in math (male and female proficiency levels were similar). In comparison, about one in four 12th grade students (26%) were proficient in math in 2013. Male 12th grade students (28%) were more likely to be proficient in math than were female 12th grade students (24%).

Note: The National Assessment of Educational Progress (NAEP) defines this measure as "Proficient is defined as solid academic performance for each grade assessed. Students reaching this level have demonstrated competency over challenging subject matter, including knowledge of the subject matter, application of such knowledge to real-world situations, and analytical skills appropriate to the subject matter."

Writing Proficiency

In 2011, among both 8th grade and 12th grade students, more than one in four students (27%) were at the proficient or advanced writing level. In both grade levels, female students were more likely to be proficient in writing than were male students.

Note: The National Assessment of Educational Progress defines this measure as: "Proficient is defined as solid academic performance for each grade assessed. Students reaching this level have demonstrated competency over challenging subject matter, including subject-matter knowledge, application of such knowledge to real-world situations, and analytical skills appropriate to the subject matter."

Healthy Relationships

Dating Violence

Intimate partner violence is associated not only with physical injury, but also with emotional and behavioral problems.

In 2013, one in 10 high school students who had dated in the 12 months before the survey (10%) reported that they were hit, slapped, or physically hurt on purpose by their boyfriend or girlfriend. Female high school students (13%) were more likely than male high school students (7%) to experience dating violence in the past year. This number may be a conservative estimate because dating violence incidents are often not reported.

Bullying

Bullying is associated with a number of serious health issues, including substance abuse and emotional problems, and even with suicide.

In 2013, one in five high school students (20%) reported being bullied at school. Female high school students (24%) were more likely to report being bullied at school in the past 12 months than male high school students (16%).

Note: YRBS defines this measure as: "Bullying is when one or more students tease, threaten, spread rumors about, hit, shove, or hurt another student over and over again. It is not bullying when two students of about the same strength or power argue or fight or tease each other in a friendly way."

Neighborhood Safety

The actual or perceived safety of neighborhoods can influence health directly or indirectly. If safety concerns restrict opportunities to get physical exercise, for example, adolescents' health can suffer.

In 2011–12, nearly nine out of 10 parents of adolescents ages 12–17 felt that their child was usually or always safe in their neighborhood. However, 12 percent of parents of adolescents reported that their child was never or only sometimes safe in their neighborhood.

Supportive Neighborhoods

Supportive neighborhoods—where people look out for each other's well-being, and families can rely on neighbors' help—contribute to social and emotional health. In 2011–12, most parents of adolescents ages 12–17 (84%) agreed that their neighborhood was supportive, but almost one in six (16%) disagreed that their neighborhood was supportive.

Note: National Survey of Children's Health (NSCH) defines this measure as: "Supportive neighborhood information is reported by parents and is based on the statements: people in my neighborhood help each other out; we watch out for each other's children in this neighborhood; there are people I can count on in this neighborhood; if my child were outside playing and got hurt or scared, there are adults nearby who I trust to help my child. Parents were asked whether they strongly agree, somewhat agree, somewhat disagree, or strongly disagree with each statement. Choosing a 'disagree' option on more than one statement removes someone from living in a supportive neighborhood."

Chapter 2

Understanding Adolescent Health

Adolescents (ages 10 to 17) and young adults (ages 18 to 25) make up 22 percent of the U.S. population. The behavioral patterns established during these developmental periods help determine young people's current health status and their risk for developing chronic diseases during adulthood.

Although adolescence and young adulthood are generally healthy times of life, some important health and social problems either start or peak during these years. Examples include:

- Mental disorders

- Substance use

- Smoking/nicotine use

- Nutrition and weight conditions

- Sexually transmitted infections, including human immunodeficiency virus (HIV)

- Teen and unintended pregnancies

- Homelessness

This chapter includes text excerpted from "Adolescent Health," Office of Disease Prevention and Health Promotion (ODPHP), U.S. Department of Health and Human Services (HHS), September 20, 2017.

- Academic problems and dropping out of school

- Homicide

- Suicide

- Motor vehicle collisions

Because they are in developmental transition, adolescents and young adults (AYAs) are particularly sensitive to influences from their social environments. Their families, peer groups, schools, and neighborhoods can either support or threaten young people's health and well-being. Societal policies and cues, such as structural racism and media messages, can do the same. Older adolescents and young adults, including those with chronic health conditions, may face challenges as they transition from the child to the adult healthcare system, such as changes in their insurance coverage and legal status and decreased attention to their developmental and behavioral needs. Bolstering the positive development of young people facilitates their adoption of healthy behaviors and helps ensure a healthy and productive adult population.

Why Is Adolescent Health Important?

Adolescence is a critical transitional period that includes the biological changes of puberty and developmental tasks such as normative exploration and learning to be independent. Young adults who have reached the age of majority also face significant social and economic challenges with few organizational supports at a time when they are expected to take on adult responsibilities and obligations.

There are significant disparities in outcomes among racial and ethnic groups. In general, AYAs who are African American, American Indian, or Latino, especially those living in poverty, experience worse outcomes in a variety of areas such as obesity, teen, and unintended pregnancy, tooth decay, and educational achievement, compared to AYAs who are Caucasian or Asian American. In addition, sexual minority youth have a higher prevalence of many health risk behaviors.

The financial burdens of preventable health problems are large and include the long-term costs of chronic diseases resulting from behaviors begun during adolescence and young adulthood. For example, the annual adult health-related financial burden of cigarette smoking, which usually starts during these years, was calculated as $289 billion for 2009–2012.

There are many examples of effective policies and programs that address AYA health issues:

- Access to healthcare
- School-based healthcare services
- State graduated driver licensing programs
- Prevention of alcohol, marijuana, and tobacco use
- Violence prevention
- Delinquency prevention
- Mental health and substance use interventions
- Teen pregnancy prevention
- HIV prevention

Adolescent Health and Social Factors

The leading causes of illness and death among AYAs are largely preventable, and health outcomes are frequently both behaviorally mediated and linked to multiple social factors. This is shown by the following empirical examples:

Family

- Adolescents who have good communication and are bonded with a caring adult are less likely to engage in risky behaviors.
- Parents who supervise and are involved with their adolescents' activities are promoting a safe environment for them to explore opportunities.
- The children of families living in poverty are more likely to have health conditions and poorer health status, as well as lower access to and use of healthcare services.

School

- Student health and academic achievement are linked. Healthy students are more effective learners.
- Academic success and achievement strongly predicts overall adult health outcomes. Proficient academic skills are associated with lower rates of risky behaviors and higher rates of healthy behaviors.

- High school graduation leads to lower rates of health problems and risk for incarceration, as well as enhanced financial stability and socio-emotional well-being during adulthood.

- The school social environment affects student attendance, academic achievement, engagement with learning, likelihood of graduation, social relationships, behavior, and mental health.

Neighborhoods

- AYAs growing up in distressed neighborhoods with high rates of poverty are at risk for exposure to violence and a variety of negative outcomes, including poor physical and mental health, delinquency, and risky sexual behavior.

Media Exposure

- AYAs exposed to media portrayals of violence, smoking, and drinking are at risk for adopting these behaviors.

- Although social media use offers important benefits to AYAs, such as health promotion, communication, education, and entertainment, it also increases risks for exposure to cyberbullying, engagement in "sexting," and depression.

Emerging Issues in Adolescent Health

Three important issues influence how the health of AYAs will be approached in the coming decade:

- The AYA population is becoming more ethnically diverse, with rapid increases in the numbers of Latino and Asian American youth. The growing ethnic diversity will require cultural responsiveness to healthcare needs as well as sharpened attention to disparate health, academic, and economic outcomes.

- The mental health of AYAs has a profound impact on their physical health, academic achievement, and well-being. About 50 percent of lifelong mental disorders begin by age 14 and 75 percent begin by age 24. Suicide is a leading cause of death among AYAs and suicide rates climbed significantly for these age groups between 1999 and 2014. Trauma associated with common adverse childhood experiences (ACEs) contributes to mental and behavioral health issues for many youth as well as negative adult outcomes. Fortunately, at least some ACEs can be prevented and their effects improved.

• Positive youth development (PYD) interventions are intentional processes that provide all youth with the support, relationships, experiences, resources, and opportunities needed to become competent, thriving adults. Their use is growing for preventing AYA health risk behaviors. An expanding evidence base demonstrates that well-designed PYD interventions can lead to positive outcomes, including the prevention of AYA health risk behaviors. Additional evaluation is necessary to learn how to tailor successful interventions to meet the needs of different groups of AYAs.

Chapter 3

Physical and Emotional Changes in Teens

As a teenager, you go through many physical, mental, emotional, and social changes. The biggest change is puberty, the process of becoming sexually mature. It usually happens between ages 10 and 14 for girls and ages 12 and 16 for boys. As your body changes, you may have questions about sexual health.

During this time, you start to develop your own unique personality and opinions. Some changes that you might notice include:

- Increased independence from your parents

- More concerns about body image and clothes

- More influence from peers

- Greater ability to sense right and wrong

All of these changes can sometimes seem overwhelming. Some sadness or moodiness can be normal. But feeling very sad, hopeless, or worthless could be warning signs of a mental health problem.

This chapter contains text excerpted from the following sources: Text in this chapter begins with excerpts from "Teen Development," MedlinePlus, National Institutes of Health (NIH), December 27, 2016; Text beginning with the heading "Young Teens (12–14 Years of Age)" is excerpted from "Child Development—Positive Parenting Tips," Centers for Disease Control and Prevention (CDC), February 1, 2017.

If you need help, talk to your parents, school counselor, or healthcare provider.

Young Teens (12–14 Years of Age)

Developmental Milestones

This is a time of many physical, mental, emotional, and social changes. Hormones change as puberty begins. Most boys grow facial and pubic hair and their voices deepen. Most girls grow pubic hair and breasts, and start their period. They might be worried about these changes and how they are looked at by others. This also will be a time when your teen might face peer pressure to use alcohol, tobacco products, and drugs, and to have sex. Other challenges can be eating disorders, depression, and family problems. At this age, teens make more of their own choices about friends, sports, studying, and school. They become more independent, with their own personality and interests, although parents are still very important.

Emotional / Social Changes

Children in this age group might:

- Show more concern about body image, looks, and clothes.

- Focus on themselves; going back and forth between high expectations and lack of confidence.

- Experience more moodiness.

- Show more interest in and influence by peer group.

- Express less affection toward parents; sometimes might seem rude or short-tempered.

- Feel stress from more challenging schoolwork.

- Develop eating problems.

- Feel a lot of sadness or depression, which can lead to poor grades at school, alcohol or drug use, unsafe sex, and other problems.

Thinking and Learning

Children in this age group might:

- Have more ability for complex thought.

- Be better able to express feelings through talking.
- Develop a stronger sense of right and wrong.

Teenagers (15–17 Years of Age)

Developmental Milestones

This is a time of changes for how teenagers think, feel, and interact with others, and how their bodies grow. Most girls will be physically mature by now, and most will have completed puberty. Boys might still be maturing physically during this time. Your teen might have concerns about her body size, shape, or weight. Eating disorders also can be common, especially among girls. During this time, your teen is developing his unique personality and opinions. Relationships with friends are still important, yet your teen will have other interests as he develops a more clear sense of who he is. This is also an important time to prepare for more independence and responsibility; many teenagers start working, and many will be leaving home soon after high school.

Emotional / Social Changes

Children in this age group might:

- Have more interest in romantic relationships and sexuality.
- Go through less conflict with parents.
- Show more independence from parents.
- Have a deeper capacity for caring and sharing and for developing more intimate relationships.
- Spend less time with parents and more time with friends.
- Feel a lot of sadness or depression, which can lead to poor grades at school, alcohol or drug use, unsafe sex, and other problems.

Thinking and Learning

Children in this age group might:

- Learn more defined work habits.
- Show more concern about future school and work plans.
- Be better able to give reasons for their own choices, including about what is right or wrong.

Chapter 4

Understanding Adolescent Brain Development

How the Brain Develops

What we have learned about the process of brain development helps us understand more about the roles both genetics and the environment play in our development. It appears that genetics predispose us to develop in certain ways, but our experiences, including our interactions with other people, have a significant impact on how our predispositions are expressed. In fact, research now shows that many capacities thought to be fixed at birth are actually dependent on a sequence of experiences combined with heredity. Both factors are essential for optimum development of the human brain.

Early Brain Development

The raw material of the brain is the nerve cell, called the neuron. During fetal development, neurons are created and migrate to form the

This chapter contains text excerpted from the following sources: Text beginning with the heading "How the Brain Develops" is excerpted from "Understanding the Effects of Maltreatment on Brain Development," Child Welfare Information Gateway, U.S. Department of Health and Human Services (HHS), April 2015; Text under the heading "The Adolescent Brain: Basic Facts" is excerpted from "Adolescent Development E-Learning Module," Office of Adolescent Health (OAH), U.S. Department of Health and Human Services (HHS), June 13, 2017.

various parts of the brain. As neurons migrate, they also differentiate, or specialize, to govern specific functions in the body in response to chemical signals. This process of development occurs sequentially from the "bottom up," that is, from areas of the brain controlling the most primitive functions of the body (e.g., heart rate, breathing) to the most sophisticated functions (e.g., complex thought). The first areas of the brain to fully develop are the brainstem and midbrain; they govern the bodily functions necessary for life, called the autonomic functions. At birth, these lower portions of the nervous system are very well developed, whereas the higher regions (the limbic system and cerebral cortex) are still rather primitive. Higher function brain regions involved in regulating emotions, language, and abstract thought grow rapidly in the first three years of life.

The Growing Child's Brain

Brain development, or learning, is actually the process of creating, strengthening, and discarding connections among the neurons; these connections are called synapses. Synapses organize the brain by forming pathways that connect the parts of the brain governing everything we do—from breathing and sleeping to thinking and feeling. This is the essence of postnatal brain development, because at birth, very few synapses have been formed. The synapses present at birth are primarily those that govern our bodily functions such as heart rate, breathing, eating, and sleeping. The development of synapses occurs at an astounding rate during a child's early years in response to that child's experiences. At its peak, the cerebral cortex of a healthy toddler may create 2 million synapses per second. By the time children are 2 years old, their brains have approximately 100 trillion synapses, many more than they will ever need. Based on the child's experiences, some synapses are strengthened and remain intact, but many are gradually discarded. This process of synapse elimination—or pruning—is a normal part of development. By the time children reach adolescence, about half of their synapses have been discarded, leaving the number they will have for most of the rest of their lives.

Another important process that takes place in the developing brain is myelination. Myelin is the white fatty tissue that forms a sheath to insulate mature brain cells, thus ensuring clear transmission of neurotransmitters across synapses. Young children process information slowly because their brain cells lack the myelin necessary for fast, clear nerve impulse transmission. Like other neuronal growth processes, myelination begins in the primary motor and sensory areas (the brain stem and cortex) and gradually progresses to the higher order regions that control thought, memories, and feelings. Also, like other neuronal growth processes, a child's experiences affect the rate and growth of myelination, which continues into young adulthood. By 3 years of age, a baby's brain has reached almost 90 percent of its adult size. The growth in each region of the brain largely depends on receiving stimulation, which spurs activity in that region. This stimulation provides the foundation for learning.

Adolescent Brain Development

Studies using MRI techniques show that the brain continues to grow and develop into young adulthood (at least to the midtwenties). White matter, or brain tissue, volume has been shown to increase in adults as old as 32. Right before puberty, adolescent brains experience a growth spurt that occurs mainly in the frontal lobe, which is the area that governs planning, impulse control, and reasoning. During the teenage years, the brain goes through a process of pruning synapses—somewhat like the infant and toddler brain—and also sees an increase in white matter and changes to neurotransmitter systems. As the teenager grows into young adulthood, the brain develops more myelin to insulate the nerve fibers and speed neural processing, and this myelination occurs last in the frontal lobe. MRI comparisons between the brains of teenagers and the brains of young adults have shown that most of the brain areas were the same—that is, the teenage brain had reached maturity in the areas that govern such abilities as speech and sensory capabilities.

The major difference was the immaturity of the teenage brain in the frontal lobe and in the myelination of that area. Normal puberty and adolescence lead to the maturation of a physical body, but the brain lags behind in development, especially in the areas that allow teenagers to reason and think logically. Most teenagers act impulsively at times, using a lower area of their brains—their "gut reaction"—because their frontal lobes are not yet mature. Impulsive behavior, poor decisions, and increased risk-taking are all part of the normal teenage experience. Another change that happens during adolescence is the growth and transformation of the limbic system, which is responsible for our emotions. Teenagers may rely on their more primitive limbic system in interpreting emotions and reacting since they lack the more mature cortex that can override the limbic response.

Plasticity—The Influence of Environment

Researchers use the term plasticity to describe the brain's ability to change in response to repeated stimulation. The extent of a brain's plasticity is dependent on the stage of development and the particular brain system or region affected. For instance, the lower parts of the brain, which control basic functions such as breathing and heart rate, are less flexible, or plastic, than the higher functioning cortex, which controls thoughts and feelings. While cortex plasticity decreases as a child gets older, some degree of plasticity remains. In fact, this brain plasticity is what allows us to keep learning into adulthood and throughout our lives.

The developing brain's ongoing adaptations are the result of both genetics and experience. Our brains prepare us to expect certain experiences by forming the pathways needed to respond to those experiences. For example, our brains are "wired" to respond to the sound of speech; when babies hear people speaking, the neural systems in their brains responsible for speech and language receive the necessary stimulation to organize and function. The more babies are exposed to people speaking, the stronger their related synapses become. If the appropriate exposure does not happen, the pathways developed in anticipation may be discarded. This is sometimes referred to as the concept of "use it or lose it." It is through these processes of creating, strengthening, and discarding synapses that our brains adapt to our unique environment.

The ability to adapt to our environment is a part of normal development. Children growing up in cold climates, on rural farms, or in large sibling groups learn how to function in those environments. Regardless of the general environment, though, all children need stimulation and nurturance for healthy development. If these are lacking (e.g., if a child's caretakers are indifferent, hostile, depressed, or cognitively impaired), the child's brain development may be impaired. Because the brain adapts to its environment, it will adapt to a negative environment just as readily as it will adapt to a positive one.

Sensitive Periods

Researchers believe that there are sensitive periods for development of certain capabilities. These refer to windows of time in the developmental process when certain parts of the brain may be most susceptible to particular experiences. Animal studies have shed light on sensitive periods, showing, for example, that animals that are artificially blinded during the sensitive period for developing vision may never develop the capability to see, even if the blinding mechanism is later removed.

It is more difficult to study human sensitive periods; however, if certain synapses and neuronal pathways are not repeatedly activated, they may be discarded, and their capabilities may diminish. For example, infants have a genetic predisposition to form strong attachments to their primary caregivers, but they may not be able to achieve strong attachments, or trusting, durable bonds if they are in a severely neglectful situation with little one-on-one caregiver contact. Children from Romanian institutions who had been severely neglected had a much better attachment response if they were placed in foster care—and thus received more stable parenting—before they were 24 months old. This indicates that there is a sensitive period for attachment, but it is likely that there is a general sensitive period rather than a true cut-off point for recovery.

While sensitive periods exist for development and learning, we also know that the plasticity of the brain often allows children to recover from missing certain experiences. Both children and adults may be able to make up for missed experiences later in life, but it is likely to be more difficult. This is especially true if a young child was deprived of certain stimulation, which resulted in the pruning of synapses (neuronal connections) relevant to that stimulation and the loss of neuronal pathways. As children progress through each developmental stage, they will learn and master each step more easily if their brains have built an efficient network of pathways to support optimal functioning.

Memories

The organizing framework for children's development is based on the creation of memories. When repeated experiences strengthen a neuronal pathway, the pathway becomes encoded, and it eventually becomes a memory. Children learn to put one foot in front of the other to walk. They learn words to express themselves. And they learn that a smile usually brings a smile in return. At some point, they no longer have to think much about these processes—their brains manage these experiences with little effort because the memories that have been created allow for a smooth, efficient flow of information.

The creation of memories is part of our adaptation to our environment. Our brains attempt to understand the world around us and fashion our interactions with that world in a way that promotes our survival and, hopefully, our growth, but if the early environment is abusive or neglectful, our brains may create memories of these experiences that adversely color our view of the world throughout our life.

Babies are born with the capacity for implicit memory, which means that they can perceive their environment and recall it in certain unconscious ways. For instance, they recognize their mother's voice from an unconscious memory. These early implicit memories may have a significant impact on a child's subsequent attachment relationships.

In contrast, explicit memory, which develops around age 2, refers to conscious memories and is tied to language development. Explicit memory allows children to talk about themselves in the past and future or in different places or circumstances through the process of conscious recollection.

Sometimes, children who have been abused or suffered other trauma may not retain or be able to access explicit memories of their experiences; however, they may retain implicit memories of the physical or emotional sensations, and these implicit memories may produce flashbacks, nightmares, or other uncontrollable reactions. This may be the case with very young children or infants who suffer abuse or neglect.

The Adolescent Brain: Basic Facts

Adolescents differ from adults in the way they behave, solve problems, and make decisions. Research shows that there is a biological explanation for this difference; the brain continues to develop during adolescence and even into early adulthood.

Brain Development: The Amygdala and the Frontal Cortex

The amygdala and the frontal cortex are two key regions of the brain that develop at different times. The amygdala, which processes stress and other emotions, and is responsible for instinctual reactions like fear and aggressive behavior, matures early.

On the other hand, the frontal cortex, the area of the brain responsible for judgment, self-control, emotional regulation, rational thought, goal setting, morality, and understanding consequences, is not yet fully developed in teenagers. In fact, this area of the brain develops quite dramatically during adolescence and into the mid-20s.

What Does This Mean for Adolescents?

Pictures of the brain in action show that adolescents' brains function differently from those of adults when making decisions and solving problems. Adolescents' actions are guided more by the amygdala and less by the frontal cortex. That means that teens' responses to situations are rooted in emotion rather than rationality. In other words, the last part of the brain to fully develop is one of the most important—it's the area that gives people the ability to make rational decisions.

Because the part of the brain that helps us think before we act isn't fully developed until adulthood, in stressful situations or when faced with difficult decisions, teens are more likely to:

- Think one thing and feel another
- Act from impulses that differ from thoughts or feelings
- Misread or misinterpret social cues and emotions
- Engage in risky or inappropriate behavior

How You Can Help

There are several ways you can help teens make healthy choices. Adolescents' brains go through a "use-it-or-lose-it" pruning system: brain cells and neural connections that get used the least get pruned away and die off; whereas those that get used the most become stronger.

To help teens make healthy choices, walk them through the decision-making process before they encounter risky situations. This will help them to make life-impacting decisions with less stress. Teens who undergo learning and positive experiences help build complex, adaptive brains.

Strategies to support healthy adolescent brain development:

- Encourage teens to have healthy lifestyles and offer opportunities for positive experiences
- Provide meaningful opportunities for teens to exercise logic and apply analytical and decision-making skills to build up those brain functions.
- Encourage teens to take healthy risks. Taking such risks will help to develop a stronger frontal cortex, effectively giving the teen more valuable life skills.
- Allow teens to make mistakes so that they can learn from them.

Chapter 5

Key Indicators of Adolescent Well-Being

Demographic Background

Racial and ethnic diversity in the United States has increased dramatically in the last 35 years. This growth was first evident among children, a population projected to become even more diverse in the years to come.

- In 2020, fewer than half of all United States children ages 0–17 are projected to be White, non-Hispanic, down from 74 percent in 1980 and 52 percent in 2015. By 2050, only 39 percent of all U.S. children are projected to be White, non-Hispanic.

- Hispanic children represented 25 percent of U.S. children in 2015, up from 9 percent in 1980. By 2020, they are projected to represent 26 percent of all U.S. children and 32 percent by 2050.

- In 2015, Black, non-Hispanic children represented 14 percent of all U.S. children, down from 15 percent in 1980. By 2020, they are projected to represent 14 percent of all U.S. children and 13 percent by 2050.

This chapter includes text excerpted from "America's Children in Brief: Key National Indicators of Well Being," Federal Interagency Forum on Child and Family Statistics (ChildStats.gov), July 12, 2016.

- Since 2000, Asian, non-Hispanic children have increased from 3.5 percent of all U.S. children to 5 percent in 2015. By 2020, they are projected to represent 5 percent of all U.S. children and 7 percent by 2050.

- In 2000, non-Hispanic children of two or more races represented 2 percent of all U.S. children. By 2015, they represented 4 percent of all U.S. children. By 2020, they are projected to represent 5 percent of all U.S. children and 8 percent by 2050.

- American Indian and Alaska Native, non-Hispanic children represented 0.9 percent of all U.S. children in 2015, up from 0.8 percent in 1980. By 2020, they are projected to represent 0.8 percent of all U.S. children and 0.7 percent by 2050.

- Between 2000 and 2015, the proportion of Native Hawaiian and Other Pacific Islander, non-Hispanic children remained unchanged at 0.2 percent of all U.S. children. The proportion is projected to remain unchanged at 0.2 percent between 2020 and 2050.

Family and Social Environment

Racial and Ethnic Composition of Children by Parental Nativity

The foreign born population in the United States has grown since 1970. As a result, the population of children with foreign born parents tends to be more diverse, in terms of race and Hispanic origin, than the population of children whose parents are native born. Potential language and cultural barriers confronting children and their foreign born parents may make additional language resources necessary for children, both at school and at home.

- In 2015, one quarter of all children in the United States had a parent who was foreign born. In contrast, about 71 percent of all children were native born and had native born parents.

- Among native born children with at least one foreign born parent, the majority were Hispanic in 2015, a pattern that reflects the rise of immigration from Latin America over the past few decades. In contrast, among native born children with native born parents, the majority were White, non-Hispanic in 2015

- A growing share of immigrants are coming from Asia as well as Latin America. In 2015, Asians made up just 1 percent of native born children with native born parents, but they made up a far larger proportion of the children whose parents were foreign born. Asians made up 16 percent of native born children with a foreign born parent and 23 percent of foreign born children with a foreign born parent.

Adolescent Births

Childbirth during adolescence is often accompanied by long-term difficulties for the mother and her child. Compared with babies born to older mothers, babies born to adolescent mothers, particularly younger adolescent mothers, are at higher risk of low birthweight and infant mortality. They are more likely to grow up in homes that offer lower levels of emotional support and cognitive stimulation, and they are less likely to earn high school diplomas. For mothers, giving birth during adolescence is associated with limited educational attainment, which in turn can reduce employment prospects and earnings potential. Although adolescent birth rates for all racial and ethnic groups have generally been on a long-term decline since the late 1950s, birth rates continue to vary by race and ethnicity.

- In 2014, the adolescent birth rate was 19 births per 1,000 females for American Indian or Alaska Native, non-Hispanic and Hispanic adolescents; 17 for Black, non-Hispanic; for White, non-Hispanic; and 3 for Asian or Pacific Islander, non-Hispanic adolescents ages 15–17.

- From 1995 to 2014, the total adolescent birth rate declined by 25 percentage points, from 36 per 1,000 to 11 per 1,000, a record low for the United States. This long-term downward trend was found for each racial and Hispanic origin group.

- The racial and ethnic disparity (the difference between the highest and lowest rates) in adolescent birth rates declined from 55 points in 1995 to 17 points in 2014. Yet, substantial racial and ethnic disparities remain. Adolescent birth rates among Hispanic; Black, non-Hispanic; and American Indian or Alaska Native, non-Hispanic adolescents remained higher than the rates for White, non-Hispanic and Asian or Pacific Islander, non-Hispanic adolescents throughout the entire period. Asian or Pacific Islander, non-Hispanic adolescents had the lowest birth rates.

Child Maltreatment

Child maltreatment includes physical, sexual, and psychological abuse, as well as neglect (including medical neglect). Maltreatment in general is associated with a number of negative outcomes for children, including lower school achievement, juvenile delinquency, substance abuse, and mental health problems. Certain types of maltreatment can result in long-term physical, social, and emotional problems, and even death. Child maltreatment rates vary by the race and ethnicity of the child. Understanding these variations could potentially improve prevention and intervention efforts.

- After several years of steady decreases, the national rate of substantiated child maltreatment reports increased in 2014 for the first time since 2007. Despite this recent increase, the 2014 rate of 10.2 per 1,000 children was lower than the 2007 rate of 10.6 per 1,000 children.

- The 2014 increase in national substantiated child maltreatment reports was apparent for victims of all races and ethnicities, except Asian children and children of two or more races. The victimization rates in those categories remained the same as in the previous year.

- From 2001 to 2014, Black, non-Hispanic and American Indian or Alaska Native children had the highest rates of substantiated child maltreatment reports (except in 2004 and 2010 when it was Native Hawaiian or Other Pacific Islander children and children of two or more races, respectively).

- In 2014, the victimization rates (per 1,000) were 16.4 for Black, non-Hispanic; 14.9 for American Indian or Alaska Native; 11.6 for two or more races; 9.5 for Hispanic; 9.2 for White, non-Hispanic; 9.1 for Native Hawaiian or Other Pacific Islander; and 1.8 for Asian children.

Economic Circumstances

Child Poverty

Children living in poverty are vulnerable to environmental, educational, health, and safety risks. Compared with their peers, children living in poverty, especially young children, are more likely to have cognitive, behavioral, and socioemotional difficulties. Additionally, throughout their lifetimes, they are more likely to complete fewer years of school and experience more years of unemployment. Child poverty rates in the United States vary considerably by race and Hispanic origin, a pattern that is important given the links between poverty and other economic and social outcomes.

- In 2014, 21 percent (15.5 million) of all U.S. children ages 0–17 lived in poverty.

- Overall, the poverty rate was much higher for Black, non-Hispanic and Hispanic children than for White, non-Hispanic children in 2014. Some 12 percent of White, non-Hispanic children lived in poverty, compared with 37 percent of Black, non-Hispanic children and 32 percent of Hispanic children.

- In 2014, children in married couple families were much less likely to be living in poverty than children living in female householder families (no spouse present). About 11 percent of children in married couple families were living in poverty, compared with 46 percent in female householder families.

Supplemental Poverty Measure

Since the publication of the first official poverty estimates in 1964, there has been continuing debate about the best approach to measuring poverty in the United States. Recognizing that alternative estimates of poverty can provide useful information to the public as well as to the Federal Government, the U.S. Census Bureau publishes alternative poverty estimates using the new supplemental poverty measure (SPM). The SPM does not replace the official poverty measure but serves as an additional indicator of economic well-being and provides a deeper understanding of economic conditions and policy effects. The SPM is based on the suggestions of an interagency technical working group. In contrast to the official poverty measure, which compares pre-tax cash income to a set of thresholds derived in the early 1960s, the SPM creates a more complex statistical picture by incorporating additional items such as tax payments, work expenses, medical out of pocket expenditures, and the value of noncash nutritional, energy, and housing assistance. Thresholds used in the new measure were derived by staff at the U.S. Bureau of Labor Statistics (BLS) from Consumer Expenditure Survey expenditure data on basic necessities (food, shelter, clothing, and utilities) and are adjusted for geographic differences in the cost of housing.

- For all children, the 2014 SPM rate was 17 percent, 4 percentage points lower than the official poverty rate of 21 percent.

- In 2014, the SPM rate was lower than the official poverty rate for White, non-Hispanic; Black, non-Hispanic; and Hispanic children. The difference between the two poverty rates for Asian, non-Hispanic children was not statistically significant.

- While the official poverty rate was higher for Black, non-Hispanic children than for Hispanic children in 2014, the difference between the SPM rates for these two groups was not statistically significant.

- The SPM rate was higher for Asian, non-Hispanic children than for White, non-Hispanic children in 2014. The difference in official poverty rates between these two groups was not statistically significant, however.

Secure Parental Employment

Secure parental employment is a major factor in the financial well-being of families. It is associated with higher family income and greater access to health insurance. It also has been linked to a number of positive outcomes for children, including better health, education and social/emotional development. One measure of secure parental employment is the percentage of children whose resident parent or parents were employed full time throughout a given year. Since 2000, the percentage of children living with a securely employed parent has declined for all children, regardless of race and Hispanic origin.

- In 2014, White, non-Hispanic children were most likely to live with a parent who was securely employed (82%), meaning a parent who worked year round, full time. Hispanic children were less likely to have a securely employed parent (69%) and Black, non-Hispanic children were least likely (60%).

- The pattern varied by family structure. Children with two married parents were most likely to have a securely employed parent in 2014, regardless of race and Hispanic origin, while children with a single mother were least likely.

Food Insecurity

A family's ability to provide for its children's nutritional needs is linked to the family's food security—that is, to its access at all times to adequate food for an active, healthy life for all household members. The food security status of households is based on self-reports of difficulty in obtaining enough food, reduced food intake, reduced diet quality, and anxiety about an adequate food supply. In some households classified as food insecure, only adults' diets and food intakes were affected, but in a majority of such households, children's eating patterns were also disrupted to some extent, and the quality and variety of their diets were adversely affected. In a subset of food insecure households—those classified as having very low food security among children—a parent or guardian reported that at some time during the year one or more children were hungry, skipped a meal, or did not eat for a whole day because the household could not afford enough food.

- In 2014, the percentages of children living in food insecure households were substantially above the national average (21%) for Black, non-Hispanics (34%) and Hispanics (29%), while below the national average for White, non-Hispanics (15%).

- From 2001 to 2014, the percentage of children living in food insecure households was 18 percent in 2001, 19 percent in 2004, 17 percent in 2007, then increased to 23 percent in 2008, and has remained above pre-Great Recession levels.

- Over the same period (from 2001 to 2014), compared with all households with children, the percentages of children living in food insecure households declined more sharply for Hispanics between 2003 and 2005 following the end of the 2001 recession, and increased more sharply for Hispanics and Black, non-Hispanics in 2008 with the onset of the Great Recession.

Healthcare

Health Insurance Coverage

Health insurance is a major determinant of access to and utilization of healthcare. Children with health insurance, whether public or private, have increased access and utilization compared to children without insurance. Further, insured children are more likely to have a regular and accessible source of healthcare. The percentage of children who have health insurance is one indicator of the extent to which families can obtain preventive care or healthcare for a sick or injured child. The likelihood that children have health insurance, and the type of insurance among those insured, varies by race and ethnicity.

- In 2014, Hispanic children were more likely to be uninsured (10%) than White, non-Hispanic and Black, non-Hispanic

39

children (4% each). White, non-Hispanic children were more likely to have private insurance (68%) compared to Hispanic (31%) and Black, non-Hispanic (34%) children. In 2014, Hispanic (57%) and Black, non-Hispanic (59%) children were more likely to have public coverage than White, non-Hispanic children (25%).

- For children in each racial and ethnic group—Black, non-Hispanic; Hispanic; and White, non-Hispanic—the percentage with public coverage increased and the percentage with no health insurance and with private health insurance declined from 2000 to 2014.

- Throughout 2000 to 2014, the percentage of uninsured children was higher among Hispanic children than among White, non-Hispanic and Black, non-Hispanic children. During that same period, Black, non-Hispanic children and Hispanic children were more likely than White, non-Hispanic children to have public coverage, and White, non-Hispanic children were more likely to have private insurance.

- From 2000 to 2014, the percentage of children overall with health insurance increased by 7 percentage points to 95 percent. Although the percentage of children with private coverage declined by 13 percentage points during this period to 54 percent, public coverage increased by 20 percentage points to 38 percent.

Immunization

Vaccination can prevent or lessen the severity of vaccine preventable diseases and is regarded as one of the greatest public health achievements in the United States in the 20th century. For children ages 19–35 months, receipt of the combined seven vaccine series (4:3:1:3:3:1:4) is used to evaluate the proportion of children meeting the current vaccination guidelines. Data on vaccination coverage are used to identify groups at risk of vaccine preventable diseases and to evaluate the effectiveness of programs designed to increase coverage. Black, non-Hispanic children generally have had lower vaccination coverage relative to their White, non-Hispanic counterparts; poverty status accounts for much of this difference in vaccination coverage.

- In 2014, vaccination coverage for the combined seven vaccine series (4:3:1:3:3:1:4) was higher for Hispanic (74%) and White, non-Hispanic children (73%) than for Black, non-Hispanic children (65%) ages 19–35 months.

- Between 2009 and 2014, vaccination coverage among children ages 19–35 months receiving the combined vaccine series increased for White, non-Hispanic (from 45 to 73%); Black, non-Hispanic (from 40 to 65%); and Hispanic (from 46 to 74%) children.

- During that same period, the percentage of White, non-Hispanic children ages 19–35 months receiving the combined vaccine series was higher than the percentage of Black, non-Hispanic children, except for 2010, when coverage did not differ. Vaccination coverage for the combined series between White, non-Hispanic and Hispanic children was not significantly different.

Oral Health

Oral health is an essential component of overall health. Tooth decay is one of the most common chronic conditions among children. If untreated, decay may cause pain, infection, and problems with eating, speaking, and concentrating. Regular dental visits provide an opportunity for prevention, early diagnosis, and treatment of tooth decay and other oral and craniofacial diseases and conditions. Low income and minority children are at the greatest risk of inadequate access to oral healthcare. The prevalence of untreated tooth decay varies by race and ethnicity.

- During 2013–2014, 89 percent of children ages 5–11 had a dental visit in the past year, an 8 percentage point increase from 1999–2000. During 2013–2014, 87 percent of adolescents ages 12–17 had a dental visit in the past year, a 7 percentage point increase from 1999–2000.

- Between 1999–2000 and 2013–2014, the percentage of children and adolescents with a dental visit in the past year increased for all racial and ethnic groups, except Asian, non-Hispanic children and adolescents.

- Among children in 2013–2014, White, non-Hispanic children (90%) were more likely to have had a dental visit in the past year than Black, non-Hispanic (88%) and Hispanic (87%) children. The percentages of dental visits in the past year for American Indian or Alaska Native, non-Hispanic (93%) and Asian, non-Hispanic (87%) children were not different from those of other racial and ethnic groups.

41

- Among adolescents in 2013–2014, White, non-Hispanic adolescents (90%) were more likely to have had a dental visit in the past year than Black, non-Hispanic (84%); Asian, non-Hispanic (84%); and Hispanic (81%) adolescents. The percentage of dental visits in the past year for American Indian or Alaska Native, non-Hispanic adolescents (89%) was not significantly different from other racial and ethnic groups.

Physical Environment and Safety

Outdoor Air Quality

One important children's environmental health measure is the percentage of children living in areas in which air pollution levels are higher than the allowable levels of the Primary National Ambient Air Quality Standards (NAAQS). The Environmental Protection Agency (EPA) sets these standards to protect public health, including susceptible groups such as children. Ozone and particulate matter (PM) are air pollutants associated with increased asthma episodes, and other respiratory illnesses in children, all of which can lead to increased emergency room visits and hospitalizations. PM, especially fine PM (PM2.5), contains microscopic solids or liquid droplets that are so small that they can get deep into lungs and cause serious health problems. Studies indicate the possibility of race related increases in risk for some health effects resulting from exposure to ozone and PM, although the understanding of potential differences by race is limited by the small number of studies and possibly confounded by other factors.

- In 2014, about 54 percent of all U.S. children lived in counties with measured pollutant concentrations above the level of the 8 hour ozone Primary National Ambient Air Quality Standard (NAAQS) at least once during the year.

- In 2014, approximately 68 percent of Asian or Pacific Islander, non-Hispanic and 67 percent of Hispanic children lived in counties that exceeded the level of the allowable air quality standard for ozone, compared with 57 percent of Black, non-Hispanic; 46 percent of White, non-Hispanic; and 34 percent of American Indian or Alaska Native, non-Hispanic children.

- From 2000 to 2014, the percentage of children living in counties with measured ozone concentrations above the level of the current standard at least one day per year declined from 67 to 54 percent.

- In 2014, about 28 percent of all children lived in counties with measured concentrations of PM2.5 above the level of the 24 hour Primary National Ambient Air Quality Standard at least once during the year.

- In 2014, approximately 38 percent of Asian or Pacific Islander, non-Hispanic and 42 percent of Hispanic children lived in counties that exceeded the level of the allowable air quality standard for PM2.5 compared with 25 percent of Black, non-Hispanic; 21 percent of White, non-Hispanic; and 20 percent of American Indian or Alaska Native, non-Hispanic children.

- From 2000 to 2014, the percentage of children living in counties with measured PM2.5 concentrations above the level of the current standard at least one day per year declined from 62 to 28 percent.

Secondhand Smoke

The U.S. Surgeon General has determined that there is no safe level of exposure to secondhand tobacco smoke. Children who are exposed to secondhand smoke have an increased risk of adverse health effects, such as respiratory symptoms, lower respiratory tract infections, bronchitis, pneumonia, middle ear disease, and sudden infant death syndrome. Further, secondhand smoke can play a role in the development and exacerbation of asthma. Cotinine, a breakdown product of nicotine, is used as a marker for exposure to secondhand smoke in nonsmokers. Cotinine levels at or above 0.05 nanograms per milliliter (ng/mL) are often used as an indicator of secondhand smoke exposure in the previous 1 to 2 days. Previous research has found that the likelihood of exposure to secondhand smoke varies by the race and ethnicity of the child.

- In 2011–2012, 69 percent of Black, non-Hispanic; 37 percent of White, non-Hispanic; and 30 percent of Mexican American children ages 4–11 had detectable levels of cotinine, indicating that they had been exposed to secondhand smoke (defined as cotinine levels at or above 0.05 ng/mL) in the previous day or two.

- From 1999–2000 through 2011–2012, the percentage of all children ages 4–11 with exposure to secondhand smoke declined by 24 percentage points. There were significant declines in secondhand smoke exposure for each racial and ethnic group—25 percentage points among White, non-Hispanic; 18 percentage points among Black, non-Hispanic; and 19 percentage points among Mexican American children.

- Throughout the period, the percentage of Black, non-Hispanic children exposed to secondhand smoke was approximately 2 to 2½ times higher than that of Mexican American children. For most of the period, the percentage of Black, non-Hispanic children ages 4–11 with secondhand smoke exposure was also higher than that of White, non-Hispanic children. In 2003–2004 and 2007–2008, there were no significant differences between the secondhand smoke exposure rates of Black and White, non-Hispanic children.

Lead in the Blood of Children

Lead is a major environmental health hazard for children. Childhood exposure to lead contributes to reduced intelligence quotient (IQ) and academic achievement and behavioral problems. The chief sources of exposure for children are deteriorating lead based paint in homes, water from leaded pipes, and consumer products. Young children are particularly vulnerable to lead because of their developing nervous systems and their hand to mouth behavior. A blood lead level of 5 micrograms per deciliter (μg/dL) is defined as "elevated" for purposes of identifying children for follow-up, but no level of lead exposure can be considered safe. Blood lead levels have declined since the 1970s, due largely to the removal of lead from gasoline and paint. Yet in 2005–2006, 15 percent of U.S. homes with young children had indoor lead hazards, including lead based paint.4 Children with nutritional deficiencies or living in poverty or older housing are more likely to have elevated blood lead levels.

- In 2007–2014, 1.9 percent of children ages 1–5 (approximately 390,000 children) had blood lead levels at or above 5 μg/dL. Among Black, non-Hispanic children ages 1–5, 4.0 percent had elevated blood lead levels, compared with 1.9 percent of White, non-Hispanic children and 1.1 percent of Mexican American children. In 2007–2014, Black, non-Hispanic children ages 1–5 were twice as likely as White, non-Hispanic children and three times as likely as Mexican American children to have elevated blood lead levels.

- Between 1999–2006 and 2007–2014, the percentage of all children ages 1–5 with blood lead levels at or above 5 μg/dL declined by approximately 4 percentage points. Black, non-Hispanic and

Mexican American children also had large declines in the percentage with elevated blood lead levels between these two time periods, by 10 percentage points and 3 percentage points, respectively. However, the percentage of White, non-Hispanic children ages 1–5 with elevated blood lead levels was not statistically different between 1999–2006 and 2007–2014.

- In both 1999–2006 and 2007–2014, Black, non-Hispanic children were more likely to have elevated blood lead levels than White, non-Hispanic and Mexican American children.

Youth Victims of Serious Violent Crimes

Violence frequently has dire and long-lasting impacts on young people who experience, witness, or feel threatened by it. In addition to causing direct physical harm to young victims, serious violence can adversely affect their mental health and development and increase the likelihood that they themselves will commit acts of serious violence. Examining violent victimization rates by race and ethnicity is important for understanding whether the risk for victimization differs for youth from different racial and ethnic backgrounds.

- For all youth ages 12–17, the rate of serious violent victimization declined sharply from the early 1990s through the early 2000s and has declined more slowly since then. In 1993, youth ages 12–17 experienced 40 serious violent crimes per 1,000 youth, compared with 18 crimes per 1,000 youth in 2000 and 8 crimes per 1,000 youth in 2014.

- From 1993 to 2014, the rate at which White, non-Hispanic youth were victims of serious violent crimes decreased from 36 crimes per 1,000 youth to 7 crimes per 1,000 youth.

- Over the same period, the serious violent victimization rate for Black, non-Hispanic youth decreased from 54 crimes per 1,000 youth in 1993 to 11 crimes per 1,000 youth in 2014.

- Serious violent victimization rates decreased for Hispanic youth from 52 crimes per 1,000 youth in 1993 to 9 crimes per 1,000 youth in 2014.

- In 2014, there were no significant differences in the rates at which White, non-Hispanic, Black, non-Hispanic, and Hispanic youth ages 12–17 were victims of serious violent crimes.

45

Child and Adolescent Injury and Mortality

Unintentional injuries are the leading cause of death for children and adolescents. In 2014, 35 percent of deaths among adolescents ages 15–19 and 30 percent of deaths among children ages 1–14 were due to unintentional injuries.50 For both age groups, motor vehicle related (MVR) injury deaths are the leading type of unintentional injury death. Compared with younger children, adolescents have much higher death rates overall and from injuries, and are much more likely to die from injuries sustained in motor vehicle traffic crashes. In 2014, the reported MVR deaths rates for American Indian or Alaska Native children under age 20 were more than double the rates for White, non-Hispanic; Black, non-Hispanic; Asian or Pacific Islander, non-Hispanic; and Hispanic children under age 20. Research has found that the race and ethnicity of Hispanic, American Indian or Alaska Native, and Asian or Pacific Islander decedents is often misclassified on death certificates, resulting in an underestimate of death rates. Therefore, death rates cannot be accurately reported for all racial and ethnic groups.

- In 2014, the MVR death rate for children ages 1–14 was 2.2 deaths per 100,000 population, representing 1,234 deaths. MVR death rates for Black, non-Hispanic (2.8); White, non-Hispanic (2.0); and Hispanic (2.2) children ranged from 2 to 3 deaths per 100,000 population.

- During most of 1999 to 2014, Black, non-Hispanic children had a higher MVR death rate than White, non-Hispanic children. Death rates for Black, non-Hispanic; White, non-Hispanic; and Hispanic children differed by 1 to 2 points throughout the period.

- Among adolescents, the MVR death rate in 2014 was 11.9 deaths per 100,000 population, a total of 2,515 deaths. The MVR death rate for White, non-Hispanic (13.0) adolescents was higher than the rates for Black, non-Hispanic (11.4) and Hispanic (10.6) adolescents.

- Between 1999 and 2014, the total MVR death rate for adolescents ages 15–19 declined from 26 deaths per 100,000 population to 12 deaths per 100,000 population. The MVR death rates for each racial and ethnic group declined throughout the period.

- Throughout 1999 to 2014, White, non-Hispanic adolescents had a higher MVR death rate than Black, non-Hispanic and

Hispanic adolescents. This disparity in death rates declined from an 11 point difference in 1999 to about a 2 point difference in 2014.

Behavior

Illicit Drug Use

The adolescent years can be a critical period for both substance use—including alcohol, tobacco, and illegal and prescription drugs—and the development of substance use disorders. When substance use disorders occur in adolescence, they may affect key developmental and social transitions, and they can interfere with normal brain maturation. Chronic and heavy marijuana use in adolescence, for example, has been shown to lead to a loss of IQ that is not recovered even if the individual quits using in adulthood. The abuse of prescription and over-the-counter drugs can be addictive and puts users at risk of other adverse health effects, including overdose—especially when taken along with other drugs or alcohol. Impaired memory or thinking ability and other problems caused by drug use can derail a young person's social and educational development and hold him or her back in life. Examining illicit drug use among adolescents by race and ethnicity can provide us with a fuller picture of who is at risk.

- Between 2014 and 2015, illicit drug use in the past 30 days remained stable at 8 percent among 8th grade students and 24 percent among 12th grade students. However, among 10th grade students, illicit drug use declined from 19 percent to 17 percent.

- Among 12th graders, 23 percent of both White, non-Hispanic and Hispanic students and 24 percent of Black, non-Hispanic students reported using illicit drugs in the past 30 days in 2015. Among 10th grade students, the percentages were 16 percent for White, non-Hispanics and 20 percent for both Black, non-Hispanics and Hispanics. Among 8th grade students, the percentages were 6 percent for White, non-Hispanic students; 9 percent for Black, non-Hispanic students; and 10 percent for Hispanic students.

- Over the past several decades, 12th grade White non-Hispanics and Hispanics reported similar rates of past month illicit drug use with rates consistently above those reported by Black non-Hispanics. Since 2012, there has been a narrowing of this gap and in 2015 there was no significant difference in the rate of past month illicit drug use reported by White non-Hispanics, Hispanics or Black non-Hispanics.

Sexual Activity

Early sexual activity is associated with emotional and physical health risks. Youth who engage in sexual activity are at risk of contracting sexually transmitted infections (STIs) and becoming pregnant. STIs, including human immunodeficiency virus (HIV), can infect a person for a lifetime and have consequences including disability and early death. Delaying sexual initiation is associated with a decrease in the number of lifetime sexual partners, and decreasing the number of lifetime partners is associated with a decrease in the rate of STIs. Additionally, teen pregnancy is associated with a number of negative risk factors, not only for the mother but also for her child. Examining sexual activity by race and ethnicity can help us determine who is at highest risk for negative emotional and physical consequences.

- In 2013, 47 percent of high school students in grades 9 through 12 reported ever having had sexual intercourse.

- The percentage of students who reported ever having had sexual intercourse declined from 1991 (54%) to 2001 (46%) and remained stable from 2001 to 2013.

- The percentage of students who reported ever having had sexual intercourse differed by race and Hispanic origin. In 2013, 61 percent of Black, non-Hispanic students reported ever having had sexual intercourse, compared with 49 percent of Hispanic students and 44 percent of White, non-Hispanic students.

Regular Cigarette Smoking

Smoking has serious long-term consequences, including the risk of smoking related diseases and premature death, as well as the increased healthcare costs related to treating associated illnesses. Over 480,000 deaths are attributable annually to tobacco use, making tobacco more lethal than all other addictive drugs. Nearly 87 percent of smokers start smoking by age 18. Each day in the United States, approximately 2,300 young people under 18 years of age smoke their first cigarette, and an estimated 450 youth in that age group become daily cigarette smokers.63 Smoking rates vary greatly by race and ethnicity. The high rate of use and the consequences of cigarette smoking underscore the importance of studying patterns of smoking among adolescents.

- In 2015, the percentage of 8th, 10th, and 12th grade students who reported smoking cigarettes daily in the past 30 days has continued to be the lowest since data collection began in 1980. In 2015, 1 percent of 8th grade students, 3 percent of 10th grade students, and 6 percent of 12th grade students—down from 9 percent, 16 percent, and 22 percent, respectively, in 1995— reported smoking in the past 30 days.

- In 2015, among 12th graders, an estimated 7.3 percent of White, non-Hispanic students reported daily cigarette use in the past month—this is nearly twice as many as the 4 percent of Black, non-Hispanic and 3.7 percent of Hispanic students that reported regular cigarette use.

- Since 2000, the largest decline in regular cigarette use among 12th graders was a 76 percent drop reported by Hispanic students—from 16 to 4 percent. Among Whites, there was a 70 percent decline in the same time period—from 26 to 7 percent. Among Black, non-Hispanics, the rate of regular cigarette use dropped by 50 percent—from 8 percent to 4 percent.

Alcohol Use

Alcohol is the most common illicit substance used during adolescence. Heavy use is associated with negative outcomes such as problems in school and the workplace, being involved in fights, criminal activities, or motor vehicle crashes, resulting in injuries as well as death. Binge drinking, defined here as five or more alcoholic beverages in a row or during a single occasion in the previous two weeks, is a common pattern of alcohol abuse. Early onset of binge drinking may be especially problematic, potentially increasing the likelihood of negative outcomes including alcohol use disorder. While overall trends of binge drinking continue to decline among adolescents, examining alcohol use by race and ethnicity can help us to better understand who is at greatest risk for negative consequences.

- In 2015, the percentages of 10th, and 12th grade students who reported binge drinking were the lowest since the survey began in 1980.

- In 2015, 5 percent of 8th graders reported binge drinking down from 11 percent in 1991, the first year the survey reported on 8th and 10th grade alcohol use. Among, 10th graders, there was a decline from 21 percent in 1991 to 11 percent in 2015.

- Twelfth graders were first surveyed in 1980 and have also reported a long-term decline from 41 percent in 1980 to 17 percent in 2015.

- Among 12th grade students, 21 percent of White, non-Hispanics and 19 percent of Hispanics reported binge drinking. This was two times the rate of Black, non-Hispanic 12th graders who reported binge drinking (10%) in 2015.

- Among 12th graders, long-term trends of reported binge drinking have declined among White, non-Hispanics; Black, non-Hispanics; and Hispanics. Since 1980, reported use among White, non-Hispanics declined from 44 percent in that year to 21 percent in 2015. Among Black, non-Hispanics, binge drinking dropped from 18 percent in 1980 to 10 percent in 2015 and among Hispanics binge drinking decreased from 33 percent in 1980 to 19 percent in 2015.

Education

Mathematics and Reading Achievement

The extent of children's knowledge, as well as their ability to think, learn, and communicate, affects their likelihood of becoming productive adults and active citizens. Mathematics and reading achievement test scores measure students' skills in these subjects and are good indicators of overall achievement in school. Students with lower levels of academic achievement tend to have less favorable educational outcomes. In addition, differences in academic performance between groups of students, or achievement gaps, have long been documented for students from different racial and ethnic backgrounds.

- At grade 4, the average mathematics scores for non-Hispanic White, Black, and Asian or Pacific Islander students were all higher in 2015 than in 1990; this finding also held for Hispanic students.

- In 2015 and in all previous assessment years, the average mathematics score for White, non-Hispanic 4th grade students was higher than the scores for their Black, non-Hispanic and Hispanic peers. However, there has been some narrowing of racial and ethnic achievement gaps for 4th grade students over time. For example, the White Black mathematics achievement gap at grade 4 narrowed from 32 points in 1990 to 24 points in 2015.

- Despite increases over time, in 2015, for the first time, the average mathematics scale score for 4th grade students was lower than in the previous assessment year, 2013 (240 vs 242).

- The 2015 average mathematics score for 4th grade students (240) translates into a Basic level of proficiency, but patterns in mathematics achievement varied among racial and ethnic groups. For example, the average mathematics score for 4th grade Asian or Pacific Islander students (257) was higher than the scores for their counterparts. The score for White, non-Hispanic students (248) at grade 4 was also higher than the scores for non-Hispanic students who were Black (224) and American Indian or Alaska Native (227), as well as Hispanic students (230).

- At grade 8, the average mathematics scores for non-Hispanic White, Black, and Asian or Pacific Islander students were all higher in 2015 than in 1990; the same was true for Hispanic students.

- In 2015 and in all previous assessment years, the average mathematics scores for White, non-Hispanic students at grade 8 have been higher than the scores for their Black, non-Hispanic and Hispanic peers. At grade 8, the 2015 achievement gaps between White, non-Hispanic and Black, non-Hispanic students and between White, non-Hispanic and Hispanic students were not statistically different from the gaps in 1990.

- As was the case for 4th grade students, in 2015, the average mathematics score for 8th grade students was lower than the average score for the previous assessment year for the first time (282 in 2015 vs 285 in 2013). Nonetheless, the 8th grade average mathematics score in 2015 was higher than in 1990 (263).

- At grade 8, the average mathematics score in 2015 (282) aligned with a Basic level of proficiency.65 However, mathematics performance varied among students. The average mathematics score at grade 8 was higher for Asian or Pacific Islander, non-Hispanic students (306) than for their peers in the other racial and ethnic groups. In addition, the average 8th grade mathematics score was higher for White, non-Hispanic (292) students than for non-Hispanic students who were Black (260) and American Indian or Alaska Native (267) as well as Hispanic students (270).

High School Completion

Attainment of a high school diploma or its equivalent is an indicator that a person has acquired the basic academic skills needed to function in today's society. The percentage of young adults ages 18–24 with a high school diploma or an equivalent credential is a measure of the extent to which young adults have completed a basic prerequisite for many entry level jobs and for higher education. Persons with higher levels of education tend to have better economic outcomes than their peers with lower levels of education.

- In 2014, 92 percent of young adults ages 18–24 had completed high school with a diploma or an alternative credential, such as a General Educational Development (GED) certificate. The high school completion rate has increased from 84 percent in 1980.

- The high school completion rate for Black, non-Hispanic young adults increased from 75 percent in 1980 to 92 percent in 2014. Among White, non-Hispanic young adults, this rate increased from 87 percent in 1980 to 94 percent in 2014. While the high school completion rate for Hispanic young adults has consistently been lower during this period than for their White, non-Hispanic and Black, non-Hispanic peers, the rate for Hispanic young adults increased 30 percentage points between 1980 and 2014, from 57 percent to 87 percent.

- High school completion rates increased between 2003 (when separate data became available for all race groups) and 2014 for Asian, non-Hispanic young adults (from 95 to 99%) and non-Hispanic young adults of two or more races (from 92 to 97%). During this period, the completion rates also increased for young adults who were Hispanic (from 69 to 87%); Black, non-Hispanic (from 85 to 92%); and White, non-Hispanic (from 92 to 94%). In contrast, 2014 completion rates for non-Hispanic American Indian or Alaska Native (79%) and Pacific Islander young adults (99%) were not statistically different from the rates in 2003.

- In 2014, the high school completion rate was higher for non-Hispanic young adults who were White (94%), Asian (99%), and of two or more races (97%) than for those who were Black, non-Hispanic (92%); Hispanic (87%); and American Indian or Alaska Native, non-Hispanic (79%). The completion rate was also higher for Black, non-Hispanic young adults than for their Hispanic and American Indian or Alaska Native, non-Hispanic peers.

College Enrollment

A college education generally enhances a person's employment prospects and increases his or her earning potential. The percentage of high school completers who enroll in college in the fall immediately after high school is one measure of the accessibility and perceived value of a college education by high school completers. Research shows that high school completers who delay enrollment in postsecondary education are less likely to persist in their education and to attain a postsecondary credential.

- In 2014, 68 percent of high school completers enrolled in a 2 year or 4 year college in the fall immediately after high school. Between 1980 and 2014, the rate of immediate college enrollment trended upward nearly 20 percentage points, from 49 percent to 68 percent.

- In 1980, some 52 percent of White, non-Hispanic high school completers immediately enrolled in college; this rate increased to 68 percent in 2014. The immediate college enrollment rate for Black, non-Hispanic high school completers increased from 44 percent in 1980 to 63 percent in 2014.

- The immediate college enrollment rate for Hispanic high school completers also increased, from 50 percent in 1980 to 62 percent in 2014.

- In 2014, the immediate college enrollment rates for White, non-Hispanic high school completers (68%); Black, non-Hispanic high school completers (63%); and Hispanic high school completers were not statistically different (62%), due in part to large standard errors for Black, non-Hispanic and Hispanic high school completers. In 1980, the immediate college enrollment rate was higher for White, non-Hispanic high school completers (52%) than for their Black, non-Hispanic peers (44%).

Youth Neither Enrolled in School nor Working

Youth ages 16–19 who are neither enrolled in school nor working are detached from these core activities, both of which play an important role in one's transition from adolescence to adulthood. If this detachment lasts for several years, it can hinder a youth's opportunity to build a work history that contributes to future higher wages and employability. The percentage of youth who are not enrolled in school and not working is one measure of the proportion of young people who are at risk of limiting their future prospects. Analysis done by the Congressional Research Service (CRS) finds that a greater share of minority youth, particularly Black males, are disconnected, and that their rates of disconnection have been higher over time. Disconnected youth are also twice as likely to be poor as their connected peers.

- In 2015, 9 percent of youth ages 16–19 were neither enrolled in school nor working. This figure was unchanged from 2014 and little different over the past 20 years.

- The percentage of Black, non-Hispanic youth and Hispanic youth neither enrolled in school nor working has declined since 1985.

- Black, non-Hispanic youth had a higher rate of detachment from work and school, at 12 percent, than Hispanic youth (10%) and White, non-Hispanic youth (7%) in 2015.

- For youth ages 16–17, the rate of detachment was less than half the rate of older youth ages 18–19. In 2015, 5 percent of both Black, non-Hispanic youth and Hispanic youth ages 16–17 were neither enrolled in school nor working, compared with 4 percent of White, non-Hispanic youth in this age group.

- Older youth, ages 18–19, had a higher rate of detachment from work and school at 13 percent. Black, non-Hispanic youth in this age group saw a detachment rate of 19 percent in 2015, compared with 16 percent for Hispanic youth and 11 percent for White, non-Hispanic youth. These figures were either the same as or almost unchanged from 2014.

Health

Infant Mortality

Infant mortality is defined as the death of an infant before his or her first birthday. Infant mortality is related to the underlying health of the mother, public health practices, socioeconomic conditions, and availability and use of appropriate healthcare for infants and pregnant women. Despite medical advances and public health efforts, the mortality rates of Black, non-Hispanic and American Indian or Alaska Native infants have been consistently higher than the rates of other racial and ethnic groups. A higher percentage of preterm births accounts for most of the higher infant mortality for Black, non-Hispanic infants. Higher rates of sudden infant death syndrome (SIDS), birth defects, preterm births, and injuries account for much of the higher infant mortality among American Indian or Alaska Native infants.

- In 2013, the infant mortality rates were 11.1 infant deaths per 1,000 live births for Black, non-Hispanics; 7.7 infant deaths per 1,000 live births for American Indian or Alaska Native, non-Hispanics; 5.1 infant deaths per 1,000 live births for White, non-Hispanics; 5.0 infant deaths per 1,000 live births for Hispanics; and 3.9 infant deaths per 1,000 live births for Asian or Pacific Islander, non-Hispanics.

- From 1999 to 2013, the total infant mortality rate declined by 1 percentage point. During the same time period, the infant mortality rate declined by 3 points for Black, non-Hispanic infants and 1 point for White, non-Hispanic; Asian or Pacific Islander, non-Hispanic; and Hispanic infants. Infant mortality for American Indian or Alaska Native, non-Hispanic infants was stable from 1999 to 2013.

- Despite the declines in infant mortality between 1999 and 2013, rates for Black, non-Hispanic and American Indian or Alaska Native, non-Hispanic infants remained higher than the rates for White, non-Hispanic; Hispanic; and Asian or Pacific Islander, non-Hispanic infants throughout the entire period.

Adolescent Depression

Depression has a significant impact on adolescent development and well-being. Adolescent depression can adversely affect school and work performance, impair peer and family relationships, and exacerbate the severity of other health conditions such as asthma and obesity. Major depressive episodes (MDE) often persist, recur, or continue into adulthood. Youth with MDE are at greater risk for suicide and are more likely to initiate alcohol and other drug use compared with youth without MDE. The majority of youth with MDE do not receive depression care. Moreover, racial/ethnic minority youth with MDE are less likely to receive depression care compared with their White counterparts.

- In 2014, about 11 percent of youth ages 12–17 had a major depressive episode (MDE) during the past year, a higher prevalence than that reported in 2004 (9%). The prevalence of MDE in the past year among White, non-Hispanic youth in 2014 (12%) was higher than among Black, non-Hispanic youth (9%) and among American Indian or Alaska Native, non-Hispanic youth (7%).

- However, in 2014, the prevalence of MDE in the past year among White, non-Hispanic youth (12%) was similar to that among non-Hispanic youth of two or more races (13%), among Hispanic youth (12%), and among Asian, non-Hispanic youth (10%).

- Among White, non-Hispanic youth as well as among Hispanic youth, the prevalence of MDE in the past year increased from 9 percent in 2004 to 12 percent in 2014. However, the prevalence of MDE in the past year in 2004 did not differ from that in 2014 among the other youth by race and ethnicity.

Obesity

Children with obesity often become adults with obesity, with increased risks for a wide variety of poor health outcomes, including diabetes, stroke, heart disease, arthritis, and certain cancers. The consequences of obesity for children and adolescents are often psychosocial but also include high blood pressure, diabetes, early puberty, and asthma. The prevalence of obesity among U.S. children changed relatively little from the early 1960s through 1980; however, after 1980 it increased sharply. In addition to individual factors such as diet and physical activity, other factors, including social, economic, and environmental forces (e.g., trends in eating out), may have contributed to the increased prevalence of obesity. Previous research has found that the prevalence of obesity among children varies by race and ethnicity.

- From 1988–1994 to 2011–2014, the percentage of children ages 6–17 with obesity increased by 8 percentage points from 11 to 19 percent. During the same time period, the percentage of children with obesity increased by 7 percentage points for White, non-Hispanic; 9 percentage points for Black, non-Hispanic; and 10 percentage points for Mexican American children.

- From 1988–1994 to 2011–2014, White, non-Hispanic children were less likely to have obesity than Black, non-Hispanic and Mexican American children. During the same period, the percentages of Black, non-Hispanic and Mexican American children with obesity were similar.

- Between 2007–2010 and 2011–2014, the percentage of children ages 6–17 with obesity was not measurably different for each racial and ethnic group.

- In 2011–2014, 19 percent of children ages 6–17 had obesity.

- Asian, non-Hispanic children ages 6–17 (10%) were least likely to have obesity, followed by White, non-Hispanic children (17%). The prevalence of obesity was highest among Black, non-Hispanic (23%) children and Hispanic (24%) children.

Asthma

Asthma is one of the most common childhood chronic diseases. It causes wheezing, difficulty in breathing, and chest tightness. Some children diagnosed with asthma may not experience any serious respiratory effects. Others may have mild symptoms or may respond well to management of their asthma, typically through the use of medication. However, some children with asthma may suffer serious attacks that limit their activities, result in visits to emergency rooms or hospitals, or, in rare cases, cause death. Air pollution and secondhand tobacco smoke, along with infections, exercise, and allergens, can trigger asthma attacks in children with asthma. The prevalence of asthma among children doubled from 1980 to 1995 and then increased more slowly during the 2000s. Racial disparities in childhood asthma prevalence have emerged since 1996. Higher asthma prevalence among children has been observed by poverty level and geographic region of residence.

- In 2014, 13 percent of Black, non-Hispanic children were reported to currently have asthma, compared with 8 percent of White, non-Hispanic; 8 percent of Hispanic; and 6 percent of Asian, non-Hispanic children.

- From 2001 to 2014, the percentage of Hispanic; White, non-Hispanic; and Asian, non-Hispanic (trend from 2004 to 2014) children with current asthma was stable. The percentage of Black, non-Hispanic children with current asthma increased from 2001 to 2010 and then declined from 2011 to 2014.

- Throughout this period, the percentage of Black, non-Hispanic children with current asthma was higher than the corresponding percentages for Hispanic; White, non-Hispanic; and Asian, non-Hispanic children with current asthma.

Chapter 6

For Parents: Talking to Teens about Health Issues

Chapter Contents

Section 6.1—Positive Parenting.. 60

Section 6.2—Communicating with Your Child 63

Section 6.3—Talking about Substance Abuse............................ 67

Section 6.4—Talking about Healthy Relationships 72

Section 6.5—Talking about Sex 75

Section 6.6—Monitoring Your Teen's Activities........................ 80

Section 6.1

Positive Parenting

This section includes text excerpted from "Positive Parenting— Building Healthy Relationships with Your Kids," *NIH News in Health*, National Institutes of Health (NIH), September 2017.

Parents have an important job. Raising kids is both rewarding and challenging. You're likely to get a lot of advice along the way, from doctors, family, friends, and even strangers. But every parent and child is unique. Being sensitive and responsive to your kids can help you build positive, healthy relationships together.

"Being a sensitive parent and responding to your kids cuts across all areas of parenting," says Arizona State University's Dr. Keith Crnic, a parent child relationship expert. "What it means is recognizing what your child needs in the moment and providing that in an effective way."

This can be especially critical for infants and toddlers, he adds. Strong emotional bonds often develop through sensitive, responsive, and consistent parenting in the first years of life. For instance, holding your baby lovingly and responding to their cries helps build strong bonds.

Building Bonds

Strong emotional bonds help children learn how to manage their own feelings and behaviors and develop self-confidence. They help create a safe base from which they can explore, learn, and relate to others.

Experts call this type of strong connection between children and their caregivers "secure attachment." Securely attached children are more likely to be able to cope with challenges like poverty, family instability, parental stress, and depression.

A analysis shows that about 6 out of 10 children in the United States develop secure attachments to their parents. The 4 out of 10 kids who lack such bonds may avoid their parents when they are upset or resist their parents if they cause them more distress. Studies suggest that this can make kids more prone to serious behavior problems. Researchers have been testing programs to help parents develop behaviors that encourage secure attachment.

Being Available

Modern life is full of things that can influence your ability to be sensitive and responsive to your child. These include competing priorities, extra work, lack of sleep, and things like mobile devices. Some experts are concerned about the effects that distracted parenting may have on emotional bonding and children's language development, social interaction, and safety.

If parents are inconsistently available, kids can get distressed and feel hurt, rejected, or ignored. They may have more emotional outbursts and feel alone. They may even stop trying to compete for their parent's attention and start to lose emotional connections to their parents.

"There are times when kids really do need your attention and want your recognition," Crnic explains. Parents need to communicate that their kids are valuable and important, and children need to know that parents care what they're doing, he says.

It can be tough to respond with sensitivity during tantrums, arguments, or other challenging times with your kids. "If parents respond by being irritable or aggressive themselves, children can mimic that behavior, and a negative cycle then continues to escalate," explains Dr. Carol Metzler, who studies parenting at the Oregon Research Institute (ORI).

According to Crnic, kids start to regulate their own emotions and behavior around age three. Up until then, they depend more on you to help them regulate their emotions, whether to calm them or help get them excited. "They're watching you to see how you do it and listening to how you talk to them about it," he explains. "Parents need to be good self-regulators. You're not only trying to regulate your own emotions in the moment, but helping your child learn to manage their emotions and behavior."

As kids become better at managing their feelings and behavior, it's important to help them develop coping skills, like active problem solving. Such skills can help them feel confident in handling what comes their way.

"When parents engage positively with their children, teaching them the behaviors and skills that they need to cope with the world, children learn to follow rules and regulate their own feelings," Metzler says.

"As parents, we try really hard to protect our kids from the experience of bad things," Crnic explains. "But if you protect them all the time and they are not in situations where they deal with difficult or adverse circumstances, they aren't able to develop healthy coping skills."

He encourages you to allow your kids to have more of those experiences and then help them learn how to solve the problems that emerge. Talk through the situation and their feelings. Then work with them to find solutions to put into practice.

Meeting Needs

As children grow up, it's important to remember that giving them what they need doesn't mean giving them everything they want. "These two things are very different," Crnic explains. "Really hone in on exactly what's going on with your kid in the moment. This is an incredibly important parenting skill and it's linked to so many great outcomes for kids."

Think about where a child is in life and what skills they need to learn at that time. Perhaps they need help managing emotions, learning how to behave in a certain situation, thinking through a new task, or relating to friends.

"You want to help kids become confident," Crnic says. "You don't want to aim too high where they can't get there or too low where they have already mastered the skill." Another way to boost confidence while strengthening your relationship is to let your kid take the lead.

"Make some time to spend with your child that isn't highly directive, where your child leads the play," advises Dr. John Bates, who studies children's behavior problems at Indiana University Bloomington. "Kids come to expect it and they love it, and it really improves the relationship."

Bates also encourages parents to focus on their child's actual needs instead of sticking to any specific parenting principles.

It's never too late to start building a healthier, more positive relationship with your child, even if things have gotten strained and stressful. "Most importantly, make sure that your child knows that you love them and are on their side," Metzler says. "For older children, let them know that you are genuinely committed to building a stronger relationship with them and helping them be successful."

By being a sensitive and responsive parent, you can help set your kids on a positive path, teach them self-control, reduce the likelihood of troublesome behaviors, and build a warm, caring parent child relationship.

Section 6.2

Communicating with Your Child

This section includes text excerpted from "Conversation Tools," Office of Adolescent Health (OAH), U.S. Department of Health and Human Services (HHS), October 14, 2016.

Every parent of a teen has experienced it: that rare moment when your teen opens up and shares information with you about his or her life. It's a joy.

But every parent also knows that much of the time, talking to a teen can be a bit of a struggle. In fact, parents often think that teens don't listen and what a parent says doesn't matter.

Parents do matter. What you say does make a difference. Research shows that nearly four in 10 teens (38%) report that parents most influence their decisions about sex, compared to only 22 percent reporting that friends most influence their decision.

The first step in having good conversations with your teen is to think, in a quiet moment, how you feel about whatever it is you want to talk about with your teen. It is important to be honest with yourself so that you can be honest with your teen. Then, take advantage of the teachable moments in your lives and take some conversation tips from parents who've been in your shoes.

Teachable Moments

Choosing Your Moment

Everyday situations can offer a natural way to ease into a conversation with a teen. That can be a lot easier than telling your teen, "We need to talk." And better received too. Many parents report, for example, that they often talk to their teen when they are driving in their car. Perhaps it's because there is very little eye contact when driving, something a teen may find a bit less nerve-wracking. Maybe it's the fact that the conversation can end and the radio can be turned back up, offering an easy transition back into less stressful topics.

Remember, your goal is not to deliver a lecture or scare either one of you. Your goal is to have a conversation. And that conversation takes place over time, sometimes in bits and pieces.

Conversation Starters

Maybe it's a scene from a movie or TV show. Perhaps it's a song lyric or a news story. Or it could be something that has happened in the neighborhood. These, or anything else that seems timely, can be effective conversation starters.

A good way to start is simply to ask, "What do you think about that?" And "that" might be:

- A peer or family member learns she is pregnant

- A television show discusses teen relationships

- A news report on something involving teens

- A popular song on the radio that talks about relationships

If your son or daughter answers, "I dunno" or something like that, say, "Well, let me share what I think." Don't lecture. Just use it as a jumping-off point to talk about your views and feelings.

You might also ask, "Do you know anybody that has happened to?"

Conversation Tips

Teens say that they are uncomfortable talking about sex with their parents because they worry it will make their parents angry, or that their parents will assume they are doing some things they might not actually be doing. In other words, teens say they are afraid their parents will "freak out." So that's the first conversation tip—don't freak out. You may be freaking out on the inside, but on the outside, try to keep calm.

Keep your composure. Remain calm. Becoming angry or overreacting to a question or mistake can upset your teen, or worse, silence any hope of future dialogue. Instead, listen and ask open-ended questions.

Be present. Parents have a lot going on these days. When you have a chance to talk with your teen though, try to put some of those worries and activities aside. Pay attention to the conversation and don't do too many other things at the same time. You don't have to drop everything; you can cook or do laundry while you talk. Just be sure to listen and make certain your teen knows you are hearing every word.

Be sympathetic. Let your teen know you understand how challenging life as an adolescent can be. Your teen may not believe you can really relate. Help teens know that you understand that the social pressures and obligations of a teen can feel like a lot. Encourage them to stay focused on school and other priorities.

Stress safety. Regardless of your views on the timing of sex, safety is an important part of the message to give your teen. Stress the absolute necessity of using a condom every single time. And stress the importance of using birth control. Don't lecture or nag, but don't be too shy to emphasize this point.

Provide the facts. Give teens complete and honest information. Make sure they understand that condoms aren't just for preventing pregnancy, but also for reducing the likelihood of contracting sexually transmitted diseases (STD) and human immunodeficiency virus (HIV). Make sure they know that birth control methods do not necessarily provide protection against STDs and HIV.

Talk with them, instead of preaching. Resist the urge to talk AT them. Instead, share with them. Let them know how you felt and the challenges you faced when you were their age.

Have lots of discussions. Don't look at this as one huge, overwhelming moment. Keep in mind that talking to your teen is an ongoing conversation. It takes place in bits and pieces over time. It's not one big talk. Truth be told, when it comes to important topics like relationships, your teen does want to hear from you, but might find talking comfortable for only a few minutes at a time. Give your opinion over time, instead of just unloading one large lecture, and allow your teen to think through what you are sharing.

Keep tabs on TV. More than 75 percent of prime-time programs contain sexual content, yet only 14 percent of sexual incidents mention risks or responsibilities of sexual activity.

Make media matter. Eight in 10 teens say the media is a good way to start conversations with parents about sex, love, and relationships. Spend time watching TV or a movie with your teen and use what happens to the characters as a way to start talking about your own values. Movies and TV shows are great conversation starters because they shift the focus away from teens to characters they might identify with.

Chat in the car. You may find the car to be a good place for having conversations that are slightly uncomfortable. You don't have to look at each other and it can be a private setting. Although teens might prefer to listen to music or look out the window, remember they're listening to you.

Text your teen. The average teen sends and receives 50 text messages a day, but makes and receives just five phone calls. For teens, and even younger children, real-time text-based communications on a cell phone or other mobile device now are the norm. Send positive text messages to your teen or follow up a conversation with a text that reinforces what you just talked about. And if the popular texting abbreviations don't come naturally to you, don't sweat it. Just write the way you talk.

Your text might say something like:

- It means a lot to me that you told me about the problem you're having with your friends. Being a teen is tough sometimes. But you are doing great. Remember, I'm here to talk more about it if you want to.

- Good luck on your math exam today. Proud of you for all the time you spent studying!

- Your performance yesterday at the concert/in the game was amazing. Let's go out tonight and celebrate!

- Have fun at the dance! Remember, I'm always happy to give you a ride—call me or text me if your ride home has been drinking.

- Hope you'll think more about what we talked about yesterday, and that you'll wait until you're a bit older to have sex. There is no rush and I want to make sure you are ready for it.

- Thanks for making dinner with me last night. It was great to get to hear about what's going on with your friends and to spend time with you one-on-one. Love you!

- It was great meeting your boyfriend last night! It felt great that you wanted me to get to know him. I'm always here to talk about the relationships in your life.

- You have always done things when you were ready for them, not on anyone else's agenda. Keep being true to yourself! Thanks for being honest with me about trying cigarettes. I think it's important to have open communication but for you to remember that smoking is really harmful.

Section 6.3

Talking about Substance Abuse

This section contains text excerpted from the following sources: Text under the heading "Could Your Kids Be at Risk for Substance Abuse?" is excerpted from "Family Checkup: Positive Parenting Prevents Drug Abuse," National Institute on Drug Abuse (NIDA), August 2015; Text beginning with the heading "The Basics: Overview" is excerpted from "Talk to Your Kids about Tobacco, Alcohol, and Drugs," Office of Disease Prevention and Health Promotion (ODPHP), U.S. Department of Health and Human Services (HHS), June 29, 2017.

Could Your Kids Be at Risk for Substance Abuse?

Families strive to find the best ways to raise their children to live happy, healthy, and productive lives. Parents are often concerned about whether their children will start or are already using drugs such as tobacco, alcohol, marijuana, and others, including the abuse of prescription drugs. Research supported by the National Institute on Drug Abuse (NIDA) has shown the important role that parents play in preventing their children from starting to use drugs.

The Basics: Overview

Talk to your child about the dangers of tobacco, alcohol, and drugs. Knowing the facts will help your child make healthy choices.

What Do I Need to Say?

When you talk about tobacco, alcohol, and drugs:

- Teach your child the facts.
- Give your child clear rules.

- Find out what your child already knows.

- Be prepared to answer your child's questions.

- Talk with your child about how to say "no."

When Should I Start Talking with My Child?

Start early. By preschool, most children have seen adults smoking cigarettes or drinking alcohol, either in real life, on TV, or online.

Make sure your child knows right from the start that you think it's important to stay safe and avoid drugs.

Here are more reasons to start the conversation early:

- Almost 9 out of 10 smokers start smoking before they turn 18.

- Many kids start using tobacco by age 11 and are addicted by age 14.

- By the time they are in 8th grade, most children think that using alcohol is okay.

- At age 12 or 13, some kids are already using drugs like marijuana or prescription pain relievers.

What If My Child Is Older?

It's never too late to start the conversation about avoiding drugs. Even if your teen may have tried tobacco, alcohol, or drugs, you can still talk about making healthy choices and how to say "no" next time.

What Do I Need to Know about Prescriptions and Other Medicines?

When you talk to your child about the dangers of drugs, don't forget about drugs that may already be in your home. Prescription drugs are the third most commonly abused substances by teens age 14 and older (after marijuana and alcohol).

Prescription or over-the-counter (OTC) drug abuse is when a person:

- Takes too much of a prescription or OTC drug

- Takes a prescription drug prescribed to someone else

- Uses a prescription or OTC drug to get high

When not taken safely, prescription and OTC medicines can be just as addictive and dangerous as other drugs.

Commonly abused prescription or OTC drugs include:

- Painkillers, like Vicodin, OxyContin, or codeine
- Medicines used for anxiety or sleep problems, like Valium or Xanax
- Medicines that treat ADHD (attention deficit hyperactivity disorder), like Adderall or Ritalin

Make sure to talk to your kids about the dangers of prescription drug abuse.

Set a good example for your kids—never take someone else's prescription medicine or give yours to anyone else. Keep track of the medicines in your home and store them in a locked cabinet.

Why Do I Need to Talk to My Child?

Research shows that kids do listen to their parents. Children who learn about drug risks from their parents are less likely to start using drugs.

When kids choose not to use alcohol or drugs, they are also less likely to:

- Have serious trouble in school
- Get hurt in a car accident
- Be a victim of crime
- Have a problem with addiction as an adult

If you don't talk about it, your child may think it's okay to use alcohol and other drugs.

Take Action!

Talk with your child about tobacco, alcohol, and drugs today—and keep the conversation going.

Talk with Your Child Early and Often

Start conversations about your values and expectations while your child is young. Your child will get used to sharing information and opinions with you. This will make it easier for you to continue talking as your child gets older.

Here are some tips:

- Use everyday events to start a conversation. For example, if you see a group of kids smoking, talk about how tobacco harms the body.

- Give your child your full attention. Turn off your TV, radio, cell phone, and computer, and really listen.

- Try not to "talk at" your child. Encourage your child to ask questions. If you don't know the answer to a question, look it up together.

- Find age appropriate ways to talk to your child about drugs.

Teach Your Child the Facts

Your child needs to know how drugs can harm the brain, affect the body, and cause problems at home and in school. Kids who know the facts are more likely to make good choices.

- If your child likes sports, focus on how smoking can affect athletic performance. Or you can say that tobacco causes bad breath and yellow teeth. Get the facts on tobacco.

- Remind your child that alcohol is a powerful drug that slows down the body and brain. Get the facts on alcohol.

- Tell your child how other drugs—like steroids, marijuana, and prescription medicines—affect the brain and body. Get the facts on other drugs.

Set Clear Rules for Your Child

Not wanting to upset their parents is the number one reason kids give for not using drugs. Your child will be less tempted to use tobacco, alcohol, and drugs if you explain your rules clearly.

Here are some things to keep in mind when you talk to your child:

- Explain that you set rules to keep your child safe.

- Tell your child you expect her not to use tobacco, alcohol, or drugs.

- Let your child know what will happen if he breaks the rules.

- Praise your child for good behavior.

Help Your Child Learn How to Say "No"

Kids say that they use alcohol and other drugs to "fit in and belong" with other kids. That's why it's important for parents to help children build the confidence to make a healthy choice when someone offers tobacco, drugs, or alcohol.

Set a Good Example

- If you smoke, try to quit.
- If you drink alcohol, don't drink too much or too often.
- If you use drugs, find a treatment program near you.
- Use prescription and over-the-counter medicines safely.
- Never drink or use drugs and drive.

What If I've Used Drugs in the Past?

Be honest with your child, but don't give a lot of details.

Get Help If You Need It

If you think your child may have a drug or alcohol problem, get help. Don't wait.

What about Cost?

Drug and alcohol assessments for teens are covered under the Affordable Care Act (ACA), the healthcare reform law passed in 2010. Depending on your insurance plan, your child may be able to get an assessment at no cost to you.

Section 6.4

Talking about Healthy Relationships

This section includes text excerpted from "Talk with Your Teen about Healthy Relationships," Office of Disease Prevention and Health Promotion (ODPHP), U.S. Department of Health and Human Services (HHS), January 28, 2017.

The Basics

You can help your teen build strong, respectful relationships. Start by teaching your son or daughter about healthy relationships.

Unfortunately, many teens have relationships that are unhealthy. More than 1 in 10 teens who have been on a date have also been:

- Physically abused (hit, pushed, or slapped) by someone they've gone out with

- Sexually abused (kissed, touched, or forced to have sex without wanting to) by someone they've dated

You can help your kids:

- Develop skills for healthy and safe relationships
- Set expectations for how they want to be treated
- Recognize when a relationship is unhealthy
- Support friends dealing with unhealthy relationships

Talking about healthy relationships is a great way to show that you are available to listen and answer questions—so make sure to check in often with your teen. Together, you can agree on clear rules about dating to help keep your teen safe.

Take Action!

Help Your Teen Develop Problem Solving Skills

Help your teen think about healthy relationships by asking how he'd handle different situations. You might ask, "What would you do if:

- you think your friend's partner isn't treating him right?"

- your partner calls you to come over whenever you try to hang out with your friends?"

- your friend yells at his girlfriend in front of everyone at a party?"

It may help to use examples from TV shows, movies, or songs to start the conversation.

Be sure to listen respectfully to your teen's answer, even if you don't agree. Then you can offer your opinion and explore other options together.

Help Your Teen Support a Friend

It's also a good idea to talk with your teen about what she can do if a friend is in an unhealthy relationship. Suggest that your teen talk to you or another adult, like a school counselor, if she notices signs of dating violence.

Set Rules for Dating

As kids get older, they gain more independence and freedom. But teens still need parents to set boundaries and expectations for behavior.

Here are some things to talk about with your teen:

- Are friends allowed to come over when you aren't home?

- Can your son go on a date with someone you haven't met?

- How can your daughter reach you if she needs a ride home?

Be a Role Model

You can teach your kids a lot by treating them and others with respect. As you talk with your teen about healthy relationships, think about your own behavior. Does it match the values you are talking about?

Treating your kids with respect also helps you build stronger relationships with them. This can make it easier to communicate with your teen about important issues like staying safe.

Talk to Your Kids about Sex

Teens who have sex with more than one person are at higher risk of being in an unhealthy relationship.

73

Talk to Your Kids about Preventing STDs

About half of all STD cases in the United States happen in teens and young adults ages 15 to 24.

Talk with Your Kids about Alcohol and Other Drugs

Alcohol and drugs don't cause violence or unhealthy relationships—but they can make it harder to make healthy choices.

If You Are Worried, Talk to Your Teen

If you think your teen's relationship might be violent, take these steps:

- Write down the reasons you are worried.

- Tell your teen why you are concerned. Point out specific things that don't seem right to you.

- Listen to your teen calmly, and thank her or him for opening up.

Get Help If You Need It

If you are worried about your teen's safety, there are people who can help.

Loveisrespect is an organization that offers support and information for teens and their parents or friends who have concerns about dating relationships. To get in touch with a trained peer advocate, you can:

- Call 866-331-9474

- Text "loveis" to 22522

- www.loveisrespect.org

Section 6.5

Talking about Sex

This section includes text excerpted from "Talk to Your Kids about Sex," Office of Disease Prevention and Health Promotion (ODPHP), U.S. Department of Health and Human Services (HHS), January 4, 2017.

The Basics

Teach your children the facts about their bodies, sex, and relationships. Talking with your kids about sex may not be easy, but it's important—and it's never too early to start. You can make a big difference in helping them stay healthy and make good choices as they grow up.

It may be hard to know where to start, especially if your parents didn't talk to you about sex when you were growing up. The following tips and strategies can help.

What Do I Say?

Kids will have different questions and concerns about sex at different ages. As your child gets older, the things you talk about will change. Remember to:

- Talk early and often. You don't have to fit everything into one conversation.

- Be ready to answer questions. Children's questions can tell you a lot about what they already know.

- Listen carefully, even if you don't agree with your child's opinion.

- Try using things that come up on TV or in music to start a conversation.

- Be honest about how you are feeling. For example, if you are embarrassed or uncomfortable, it's okay to say so.

Will Talking to My Child Really Make a Difference?

Parents are the most important influence on a teen's decisions about sex and relationships. Your child may want to talk to you about sex and dating, but may not know how to start the conversation.

Teens who talk with their parents about sex are more likely to put off having sex until they are older. They are also more likely to make healthy choices, like using condoms to prevent pregnancy and sexually transmitted diseases (STD), if they do choose to have sex.

When Is the Right Time to Start Talking?

It's never too early to start talking to children about their bodies. Use the correct names for private body parts.

What Do I Tell My Child about Puberty?

Puberty is when your child's body starts to change into an adult's body. Puberty is different for each child.

- For girls, puberty usually starts between ages 9 and 13.

- For boys, it usually begins between ages 10 and 13.

Puberty can be a confusing and overwhelming time for many kids. You can help your kids by:

- Telling them that puberty is a normal part of growing up

- Sharing facts to help them understand their changing bodies and feelings

- Talking about your own experiences when you were a kid

As your kids get older, they may be less likely to ask you questions, so it's a good idea for you to start conversations with them.

What If My Child Has Questions about Being a Boy or Girl?

Some children act or feel like they are a different gender than the sex that's listed on their birth certificate. For example, a child who was born male may feel like a girl, not a boy. And some kids don't feel like a boy or a girl.

When people act or feel like they are a different gender than their birth sex, this is called being "gender nonconforming." Some children may feel this way from very early on, while others may start to feel this way during puberty.

It's important to let your child know that you love and accept him or her—no matter what.

How Can I Help My Child Build Healthy Relationships?

Families have different rules about when it's okay for kids to start dating. Whatever your family rules are, the best time to start talking about healthy relationships is before your child starts dating.

Start conversations about what to look for in a romantic partner. Help your kids develop realistic and healthy expectations for their relationships.

Talk about Opposite Sex and Same Sex Relationships

When you talk about sex and relationships, don't assume that your teen is only interested in opposite sex relationships. Some teens may be interested in same sex relationships or identify as lesbian, gay, or bisexual.

No matter what, it's important to let your child know that you love and accept him or her. Lesbian, gay, and bisexual teens whose parents are supportive are less likely to be depressed, and more likely to make healthy choices about sex and relationships.

What Do I Tell My Child about Preventing Pregnancy and STDs?

Make sure your kids have the facts they need to make healthy decisions. This includes information about pregnancy and STDs like human immunodeficiency virus (HIV)/acquired immunodeficiency syndrome (AIDS) and chlamydia.

Both boys and girls need to know how to stay safe. Even if you think your child isn't dating or having sex, talk about ways to prevent pregnancy and STDs.

Tell your child about different birth control methods, like birth control pills. It's also important to make sure your child knows how to use condoms to prevent STDs—even if he or she is also using another method to prevent pregnancy.

Take Action!

Kids need information from an adult they trust. Use these tips to start a conversation with your child today.

Talk Early and Often

Start having conversations about your values and expectations while your child is young. Your child will get used to sharing information and opinions with you. This will make it easier for you to keep talking as your child gets older.

There's more than one way to talk to kids about sex. Try having lots of little conversations about sex instead of one big talk. And remember, if you've been putting it off, it's never too late to start a conversation about sex.

Start Small

Try not to give your kids too much information at one time. Give them time between conversations to think. They may come back later and ask questions.

Practice Active Listening

Active listening is a way to show your kids that you are paying attention and trying to understand their thoughts and feelings. Try these tips:

- Nod your head

- Repeat back what your child says in your own words. For example, "So you are feeling frustrated with our rules. You feel that you are old enough to make your own decisions."

Ask Questions

Give your kids time and space to talk about their feelings and thoughts. Ask for their opinions. Be sure to listen, even if you don't agree with your child's opinion.

Try asking questions like:

- When do you think it's okay to start dating?

- Have you talked about puberty or sex in school? Do you have any questions?

- When do you think a person is ready to have sex?

Always take your child's values and opinions seriously. This will show that you respect what your child has to say and it can help your child feel more comfortable talking to you.

Be Ready to Answer Questions

When your kids ask you questions, ask them what they think first. Their answers will tell you more about what they are asking and why. This will also give you time to think about your answer.

Do your best to answer questions honestly and correctly. If you don't know the answer to a question, you could say, "I'm not sure. Let's look that up together."

Keep in mind that kids get information about sex from lots of different sources—like friends, the Internet, and TV. This can be confusing for your child. That's another reason why it's important for you to answer questions clearly and accurately.

Use Media to Start a Conversation

Kids see and hear messages about sex every day in the media—like on TV, in music, and online. When something comes up in a TV show or song, use it as an opportunity to start a conversation with your child.

Talk in the Car or in the Kitchen

It can sometimes be easier to talk about sex if you are doing something else at the same time. Try asking a question when you are driving in the car or busy cooking dinner.

You can still show your child that you are listening by nodding your head or repeating what your child says to you.

Be Honest

It's okay to feel embarrassed or uncomfortable. Be honest with your child about how you are feeling. Remember, when you are honest with your child, your child is more likely to be honest with you.

Talk with Other Parents

Remember that you are not the only parent thinking about how to talk to kids about sex. Ask other parents how it's going for them. You may be able to get useful tips and ideas.

Talking to parents is also a great way to learn more about the messages other kids are getting about sex and relationships.

Section 6.6

Monitoring Your Teen's Activities

This section includes text excerpted from "Monitoring
Your Teen's Activities: What Parents and Families Should Know,"
Centers for Disease Control and Prevention (CDC),
December 2012. Reviewed November 2017.

What Is Parental Monitoring?

Parental monitoring includes:

• the expectations parents have for their teen's behavior;

• the actions parents take to keep track of their teen; and

• the ways parents respond when their teen breaks the rules.

You are using parental monitoring when you ask your teen :

• Where will you be?

• Whom will you be with?

• When will you be home?

You are also monitoring when you:

• Check in with your teen by phone.

• Get to know his or her friends and their parents.

• Talk with your teen about how he or she spends time or whether
he or she is making safe choices.

• Set and enforce rules for your teen's behavior by clearly explaining the rules and consequences and following through with
appropriate consequences when the rules are broken.

Monitoring should start in early childhood and continue throughout the teen years, evolving as children grow and mature. As children
develop into teenagers, adults might view them as more independent
and less in need of monitoring. But, consistent monitoring throughout

the teen years is critical—teens' desire for independence can bring opportunities for unhealthy or unsafe behaviors.

Does Parental Monitoring Make a Difference?

Yes. Research shows that teens whose parents use effective monitoring practices are less likely to make poor decisions, such as having sex at an early age, smoking cigarettes, drinking alcohol, being physically aggressive, or skipping school. Clear communication about your expectations is especially important. Research shows that teens who believe their parents disapprove of risky behaviors are less likely to choose those behaviors.

What Can Parents Do to Monitor Their Teens Effectively?

The following are some steps you can take to monitor your teen and help protect him or her from risky behaviors:

- Talk with your teen about your rules and expectations, and explain the consequences for breaking the rules.
- Talk and listen to your teen often about how he or she feels and what he or she is thinking.
- Know who your teen's friends are.
- Talk with your teen about the plans he or she has with friends, what he or she is doing after school, and where he or she will be going.
- Set expectations for when your teen will come home, and expect a call if he or she is going to be late.
- Ask whether an adult will be present when your teen is visiting a friend's home.
- Get to know your teen's boyfriend or girlfriend.
- Get to know the parents of your teen's friends.
- Talk with your relatives, your neighbors, your teen's teachers, and other adults who know your teen. Ask them to share what they observe about your teen's behaviors, moods, or friends.
- Watch how your teen spends money.
- Keep track of how your teen spends time online, and talk about using the Internet safely.

- Pay attention to your teen's mood and behavior at home, and discuss any concerns you might have.

- If your teen does break a rule, enforce the consequences fairly and consistently.

- Make sure your teen knows how to contact you at all times.

How Can Parents Be Successful at Monitoring Their Teens?

Parental monitoring works best when parents have good, open, and caring relationships with their teens. Teens are more willing to talk to their parents if they think their parents can be trusted, have useful advice to offer, and are open and available to listen and talk. Teens who are satisfied with their relationships with their parents tend to be more willing to follow the rules. You can promote a caring relationship with your teen by listening, asking questions, asking for opinions, offering support and praise, and staying involved in your teen's life.

How Can Busy Parents Monitor Their Teens?

As a parent, you face many competing demands on your time. Work or other activities can keep you away from home and limit monitoring of your teen. To help bridge this gap, you can use e-mails, text messages, and phone calls to check in with your teen. You can also seek the support of other family members, friends, and school staff to help monitor your teen's activities and behavior. Teens who have a variety of adults supervising and monitoring their activities may be even less likely to engage in unhealthy and unsafe behaviors.

Chapter 7

For Teens: Talking to Your Parents or Guardians

Many girls have fights or tough times with the adults in their families. They can still have amazing relationships with those adults.

Talking with Parents or Guardians[1]

- **As you get older, your relationship with your parents or guardians changes.** You may want more privacy or independence, for example. That's natural, but you can still stay connected.

- **Making time to talk can help strengthen your connections.** You might just talk about simple, everyday things or talk while doing something fun together. Being in the habit of talking about small things may make it easier to talk about harder subjects.

- **If you want to share how you feel about something,** it can be easier if you use "I statements." That means you say things

This chapter includes text excerpted from documents published by two public domain sources. Text under the headings marked 1 are excerpted from "Family Relationships—Parents, Stepparents, Grandparents, and Guardians," girlshealth. gov, Office on Women's Health (OWH), September 16, 2015; Text under the heading marked 2 is excerpted from "Your Feelings—Talking to Your Parents about Emotional Problems," girlshealth.gov, Office on Women's Health (OWH), January 7, 2015.

like "I feel…" instead of criticizing the other person. Also, if you want something, try to ask politely. (Making demands is not very polite—or very effective.)

- **If you need to raise a tough topic,** keep in mind that your parents or guardians were young once, too. They may have faced very similar issues. Plus, they probably will appreciate your honesty and bravery in coming to them.

- **If you don't like your family's rules**, ask if you can discuss them. Sometimes, parents are willing to change certain rules, especially if you show you can be responsible.

Arguing with Parents or Guardians[1]

Parents and teens disagree and argue at times, even though they love each other.

Tips for handling fights with parents:

- **Talk about the rules.** Ask the reasons behind a rule so you can understand it. Consider sharing how a rule makes you feel. Ask if your parents or guardians will consider your ideas about what the rules should be.

- **Follow the rules.** Keep to your curfew if you have one. Call if you're going to be late, so your parents or guardians don't worry. If you follow the rules, your parents or guardians may be more likely to discuss them. If you don't follow the rules, you'll likely just get in trouble.

- **Pick your battles.** Cleaning your room is no fun, but it's most likely not worth fighting about.

- **Spend time with your family.** Some teens fight with their parents or guardians over how much time they spend with friends. Talk it over, and make some special family time. You might go for a walk or have dinner together.

- **Try to stay calm.** Don't yell or stomp your feet when your parents or guardians say no. If you listen and speak calmly, you may show them that you are growing up.

- **After an argument, think about what happened.** Consider your part in the problem, and apologize. Talk about how you might prevent similar fights in the future.

Handling Challenging Times[1]

Lots of teens face some really scary family issues, like illness and divorce. Over time, they usually feel better. Here are some ways you can feel better, too.

Think of ways you can cope, like going for a walk, doing something creative, or talking to a friend. Stay away from things like drugs and drinking, since they only make problems worse.

If you need support from outside your family, talk to a trusted adult, such as a teacher, religious leader, or school counselor. You also can contact a 24-hour crisis text line and a helpline for kids and teens.

- **Are you struggling because your parents are getting divorced?** Remember, divorce is never a kid's fault. With time and support, you can adjust to the changes you're facing.

- **Do you have a relative in the military?** Having a relative in the military can be scary and upsetting.

- **Is your family having money problems?** You can't solve your family's money worries, but you might suggest that your family look at a helpful website (www.usa.gov/benefits-grants-loans)..

- **Does your parent have a drug or alcohol problem?** If your parent has an addiction, you may feel scared or worried.

Talking to Your Parents about Emotional Problems[2]

It takes courage to tell a parent or guardian that you are having trouble with your feelings. But adults can help you through tough times, and it's important to get the support you need.

- **When you're ready, try to find a time when you won't get interrupted.** You may even need to schedule a time to talk. Try saying something like, "Mom and Dad, I have something I'd like to talk about. Can we sit and talk after dinner?"

- **If talking seems too hard, it might be easier to write your thoughts.** A letter, an email, or even a text message can get the conversation going. Try something as simple as "I've been feeling anxious" or "I'm worried I might be depressed." Or you might just say, "I need your help."

- **Keep in mind that if your parents or you get upset,** you can continue the conversation over time. If they ask a question about your feelings that you can't answer, you might say you'll think about it and will talk more later.

- **If you think you definitely can't talk to your parents or guardians,** reach out to another trusted adult. This might be a school counselor, teacher, religious leader, school nurse, or doctor. Definitely don't give up. You deserve to feel better!

Getting along with Stepparents[1]

A new stepparent can bring up lots of feelings. Even if you like your stepparent, you may feel sad, worried, or upset at times.
Here are some tips that can help:

- **Accept your feelings.** It's natural to have feelings like confusion, anger, and guilt when a parent remarries. Don't worry that there's something wrong with you if you have any (or all) of these feelings!

- **Sort through your feelings.** Keeping a journal might help. Friends who have gone through a similar situation may also be able to offer tips.

- **Talk honestly.** If you don't like any new rules or situations, ask calmly and respectfully about changing them. Check out tips for handling conflict.

- **Get support from your parent or another trusted adult.** Adults who care about you really want to help. If it seems too hard to turn to a family member, talk to another adult you trust. If you are struggling, a mental health professional like a school counselor can help.

- **Try to spend time with your stepparent.** This new person is going to be around, and chances are you will be happier if you can find his or her more positive sides.

Keep in mind that with patience—and some hard work—lots of stepfamilies end up feeling very close.

Part Two

Staying Healthy during Adolescence

Chapter 8

Medical Care and Your Teen

Chapter Contents

Section 8.1—What to Expect at the Doctor's Office
       (Ages 11 to 14) 90

Section 8.2—What to Expect at the Doctor's Office
       (Ages 15 to 17) 95

Section 8.3—Vaccines Teens Need 100

Section 8.1

What to Expect at the Doctor's Office (Ages 11 to 14)

This section includes text excerpted from "Make the Most of Your Child's Visit to the Doctor (Ages 11 to 14)," Office of Disease Prevention and Health Promotion (ODPHP), U.S. Department of Health and Human Services (HHS), September 22, 2017.

Kids ages 11 to 14 need to go to the doctor or nurse for a "well-child visit" once a year.

A well-child visit is when you take your child to the doctor for a full checkup to make sure she is healthy and developing normally. This is different from other visits for sickness or injury.

At a well-child visit, the doctor or nurse can help catch any problems early, when they may be easier to treat.

To make the most of the visit:

- Gather important information

- Make a list of questions for the doctor

- Know what to expect from the visit

- Help your child get more involved in the visit

What about Cost?

Under the Affordable Care Act, the healthcare reform law passed in 2010, insurance plans must cover well-child visits. Depending on your insurance plan, your child may be able to get well-child checkups at no cost to you. Check with your insurance company to learn more.

How Do I Know If My Child Is Growing and Developing on Schedule?

Your child's doctor or nurse can help you identify "developmental milestones," the new skills that children usually develop by a certain age. This is an important part of the well-child visit.

Some developmental milestones are related to your child's behavior and learning, and others are about physical changes in your child's body.

What Are Some Changes I Might See in My Child's Feelings, Relationships, and Behavior?

Developmental milestones for preteens and teens ages 11 to 14 include:

- More interest in their looks and clothes
- Mood swings (going quickly from happy to sad or sad to happy)
- More concern about what their friends and classmates think
- Stronger problem-solving skills
- Clearer sense of right and wrong
- Wanting more independence
- Challenging rules and resisting advice from parents

This is also a time when some kids may start showing signs of depression or eating disorders.

- Make sure the doctor screens your teen for depression.
- Know the signs of eating disorders.

What Are Some Physical Changes My Child Will Go Through?

Many kids ages 11 to 14 are going through puberty. Puberty is when a child's body develops into an adult's body.

For girls, puberty usually starts between ages 9 and 13. For boys, it usually starts between ages 10 and 13.

You can help by giving your child information about what changes to expect during puberty. You can also encourage your child to talk about puberty with the doctor or another trusted adult, like a teacher or school nurse.

Take Action!

Take these steps to help you and your child get the most out of well-child visits.

91

Gather important information.

Take any medical records you have to the appointment, including a record of shots your child has received.

Make a list of any important changes in your child's life since the last visit, like a:

- Separation or divorce
- New school or a move to a new neighborhood
- Serious illness or death of a friend or family member

Help your child get more involved in visits to the doctor.

Once your child starts puberty, the doctor will usually ask you to leave the room during your child's physical exam. This lets your child develop a relationship with the doctor or nurse and ask questions in private. It's an important step in teaching your child to take control of his healthcare.

Your child can also:

- Call to schedule appointments
- Help you fill out medical forms
- Write down questions for the doctor or nurse

Make a list of questions you want to ask the doctor.

Before the well-child visit, write down 3 to 5 questions you have. This visit is a great time to ask the doctor or nurse any questions about:

- A health condition your child has (like an allergy, asthma, or acne)
- Changes in behavior or mood
- Loss of interest in favorite activities
- Problems at school (like learning challenges or not wanting to go to school)

Here are some questions you may want to ask:

- How can I make sure my child is getting enough physical activity?
- How can I help my child eat healthy?
- Is my child at a healthy weight?

- Is my child's body developing normally?
- Is my preteen up to date on shots?
- How can I talk with my child about sex?
- How can I talk with my child about tobacco, alcohol, and drugs?
- How can I teach my child to use the Internet safely?
- How can I talk with my child about bullying?

Take a notepad and write down the answers so you can remember them later.

Ask what to do if your child gets sick.

Make sure you know how to get in touch with a doctor or nurse when the office is closed. Ask how to get hold of the doctor on call, or if there's a nurse information service you can call at night or on the weekend.

Know what to expect.

During each well-child visit, the doctor or nurse will ask you questions, do a physical exam, and update your child's medical history. You'll also be able to ask your questions and discuss any problems.

The doctor or nurse will ask you and your child questions.

The doctor or nurse may ask about:

- Behavior—Does your child have trouble following directions at home or at school?
- Health—Does your child often complain of headaches or other pain?
- Safety—Does anyone in your home have a gun? If so, is it unloaded and locked in a place where your child can't get it?
- School and activities—Does your child look forward to going to school? What does your child like to do after school?
- Eating habits—What does your child eat on a normal day?
- Family and friends—Have there been any recent changes in your family? How many close friends does your child have?
- Emotions—Does your child often seem sad or bored? Does your child have someone to talk to about problems?
- Sexuality—Have you talked with your child about puberty? Is your child dating?

The answers to questions like these will help the doctor or nurse make sure your child is healthy and developing normally.

The doctor or nurse will also check your child's body.

To check your child's body, the doctor or nurse will:

- Measure height and weight and figure out your child's body mass index (BMI)
- Check your child's blood pressure
- Check your child's vision and hearing
- Check your child's body parts (this is called a physical exam)
- Decide if your child needs any lab tests, like a blood test
- Give shots your child needs

The doctor or nurse will pay special attention to signs of certain issues.

The doctor or nurse will offer additional help if your child may be:

- Depressed
- Struggling with an eating disorder
- Using tobacco, alcohol, or drugs
- Experiencing any kind of violence

And if your child may be having sex, the doctor or nurse will talk to your child about preventing STDs (sexually transmitted diseases) and pregnancy.

The doctor or nurse will make sure you and your child have the resources you need.

This may include telling you and your child about:

- Websites or apps that have helpful health information
- Organizations in your community where you can go for help

If necessary, the doctor or nurse may also refer your child to a specialist.

Section 8.2

What to Expect at the Doctor's Office (Ages 15 to 17)

This section includes text excerpted from "Make the Most of Your Child's Visit to the Doctor (Ages 15 to 17)," Office of Disease Prevention and Health Promotion (ODPHP), U.S. Department of Health and Human Services (HHS), September 22, 2017.

Teens ages 15 to 17 need to go to the doctor or nurse for a "well-child visit" once a year.

A well-child visit is when you take your teen to the doctor for a full checkup to make sure he is healthy and developing normally. This is different from other visits for sickness or injury.

At a well-child visit, the doctor or nurse can help catch any problems early, when they may be easier to treat.

To make the most of your teen's visit:

- Gather important information

- Make a list of questions for the doctor

- Know what to expect from the visit

- Help your teen get more involved in the visit

What about Cost?

Under the Affordable Care Act, insurance plans must cover well-child visits. Depending on your insurance, your teen may be able to get well-child checkups at no cost to you. Check with your insurance company to learn more.

How Do I Know If My Teen Is Growing and Developing on Schedule?

Your teen's doctor or nurse can help you identify "developmental milestones," or signs to look for that show your teen is developing normally. This is an important part of the well-child visit.

Some developmental milestones are related to your teen's behavior and learning, and others are about physical changes in your teen's body.

What Are Some Changes I Might See in My Teen's Behavior, Feelings, and Relationships?

Developmental milestones for teens ages 15 to 17 include:

- Less time spent with parents or family, and more time spent with friends

- Less fighting with parents than during ages 13 and 14

- More worry about the future (like going to college or finding a job)

- More interest in romantic relationships and sex

- Trying new things, including experimenting with tobacco, alcohol, or drugs

This is also a time when some teens may start showing signs of depression, anxiety, or eating disorders. Your teen may also have a girlfriend or boyfriend.

What Are Some Physical Changes My Teen Is Going Through?

Teens ages 15 to 17 are usually either finished or close to finishing puberty. Puberty is when a child's body develops into an adult's body.

Although it may be different for some teens, most girls finish puberty by age 15. Most boys finish puberty by age 16.

Teens might not ask you questions about sex, their bodies, or relationships. That's why it's a good idea for you to start the conversation. You can also encourage your teen to ask the doctor or nurse questions about body changes.

Take Action!

Take these steps to help you and your teen get the most out of well-child visits.

Gather important information.

Take any medical records you have to the appointment, including a record of shots your teen has received.

Make a list of any important changes in your teen's life since the last visit, like a:

• Separation or divorce

• New school or a move to a new neighborhood

• Serious illness or death of a friend or family member

Help your teen get more involved in visits to the doctor.

The doctor will probably ask you to leave the room during part of the visit, usually the physical exam. This lets your teen develop a relationship with the doctor or nurse and ask questions in private. It's an important step in teaching your teen to take control of his healthcare.

Your teen can also:

• Call to schedule appointments

• Help you fill out medical forms

• Write down questions for the doctor or nurse

Make a list of questions you want to ask the doctor.

Before the well-child visit, write down 3 to 5 questions you have. This visit is a great time to ask the doctor or nurse any questions about:

• A health condition your teen has (like acne or asthma)

• Changes in your teen's behavior or mood

• Loss of interest in favorite activities

• Your teen's sexual development

• Tobacco, alcohol, or drug use

• Problems at school (like learning challenges or not wanting to go to school)

Here are some questions you may want to ask:

• Is my teen up to date on shots?

• How can I make sure my teen is getting enough physical activity?

• How can I help my teen eat healthy?

• Is my teen at a healthy weight?

- How can our family set rules more effectively?

- How can I help my teen become a safe driver?

Take a notepad and write down the answers so you can remember them later.

Ask what to do if your teen gets sick.

Make sure you know how to get in touch with a doctor or nurse when the office is closed. Ask how to get hold of the doctor on call, or if there's a nurse information service you can call at night or on the weekend.

Know what to expect.

During each well-child visit, the doctor or nurse will ask you questions, do a physical exam, and update your teen's medical history. You and your teen will also be able to ask your questions and discuss any problems.

The doctor or nurse will ask your teen questions.

The doctor or nurse may ask about:

- Behavior—Do you have trouble following directions at home or at school?

- Health—Do you often get headaches or have other kinds of pain?

- Safety—Do you always wear a seatbelt in the car? Do you and your friends use tobacco, alcohol, or drugs?

- School and activities—Do you look forward to going to school? What do you like to do after school?

- Eating habits—What do you eat on a regular day?

- Family and friends—Have there been any changes in your family recently? Do you have close friends?

- Emotions—Do you often feel sad or bored? Is there someone you trust who you can talk to about problems?

- Sexuality—Do you have any questions about your body? Do you have a boyfriend or girlfriend?

- The future—Have you started to think about what you want to do after high school?

The answers to questions like these will help the doctor or nurse make sure your teen is healthy and developing normally.

The doctor or nurse will also check your teen's body.

To check your teen's body, the doctor or nurse will:

- Measure height and weight and figure out your teen's body mass index (BMI)
- Check your teen's blood pressure
- Check your teen's vision and hearing
- Check your teen's body parts (this is called a physical exam)
- Decide if your teen needs any lab tests, like a blood test
- Give shots your teen needs

The doctor or nurse will pay special attention to signs of certain issues.

The doctor or nurse will offer additional help if your teen may be:

- Depressed
- Struggling with an eating disorder
- Using tobacco, alcohol, or other drugs
- Experiencing any kind of violence

And if your teen may be having sex, the doctor or nurse will talk about preventing STDs (sexually transmitted diseases) and pregnancy.

The doctor or nurse will make sure you and your teen have the resources you need.

This may include telling you and your teen about:

- Websites or apps that have helpful health information
- Organizations in your community where you can go for help

If necessary, the doctor or nurse may also refer your teen to a specialist.

Section 8.3

Vaccines Teens Need

This section contains text excerpted from the following sources:
Text beginning with the heading "Your Preteens and Teens Need
Vaccines, Too!" is excerpted from "Your Preteens and Teens Need
Vaccines Too!" Vaccines.gov, U.S. Department of Health and Human
Services (HHS), May 24, 2017; Text under the heading "Vaccines
for 13 to 18 Years" is excerpted from "Vaccines for Your Children:
Protect Your Child at Every Age—13 to 18 Years," Centers for
Disease Control and Prevention (CDC), April 15, 2016.

Your Preteens and Teens Need Vaccines, Too!

Because most preteens get their shots in the month of August before
school begins, it can be difficult to get in to see your child's doctor or
nurse. Make an appointment to get your child vaccinated earlier this
summer and beat the back to school rush!

There are four vaccines recommended for preteens to help protect
your children, as well as their friends and family members, from serious illness. While your kids should get a flu vaccine every year, the
three other preteen vaccines should be given when kids are either 11
or 12 years old.

What Vaccines Are Recommended for My Preteen?

Boys and girls should get the following vaccines at age 11 or 12
years:

- **HPV vaccine.** Human papillomavirus (HPV) vaccine helps protect against HPV infections that cause cancer. All boys and girls
should finish the HPV vaccine series before they turn 13 years old.

- **Quadrivalent meningococcal conjugate vaccine.** Quadrivalent meningococcal conjugate vaccine protects against some of
the bacteria that can cause infections of the lining of the brain
and spinal cord (meningitis) and bloodstream infections (bacteremia or septicemia). These illnesses can be very serious, even
fatal.

- **Tdap vaccine.** Tdap vaccine provides a booster to continue protection from childhood against three serious diseases: tetanus, diphtheria, and pertussis (also called whooping cough).

- **Flu vaccine.** Preteens and teens should get a flu vaccine every year, by the end of October if possible. It is very important for preteens and teens with chronic health conditions like asthma or diabetes to get the flu shot, but the flu can be serious for even healthy kids.

Be sure to check with the doctor to make sure that your preteen is up to date on all the vaccines they need. They may need to "catch up" on vaccines they might have missed when they were younger.

Some preteens and teens may faint after getting a shot or any other medical procedure. Sitting or lying down while getting shot and staying that way for about 15 minutes after the shots can help prevent fainting. Most side effects from vaccines are very minor—such as redness or soreness in the arm—especially compared with the serious diseases that these vaccines prevent.

Need Help Paying for Vaccines?

Most health insurance plans cover the cost of vaccines. If you don't have insurance, or if it does not cover vaccines, the Vaccines for Children (VFC) program may be able to help. The VFC program provides vaccines for children ages 18 years and younger, who are not insured, Medicaid eligible, or American Indian or Alaska Native.

Vaccines for 13 to 18 Years

Between 13 through 18 years old, your child should visit the doctor once each year for check-ups. This can be a great time to get any vaccines your teen may need. Below are vaccines recommended for your teen.

The following vaccines are recommended by the American Academy of Pediatrics (AAP), the American Academy of Family Physicians (AAFP), other medical societies, and CDC:

- **Flu Vaccine.** Everyone 13–18 years of age and older should get a flu vaccine every year.

- **Meningococcal Conjugate Vaccine.** A booster dose of meningococcal conjugate vaccine is needed at age 16 to maintain protection against some of the bacteria that can cause meningococcal disease, including sepsis and meningitis.

- **Serogroup B Meningococcal Vaccine.** Teens may also be vaccinated with a serogroup B meningococcal vaccine (2 or 3 doses depending on brand), preferably at 16 through 18 years old, but also up to age 23.

Catch-Up Vaccinations

If your child has not yet started or completed the HPV vaccine series, they should get those shots now. If your child has not received a one-time dose of Tdap, they should get that shot as soon as possible.

- **HPV Vaccine.** Human papillomavirus (HPV) vaccines help protect both girls and boys from HPV infection and cancers caused by HPV.

- **Tdap Vaccine.** Tdap vaccine is recommended for protection against tetanus, diphtheria and pertussis (whooping cough).

Is Your Teen Traveling?

Does your teen have an opportunity for travel outside the United States? Be sure to check Centers for Disease Control and Prevention's (CDC) Traveler's' Health Vaccinations website and to talk to your child's doctor about routine and travel-related vaccines.

Vaccines before College

Before your child enters college, check that his or her vaccinations are up to date. These include childhood, preteen and teen vaccinations. Many states recommend and several states require that some college students receive the meningococcal conjugate vaccine.

Chapter 9

Nutrition Recommendations for Teens

As you get older, you're able to start making your own decisions about a lot of things that matter most to you. You may choose your own clothes, music, and friends. You also may be ready to make decisions about your body and health.

Did You Know?

About 20 percent of kids between 12 and 19 years old have obesity. But small changes in your eating and physical activity habits may help you reach and stay a healthy weight.

How Does the Body Use Energy?

Your body needs energy to function and grow. Calories from food and drinks give you that energy. Think of food as energy to charge up your battery for the day. Throughout the day, you use energy from the battery to think and move, so you need to eat and drink to stay powered up. Balancing the energy you take in through food and beverages with the energy you use for growth, activity, and daily

This chapter includes text excerpted from "Take Charge of Your Health: A Guide for Teenagers," National Institute of Diabetes and Digestive and Kidney Diseases (NIDDK), December 2016.

living is called "energy balance." Energy balance may help you stay a healthy weight.

How Many Calories Does Your Body Need?

Different people need different amounts of calories to be active or stay a healthy weight. The number of calories you need depends on whether you are male or female, your genes, how old you are, your height and weight, whether you are still growing, and how active you are, which may not be the same every day.

How Should You Manage or Control Your Weight?

Some teens try to lose weight by eating very little; cutting out whole groups of foods like foods with carbohydrates, or "carbs;" skipping meals; or fasting. These approaches to losing weight could be unhealthy because they may leave out important nutrients your body needs. In fact, unhealthy dieting could get in the way of trying to manage your weight because it may lead to a cycle of eating very little and then overeating because you get too hungry. Unhealthy dieting could also affect your mood and how you grow.

Smoking, making yourself vomit, or using diet pills or laxatives to lose weight may also lead to health problems. If you make yourself vomit, or use diet pills or laxatives to control your weight, you could have signs of a serious eating disorder and should talk with your healthcare professional or another trusted adult right away. If you smoke, which increases your risk of heart disease, cancer, and other health problems, quit smoking as soon as possible.

If you think you need to lose weight, talk with a healthcare professional first. A doctor or dietitian may be able to tell you if you need to lose weight and how to do so in a healthy way.

Choose Healthy Foods and Drinks

Healthy eating involves taking control of how much and what types of food you eat, as well as the beverages you drink. Try to replace foods high in sugar, salt, and unhealthy fats with fruits, vegetables, whole grains, low fat protein foods, and fat free or low fat dairy foods.

Fruits and Vegetables

Make half of your plate fruits and vegetables. Dark green, red, and orange vegetables have high levels of the nutrients you need, like vitamin C, calcium, and fiber. Adding tomato and spinach—or any other available greens that you like—to your sandwich is an easy way to get more veggies in your meal.

Grains

Choose whole grains like whole wheat bread, brown rice, oatmeal, and whole grain cereal, instead of refined grain cereals, white bread, and white rice.

Protein

Power up with low fat or lean meats like turkey or chicken, and other protein rich foods, such as seafood, egg whites, beans, nuts, and tofu.

Dairy

Build strong bones with fat free or low fat milk products. If you can't digest lactose—the sugar in milk that can cause stomach pain or gas—choose lactose free milk or soy milk with added calcium. Fat free or low fat yogurt is also a good source of dairy food.

Fats

Fat is an important part of your diet. Fat helps your body grow and develop, and may even keep your skin and hair healthy. But fats have more calories per gram than protein or carbs, and some are not healthy.

Some fats, such as oils that come from plants and are liquid at room temperature, are better for you than other fats. Foods that contain healthy oils include avocados, olives, nuts, seeds, and seafood such as salmon and tuna fish.

Solid fats such as butter, stick margarine, and lard, are solid at room temperature. These fats often contain saturated and trans fats, which are not healthy for you. Other foods with saturated fats include fatty meats, and cheese and other dairy products made from whole milk. Take it easy on foods like fried chicken, cheeseburgers, and fries, which often have a lot of saturated and trans fats. Options to consider include a turkey sandwich with mustard or a lean meat, turkey, or veggie burger.

Your body needs a small amount of sodium, which is mostly found in salt. But getting too much sodium from your foods and drinks can raise your blood pressure, which is unhealthy for your heart and your body in general. Even though you're a teen, it's important to pay attention to your blood pressure and heart health now to prevent health problems as you get older.

Try to consume less than 2,300 mg, or no more than 1 teaspoon, of sodium a day. This amount includes the salt in already prepared food, as well as the salt you add when cooking or eating your food.

Processed foods, like those that are canned or packaged, often have more sodium than unprocessed foods, such as fresh fruits and vegetables. When you can, choose fresh or frozen fruits and veggies over processed foods. Try adding herbs and spices instead of salt to season your food if you make your own meals. Remember to rinse canned vegetables with water to remove extra salt. If you use packaged foods, check the amount of sodium listed on the Nutrition Facts label.

Limit Added Sugars

Some foods, like fruit, are naturally sweet. Other foods, like ice cream and baked desserts, as well as some beverages, have added sugars to make them taste sweet. These sugars add calories but not vitamins or fiber. Try to consume less than 10 percent of your daily calories from added sugars in food and beverages. Reach for an apple or banana instead of a candy bar.

Many teens need more of these nutrients:

- **Calcium,** to build strong bones and teeth. Good sources of calcium are fat free or low fat milk, yogurt, and cheese.

- **Vitamin D,** to keep bones healthy. Good sources of vitamin D include orange juice, whole oranges, tuna, and fat free or low fat milk.

- **Potassium,** to help lower blood pressure. Try a banana, or baked potato with the skin, for a potassium boost.

- **Fiber,** to help you stay regular and feel full. Good sources of fiber include beans and celery.

- **Protein,** to power you up and help you grow strong. Peanut butter; eggs; tofu; legumes, such as lentils and peas; and chicken, fish, and low fat meats are all good sources of protein.

- **Iron,** to help you grow. Red meat contains a form of iron that your body absorbs best. Spinach, beans, peas, and iron fortified cereals are also sources of iron. You can help your body absorb the iron from these foods better when you also eat foods with vitamin C, like an orange.

Control Your Food Portions

A portion is how much food or beverage you choose to consume at one time, whether in a restaurant, from a package, at school or a friend's, or at home. Many people consume larger portions than they need, especially when away from home. Ready to eat meals—from a restaurant, grocery store, or at school—may give you larger portions than your body needs to stay charged up. The Weight control Information Network (WIN) has tips to help you eat and drink a suitable amount of food and beverages for you, whether you are at home or somewhere else.

Don't Skip Meals

Skipping meals might seem like an easy way to lose weight, but it actually may lead to weight gain if you eat more later to make up for it. Even if you're really busy with school and activities, it's important to try not to skip meals. Follow these tips to keep your body charged up all day and to stay healthy:

- **Eat breakfast every day.** Breakfast helps your body get going. If you're short on time in the morning, grab something to go, like an apple or banana.

- **Pack your lunch on school days.** Packing your lunch may help you control your food and beverage portions and increases the chances that you will eat it because you made it.

- **Eat dinner with your family.** When you eat home cooked meals with your family, you are more likely to consume healthy foods. Having meals together also gives you a chance to reconnect with each other and share news about your day.

- **Get involved in grocery shopping and meal planning at home.** Going food shopping and planning and preparing meals with family members or friends can be fun. Not only can you choose a favorite grocery store, and healthy foods and recipes, you also have a chance to help others in your family eat healthy too.

Healthy Eating Tips

Try to limit foods like cookies, candy, frozen desserts, chips, and fries, which often have a lot of sugar, unhealthy fat, and salt.

- For a quick snack, try recharging with a pear, apple, or banana; a small bag of baby carrots; or hummus with sliced veggies.

- Don't add sugar to your food and drinks.

- Drink fat free or low fat milk and avoid sugary drinks. Soda, energy drinks, sweet tea, and some juices have added sugars, a source of extra calories. The *2015–2020 Dietary Guidelines* call for getting less than 10 percent of your daily calories from added sugars.

Chapter 10

Healthy Food Choices for Teens

Eat Smart and Be Active as You Grow: 10 Tips for Teen Girls

Young girls, ages 10 to 19, have a lot of changes going on in their bodies. Building healthier habits will help you—now as a growing teen—and later in life. Growing up means you are in charge of foods you eat and the time you spend being physically active every day.

1. Build Strong Bones

A good diet and regular physical activity can build strong bones throughout your life. Choose fat-free or low-fat milk, cheeses, and yogurt to get the vitamin D and calcium your growing bones need. Strengthen your bones three times a week doing activities such as running, gymnastics, and skating.

2. Cut Back on Sweets

Cut back on sugary drinks. Many 12-ounce cans of soda have 10 teaspoons of sugar in them. Drink water when you are thirsty. Sipping

---

This chapter includes text excerpted from "Students—Teens," ChooseMyPlate. gov, U.S. Department of Agriculture (USDA), August 4, 2017.

water and cutting back on cakes, candies, and sweets helps to maintain a healthy weight.

3. Power up with Whole Grain

Fuel your body with nutrient-packed whole-grain foods. Make sure that at least half your grain foods are whole grains such as brown rice, whole-wheat breads, and popcorn.

4. Choose Vegetables Rich in Color

Brighten your plate with vegetables that are red, orange or dark green. Try acorn squash, cherry tomatoes or sweet potatoes. Spinach and beans also provide vitamins like folate and minerals like potassium that are essential for healthy growth.

5. Check Nutrition Facts Labels for Iron

Read Nutrition Facts labels to find foods containing iron. Most protein foods like meat, poultry, eggs, and beans have iron, and so do fortified breakfast cereals and breads.

6. Be a Healthy Role Model

Encourage your friends to practice healthier habits. Share what you do to work through challenges. Keep your computer and TV time to less than 2 hours a day (unless it's schoolwork).

7. Try Something New

Keep healthy eating fun by picking out new foods you've never tried before like lentils, mango, quinoa or kale.

8. Make Moving Part of Every Event

Being active makes everyone feel good. Aim for 60 minutes of physical activity each day. Move your body often. Dancing, playing active games, walking to school with friends, swimming, and biking are only a few fun ways to be active. Also, try activities that target the muscles in your arms and legs.

9. Include All Food Groups Daily

Use MyPlate (www.choosemyplate.gov/MyPlate) as your guide to include all food groups each day.

10. *Everyone Has Different Needs*

Get nutrition information based on your age, gender, height, weight, and physical activity level. Use SuperTracker (www.SuperTracker. usda.gov) to find your calorie level, choose the foods you need, and track progress toward your goals.

Choose the Foods You Need to Grow: 10 Tips for Teen Guys

Feed your growing body by making better food choices today as a teen and as you continue to grow into your twenties. Make time to be physically active every day to help you be fit and healthy as you grow.

1. *Get over the Idea of Magic Foods*

There are no magic foods to eat for good health. Teen guys need to eat foods such as vegetables, fruits, whole grains, protein foods, and fat-free or low-fat dairy foods. Choose protein foods like unsalted nuts, beans, lean meats, and fish.

2. *Always Hungry?*

Whole grains that provide fiber can give you a feeling of fullness and provide key nutrients. Choose half your grains as whole grains. Eat whole-wheat breads, pasta, and brown rice instead of white bread, rice or other refined grains. Also, choose vegetables and fruits when you need to "fill-up."

3. *Keep Water Handy*

Water is a better option than many other drink choices. Keep a water bottle in your backpack and at your desk to satisfy your thirst. Skip soda, fruit drinks, and energy and sports drinks. They are sugar-sweetened and have few nutrients.

4. *Make a List of Favorite Foods*

Like green apples more than red apples? Ask your family food shopper to buy quick-to-eat foods for the fridge like mini-carrots, apples oranges, low-fat cheese slices or yogurt. And also try dried fruit; unsalted nuts; whole-grain breads, cereal, and crackers; and popcorn.

5. Start Cooking Often

Get over being hungry by fixing your own snacks and meals. Learn to make vegetable omelets, bean quesadillas or a batch of spaghetti. Prepare your own food so you can make healthier meals and snacks. Microwaving frozen pizzas doesn't count as home cooking.

6. Skip Foods That Can Add Unwanted Pounds

Cut back on calories by limiting fatty meats like ribs, bacon, and hot dogs. Some foods are just occasional treats like pizza, cakes, cookies, candies, and ice cream. Check out the calorie content of sugary drinks by reading the Nutrition Facts label. Many 12-ounce sodas contain 10 teaspoons of sugar.

7. Learn How Much Food You Need

Teen guys may need more food than most adults, teen girls, and little kids. Go to www.SuperTracker.usda.gov. It shows how much food you need based on your age, height, weight, and activity level. It also tracks progress towards fitness goals.

8. Check Nutrition Facts Labels

To grow, your body needs vitamins and minerals. Calcium and vitamin D are especially important for your growing bones. Read Nutrition Facts labels for calcium. Dairy foods provide the minerals your bones need to grow.

9. Strengthen Your Muscles

Work on strengthening and aerobic activities. Work out at least 10 minutes at a time to see a better you. However, you need to get at least 60 minutes of physical activity every day.

10. Fill Your Plate Like MyPlate

Go to www.ChooseMyPlate.gov for more easy tips and science-based nutrition from the *Dietary Guidelines for Americans* (www.DietaryGuidelines.gov).

Chapter 11

Calcium, Vitamin D, and Teens

Chapter Contents

Section 11.1—Facts about Calcium 114
Section 11.2—Facts about Vitamin D...................................... 121

Section 11.1

Facts about Calcium

This section includes text excerpted from "Calcium,"
Office of Dietary Supplements (ODS), National
Institutes of Health (NIH), November 17, 2016.

What Is Calcium and What Does It Do?

Calcium is a mineral found in many foods. The body needs calcium to maintain strong bones and to carry out many important functions. Almost all calcium is stored in bones and teeth, where it supports their structure and hardness. The body also needs calcium for muscles to move and for nerves to carry messages between the brain and every body part. In addition, calcium is used to help blood vessels move blood throughout the body and to help release hormones and enzymes that affect almost every function in the human body.

How Much Calcium Do I Need?

The amount of calcium you need each day depends on your age. Average daily recommended amounts are listed below in milligrams (mg):

Table 11.1. Calcium Consumption on Daily Basis

Life Stage	Recommended Amount
Children 9–13 years	1,300 mg
Teens 14–18 years	1,300 mg
Pregnant and breastfeeding teens	1,300 mg

What Foods Provide Calcium?

Calcium is found in many foods. You can get recommended amounts of calcium by eating a variety of foods, including the following:

- Milk, yogurt, and cheese are the main food sources of calcium for the majority of people in the United States.

- Kale, broccoli, and Chinese cabbage are fine vegetable sources of calcium.

- Fish with soft bones that you eat, such as canned sardines and salmon, are fine animal sources of calcium.

- Most grains (such as breads, pastas, and unfortified cereals), while not rich in calcium, add significant amounts of calcium to the diet because people eat them often or in large amounts.

- Calcium is added to some breakfast cereals, fruit juices, soy and rice beverages, and tofu. To find out whether these foods have calcium, check the product labels.

What Kinds of Calcium Dietary Supplements Are Available?

Calcium is found in many multivitamin mineral supplements, though the amount varies by product. Dietary supplements that contain only calcium or calcium with other nutrients such as vitamin D are also available. Check the Supplement Facts label to determine the amount of calcium provided.

The two main forms of calcium dietary supplements are carbonate and citrate. Calcium carbonate is inexpensive, but is absorbed best when taken with food. Some over-the-counter antacid products, such as Tums® and Rolaids®, contain calcium carbonate. Each pill or chew provides 200–400 mg of calcium. Calcium citrate, a more expensive form of the supplement, is absorbed well on an empty or a full stomach.

In addition, people with low levels of stomach acid (a condition more common in people older than 50) absorb calcium citrate more easily than calcium carbonate. Other forms of calcium in supplements and fortified foods include gluconate, lactate, and phosphate.

Calcium absorption is best when a person consumes no more than 500 mg at one time. So a person who takes 1,000 mg/day of calcium from supplements, for example, should split the dose rather than take it all at once.

Calcium supplements may cause gas, bloating, and constipation in some people. If any of these symptoms occur, try spreading out the calcium dose throughout the day, taking the supplement with meals, or changing the supplement brand or calcium form you take.

Am I Getting Enough Calcium?

Many people don't get recommended amounts of calcium from the foods they eat, including:

- Boys aged 9 to 13 years
- Girls aged 9 to 18 years

When total intakes from both food and supplements are considered, many people—particularly adolescent girls—still fall short of getting enough calcium, while some older women likely get more than the upper limit.

Certain groups of people are more likely than others to have trouble getting enough calcium:

- Women of childbearing age whose menstrual periods stop (amenorrhea) because they exercise heavily, eat too little, or both. They need sufficient calcium to cope with the resulting decreased calcium absorption, increased calcium losses in the urine, and slowdown in the formation of new bone.

- People with lactose intolerance cannot digest this natural sugar found in milk and experience symptoms like bloating, gas, and diarrhea when they drink more than small amounts at a time. They usually can eat other calcium rich dairy products that are low in lactose, such as yogurt and many cheeses, and drink lactose reduced or lactose free milk.

- Vegans (vegetarians who eat no animal products) and ovo vegetarians (vegetarians who eat eggs but no dairy products), because they avoid the dairy products that are a major source of calcium in other people's diets.

Many factors can affect the amount of calcium absorbed from the digestive tract, including:

- **Age.** Efficiency of calcium absorption decreases as people age. Recommended calcium intakes are higher for people over age 70.

- **Vitamin D intake.** This vitamin, present in some foods and produced in the body when skin is exposed to sunlight, increases calcium absorption.

- **Other components in food.** Both oxalic acid (in some vegetables and beans) and phytic acid (in whole grains) can reduce calcium absorption. People who eat a variety of foods don't have to consider these factors. They are accounted for in the calcium recommended intakes, which take absorption into account.

Many factors can also affect how much calcium the body eliminates in urine, feces, and sweat. These include consumption of alcohol and caffeine containing beverages as well as intake of other nutrients (protein, sodium, potassium, and phosphorus). In most people, these factors have little effect on calcium status.

What Happens If I Don't Get Enough Calcium?

Insufficient intakes of calcium do not produce obvious symptoms in the short-term because the body maintains calcium levels in the blood by taking it from bone. Over the long-term, intakes of calcium below recommended levels have health consequences, such as causing low bone mass (osteopenia) and increasing the risks of osteoporosis and bone fractures.

Symptoms of serious calcium deficiency include numbness and tingling in the fingers, convulsions, and abnormal heart rhythms that can lead to death if not corrected. These symptoms occur almost always in people with serious health problems or who are undergoing certain medical treatments.

What Are Some Effects of Calcium on Health?

Scientists are studying calcium to understand how it affects health. Here are several examples of what this research has shown:

Bone Health and Osteoporosis

Bones need plenty of calcium and vitamin D throughout childhood and adolescence to reach their peak strength and calcium content by about age 30. After that, bones slowly lose calcium, but people can help reduce these losses by getting recommended amounts of calcium throughout adulthood and by having a healthy, active lifestyle that includes weight bearing physical activity (such as walking and running).

Osteoporosis is a disease of the bones in older adults (especially women) in which the bones become porous, fragile, and more prone to fracture. Osteoporosis is a serious public health problem for more than 10 million adults over the age of 50 in the United States. Adequate calcium and vitamin D intakes as well as regular exercise are essential to keep bones healthy throughout life.

Taking calcium and vitamin D supplements reduce the risk of breaking a bone and the risk of falling in frail, elderly adults who live in nursing homes and similar facilities. But it's not clear if the supplements help prevent bone fractures and falls in older people who live at home.

Cancer

Studies have examined whether calcium supplements or diets high in calcium might lower the risks of developing cancer of the colon or rectum or increase the risk of prostate cancer. The research to date provides no clear answers. Given that cancer develops over many years, longer term studies are needed.

Cardiovascular Disease

Some studies show that getting enough calcium might decrease the risk of heart disease and stroke. Other studies find that high amounts of calcium, particularly from supplements, might increase the risk of heart disease. But when all the studies are considered together, scientists have concluded that as long as intakes are not above the upper limit, calcium from food or supplements will not increase or decrease the risk of having a heart attack or stroke.

High Blood Pressure

Some studies have found that getting recommended intakes of calcium can reduce the risk of developing high blood pressure (hypertension). One large study in particular found that eating a diet high in fat free and low fat dairy products, vegetables, and fruits lowered blood pressure.

Preeclampsia

Preeclampsia is a serious medical condition in which a pregnant woman develops high blood pressure and kidney problems that cause protein to spill into the urine. It is a leading cause of sickness and death in pregnant women and their newborn babies. For women who get less than about 900 mg of calcium a day, taking calcium supplements during pregnancy (1,000 mg a day or more) reduces the risk of preeclampsia. But most women in the United States who become pregnant get enough calcium from their diets.

Kidney Stones

Most kidney stones are rich in calcium oxalate. Some studies have found that higher intakes of calcium from dietary supplements are linked to a greater risk of kidney stones, especially among older adults. But calcium from foods does not appear to cause kidney stones. For most people, other factors (such as not drinking enough fluids) probably have a larger effect on the risk of kidney stones than calcium intake.

Weight Loss

Although several studies have shown that getting more calcium helps lower body weight or reduce weight gain over time, most studies have found that calcium—from foods or dietary supplements—has little if any effect on body weight and amount of body fat.

Can Calcium Be Harmful?

Getting too much calcium can cause constipation. It might also interfere with the body's ability to absorb iron and zinc, but this effect is not well established. In adults, too much calcium (from dietary supplements but not food) might increase the risk of kidney stones. Some studies show that people who consume high amounts of calcium might have increased risks of prostate cancer and heart disease, but more research is needed to understand these possible links.

The upper limits for calcium are listed below. Most people do not get amounts above the upper limits from food alone; excess intakes usually come from the use of calcium supplements. Surveys show that some older women in the United States probably get amounts somewhat above the upper limit since the use of calcium supplements is common among these women.

Table 11.2. Calcium Supplements in Women

Life Stage	Upper Limit
Children 9–18 years	3,000 mg
Pregnant and breastfeeding teens	3,000 mg

Are There Any Interactions with Calcium That I Should Know About?

Calcium dietary supplements can interact or interfere with certain medicines that you take, and some medicines can lower or raise calcium levels in the body. Here are some examples:

- Calcium can reduce the absorption of these drugs when taken together:
  - Bisphosphonates (to treat osteoporosis)
  - Antibiotics of the fluoroquinolone and tetracycline families
  - Levothyroxine (to treat low thyroid activity)
  - Phenytoin (an anticonvulsant)
  - Tiludronate disodium (to treat Paget disease)
- Diuretics differ in their effects. Thiazide type diuretics (such as Diuril® and Lozol®) reduce calcium excretion by the kidneys which in turn can raise blood calcium levels too high. But loop diuretics (such as Lasix® and Bumex®) increase calcium excretion and thereby lower blood calcium levels.
- Antacids containing aluminum or magnesium increase calcium loss in the urine.
- Mineral oil and stimulant laxatives reduce calcium absorption.
- Glucocorticoids (such as prednisone) can cause calcium depletion and eventually osteoporosis when people use them for months at a time.

Tell your doctor, pharmacist, and other healthcare providers about any dietary supplements and medicines you take. They can tell you if those dietary supplements might interact or interfere with your prescription or over-the-counter medicines or if the medicines might interfere with how your body absorbs, uses, or breaks down nutrients.

Calcium and Healthful Eating

People should get most of their nutrients from food, advises the federal government's *Dietary Guidelines for Americans*. Foods contain vitamins, minerals, dietary fiber and other substances that benefit health. In some cases, fortified foods and dietary supplements may provide nutrients that otherwise may be consumed in less than recommended amounts.

Section 11.2

Facts about Vitamin D

This section includes text excerpted from "Vitamin D,"
Office of Dietary Supplements (ODS), National Institutes of
Health (NIH), April 15, 2016.

What Is Vitamin D and What Does It Do?

Vitamin D is a nutrient found in some foods that is needed for health and to maintain strong bones. It does so by helping the body absorb calcium (one of bone's main building blocks) from food and supplements. People who get too little vitamin D may develop soft, thin, and brittle bones, a condition known as rickets in children and osteomalacia in adults.

Vitamin D is important to the body in many other ways as well. Muscles need it to move, for example, nerves need it to carry messages between the brain and every body part, and the immune system needs vitamin D to fight off invading bacteria and viruses. Together with calcium, vitamin D also helps protect older adults from osteoporosis. Vitamin D is found in cells throughout the body.

How Much Vitamin D Do I Need?

The amount of vitamin D you need each day depends on your age. Average daily recommended amounts from the Food and Nutrition Board (a national group of experts) for different ages are listed below in International Units (IU):

Table 11.3. Vitamin D Supplements

Life Stage	Recommended Amount
Children 1–13 years	600 IU
Teens 14–18 years	600 IU
Pregnant and breastfeeding women	600 IU

What Foods Provide Vitamin D?

Very few foods naturally have vitamin D. Fortified foods provide most of the vitamin D in American diets.

- Fatty fish such as salmon, tuna, and mackerel are among the best sources.

- Beef liver, cheese, and egg yolks provide small amounts.

- Mushrooms provide some vitamin D. In some mushrooms that are newly available in stores, the vitamin D content is being boosted by exposing these mushrooms to ultraviolet light.

- Almost all of the U.S. milk supply is fortified with 400 IU of vitamin D per quart. But foods made from milk, like cheese and ice cream, are usually not fortified.

- Vitamin D is added to many breakfast cereals and to some brands of orange juice, yogurt, margarine, and soy beverages; check the labels.

Can I Get Vitamin D from the Sun?

The body makes vitamin D when skin is directly exposed to the sun, and most people meet at least some of their vitamin D needs this way. Skin exposed to sunshine indoors through a window will not produce vitamin D. Cloudy days, shade, and having dark colored skin also cut down on the amount of vitamin D the skin makes.

However, despite the importance of the sun to vitamin D synthesis, it is prudent to limit exposure of skin to sunlight in order to lower the risk for skin cancer. When out in the sun for more than a few minutes, wear protective clothing and apply sunscreen with an sun protection factor (SPF) of 8 or more. Tanning beds also cause the skin to make vitamin D, but pose similar risks for skin cancer.

People who avoid the sun or who cover their bodies with sunscreen or clothing should include good sources of vitamin D in their diets or take a supplement. Recommended intakes of vitamin D are set on the assumption of little sun exposure.

What Kinds of Vitamin D Dietary Supplements Are Available?

Vitamin D is found in supplements (and fortified foods) in two different forms: D2 (ergocalciferol) and D3 (cholecalciferol). Both increase vitamin D in the blood.

Am I Getting Enough Vitamin D?

Because vitamin D can come from sun, food, and supplements, the best measure of one's vitamin D status is blood levels of a form known as 25-hydroxyvitamin D. Levels are described in either nanomoles per liter (nmol/L) or nanograms per milliliter (ng/mL), where 1 nmol/L = 0.4 ng/mL.

In general, levels below 30 nmol/L (12 ng/mL) are too low for bone or overall health, and levels above 125 nmol/L (50 ng/mL) are probably too high. Levels of 50 nmol/L or above (20 ng/mL or above) are sufficient for most people.

By these measures, some Americans are vitamin D deficient and almost no one has levels that are too high. In general, young people have higher blood levels of 25-hydroxyvitamin D than older people and males have higher levels than females. By race, non-Hispanic blacks tend to have the lowest levels and non-Hispanic whites the highest. The majority of Americans have blood levels lower than 75 nmol/L (30 ng/mL).

Certain other groups may not get enough vitamin D:

- Breastfed infants, because human milk is a poor source of the nutrient. Breastfed infants should be given a supplement of 400 IU of vitamin D each day.

- People with dark skin, because their skin has less ability to produce vitamin D from the sun.

- People with disorders such as Crohn's disease or celiac disease who don't handle fat properly, because vitamin D needs fat to be absorbed.

- Obese people, because their body fat binds to some vitamin D and prevents it from getting into the blood.

What Happens If I Don't Get Enough Vitamin D?

People can become deficient in vitamin D because they don't consume enough or absorb enough from food, their exposure to sunlight is limited, or their kidneys cannot convert vitamin D to its active form in the body. In children, vitamin D deficiency causes rickets, where the bones become soft and bend. It's a rare disease but still occurs, especially among African American infants and children. In adults, vitamin D deficiency leads to osteomalacia, causing bone pain and muscle weakness.

What Are Some Effects of Vitamin D on Health?

Vitamin D is being studied for its possible connections to several diseases and medical problems, including diabetes, hypertension, and autoimmune conditions such as multiple sclerosis. Two of them discussed below are bone disorders and some types of cancer.

Bone Disorders

As they get older, millions of people (mostly women, but men too) develop, or are at risk of, osteoporosis, where bones become fragile and may fracture if one falls. It is one consequence of not getting enough calcium and vitamin D over the long term. Supplements of both vitamin D3 (at 700–800 IU/day) and calcium (500–1,200 mg/day) have been shown to reduce the risk of bone loss and fractures in elderly people aged 62–85 years. Men and women should talk with their healthcare providers about their needs for vitamin D (and calcium) as part of an overall plan to prevent or treat osteoporosis.

Cancer

Some studies suggest that vitamin D may protect against colon cancer and perhaps even cancers of the prostate and breast. But higher levels of vitamin D in the blood have also been linked to higher rates of pancreatic cancer. At this time, it's too early to say whether low vitamin D status increases cancer risk and whether higher levels protect or even increase risk in some people.

Can Vitamin D Be Harmful?

Yes, when amounts in the blood become too high. Signs of toxicity include nausea, vomiting, poor appetite, constipation, weakness, and weight loss. And by raising blood levels of calcium, too much vitamin D can cause confusion, disorientation, and problems with heart rhythm. Excess vitamin D can also damage the kidneys.

The upper limit for vitamin D is 1,000 to 1,500 IU/day for infants, 2,500 to 3,000 IU/day for children 1 to 8 years, and 4,000 IU/day for children 9 years and older, adults, and pregnant and lactating teens and women. Vitamin D toxicity almost always occurs from overuse of supplements. Excessive sun exposure doesn't cause vitamin D poisoning because the body limits the amount of this vitamin it produces.

Are There Any Interactions with Vitamin D That I Should Know About?

Like most dietary supplements, vitamin D may interact or interfere with other medicines or supplements you might be taking. Here are several examples:

- Prednisone and other corticosteroid medicines to reduce inflammation impair how the body handles vitamin D, which leads to lower calcium absorption and loss of bone over time.

- Both the weight loss drug orlistat (brand names Xenical® and Alli®) and the cholesterol-lowering drug cholestyramine (brand names Questran®, LoCholest®, and Prevalite®) can reduce the absorption of vitamin D and other fat-soluble vitamins (A, E, and K).

- Both phenobarbital and phenytoin (brand name Dilantin®), used to prevent and control epileptic seizures, increase the breakdown of vitamin D and reduce calcium absorption.

Tell your doctor, pharmacist, and other healthcare providers about any dietary supplements and medicines you take. They can tell you if those dietary supplements might interact or interfere with your prescription or over-the-counter medicines, or if the medicines might interfere with how your body absorbs, uses, or breaks down nutrients.

Vitamin D and Healthful Eating

People should get most of their nutrients from food, advises the federal government's *Dietary Guidelines for Americans.* Foods contain vitamins, minerals, dietary fiber and other substances that benefit health. In some cases, fortified foods and dietary supplements may provide nutrients that otherwise may be consumed in less-than-recommended amounts.

Chapter 12

Teens and Caffeine Use

Chapter Contents

Section 12.1—Energy Drinks 128
Section 12.2—Caffeine and Its Effects on the Body 130

Section 12.1

Energy Drinks

This section contains text excerpted from the following
sources: Text in this section begins with excerpts from
"Energy Drinks," National Center for Complementary and
Integrative Health (NCCIH), October 4, 2017; Text beginning
with the heading "What Is an Energy Drink?" is excerpted from
"Healthy Schools—The Buzz on Energy Drinks," Centers for
Disease Control and Prevention (CDC), March 22, 2016.

Energy drinks are widely promoted as products that increase alertness and enhance physical and mental performance. Marketing targeted at young people has been quite effective. Next to multivitamins, energy drinks are the most popular dietary supplement consumed by American teens and young adults. Males between the ages of 18 and 34 years consume the most energy drinks, and almost one third of teens between 12 and 17 years drink them regularly.

Caffeine is the major ingredient in most energy drinks—a 24-oz energy drink may contain as much as 500 mg of caffeine (similar to that in four or five cups of coffee). Energy drinks also may contain guarana (another source of caffeine sometimes called Brazilian cocoa), sugars, taurine, ginseng, B vitamins, glucuronolactone, yohimbe, carnitine, and bitter orange.

Consuming energy drinks also increases important safety concerns.

A growing trend among young adults and teens is mixing energy drinks with alcohol. About 25 percent of college students consume alcohol with energy drinks, and they binge drink significantly more often than students who don't mix them.

What Is an Energy Drink?

- A beverage that typically contains large amounts of caffeine, added sugars, other additives, and legal stimulants such as guarana, taurine, and L-carnitine. These legal stimulants can increase alertness, attention, energy, as well as increase blood pressure, heart rate, and breathing.

- These drinks are often used by students to provide an extra boost in energy. However, the stimulants in these drinks can have a harmful effect on the nervous system.

Are Your Kids Getting These Drinks at School?

- While nationally only 1.2 percent of high schools sell energy drinks a la carte to students in the cafeteria, as many as 11.6 percent of secondary schools in some districts sell energy drinks in vending machines, school stores, and snack bars.

- Nationwide, 75 percent of school districts do not have a policy in place regarding these types of beverages that contain high levels of caffeine for sale in vending machines, schools stores, or a la carte in the cafeteria.

The Potential Dangers of Energy Drinks

Some of the dangers of energy drinks include:

- Dehydration (not enough water in your body)
- Heart complications (such as irregular heartbeat and heart failure)
- Anxiety (feeling nervous and jittery)
- Insomnia (unable to sleep)

How Much Caffeine Is Okay?

The American Academy of Pediatrics (AAP) recommends that Adolescents aged 12–18 years should not exceed 100 mg of caffeine a day, this is the amount of caffeine in a cup of coffee.

What Can You Do?

- Teachers and other school staff can educate students about the danger of consuming too much caffeine, including energy drinks.
- Coaches can educate athletes about the difference between energy drinks and sports drinks and potential dangers of consuming highly caffeinated beverages.
- School nutrition staff can provide only healthy beverages such as fat free/low fat milk, water, and 100 percent juice if extra items (i.e., a la carte items) are sold in the cafeteria

- Parents, school staff, and community members can join the school or district wellness committee that sets the policies for health and wellness and establish or revise nutrition standards to address the sale and marketing of energy drinks in school settings.

- Everyone can model good behavior by not consuming energy drinks in front of kids.

Section 12.2

Caffeine and Its Effects on the Body

This section contains text excerpted from the following sources: Text under the heading "Caffeine's Effects—Not Totally Harmless" is excerpted from "The Buzz on Caffeine," National Institute on Drug Abuse (NIDA), February 7, 2012. Reviewed November 2017; Text beginning with the heading "Caffeine: Breaking down the Buzz" is excerpted from "The Buzz on Caffeine," National Institute on Drug Abuse (NIDA), June 25, 2014. Reviewed November 2017.

Caffeine's Effects—Not Totally Harmless

Caffeine is a mild stimulant and not a drug, so its use isn't regulated like prescription drug use is. Still, consuming too much caffeine can make you feel jittery or jumpy—your heart may race and your palms may sweat. If caffeine is taken in combination with other substances, like alcohol, it can really be dangerous because mixing a stimulant and a depressant like alcohol confuses the brain. A report from the Substance Abuse and Mental Health Services Administration (SAMHSA) shows that emergency room visits for high doses of caffeine have increased sharply. The likely cause is caffeine-infused energy drinks mixed with alcohol. Those most affected? Young people between 18 and 25 years old.

Caffeine: Breaking down the Buzz

Caffeine has a perk-up effect because it blocks a brain chemical, adenosine, which causes sleepiness. On its own, moderate amounts of caffeine rarely cause harmful long-term health effects, although it is definitely possible to take too much caffeine and get sick as a result.

Consuming too much caffeine can make you feel jittery or jumpy— your heart may race and your palms may sweat, kind of like a panic attack. It may also interfere with your sleep, which is especially important while your brain is still developing.

Some caffeine drinks and foods will affect you more than others, because they contain very different amounts.

Table 12.1. Caffeine Content

Caffeine Source	Caffeine Content
8 oz black tea	14–70 milligrams (mg)
12 oz cola	23–35 mg
8.4 oz Red Bull	75–80 mg
8 oz regular coffee	95–200 mg
1 cup semi-sweet chocolate chips	104 mg
2 oz 5-Hour Energy Shot	200–207 mg

But it's more than just how much caffeine a beverage has that can make it harmful. Even though energy drinks don't necessarily have more caffeine than other popular beverages (that is, unless you take 8 ounces of 5-Hour Energy Shot, which has 400 milligrams!), it's the way they are sometimes used that worries health experts.

In 2011, of the 20,783 emergency room visits because of energy drinks, 42 percent were because the user combined them with other drugs (e.g., prescription drugs, alcohol, or marijuana).

Caffeine + Alcohol = Danger

Mixing alcohol and caffeine is serious business. As a stimulant, caffeine sort of has the opposite effect on the brain as alcohol, which is a depressant. But don't think the effects of each are canceled out! In fact, drinking caffeine doesn't reduce the intoxication effect of alcohol (that is, how drunk you become) or reduce its cognitive impairments (that is, your ability to walk or drive or think clearly). But it does reduce alcohol's sedation effects, so you feel more awake and probably drink for longer periods of time, and you may think you are less drunk than you really are.

That can be super dangerous. People who consume alcohol mixed with energy drinks are three times more likely to binge drink than people who do not report mixing alcohol with energy drinks.

Stay Away from Caffeine

Drinking a cup of coffee, or eating a bar of chocolate, is usually not a big deal. But there are alternatives to caffeine if you're looking for an energy burst but don't want to get that jittery feeling caffeine sometimes causes. Here are a few alternatives you can try to feel energized without overdoing the caffeine:

- **Sleep.** This may sound obvious, but getting enough sleep is important. Teens need nine hours of sleep a night.

- **Eat regularly.** When you don't eat, your glucose (sugar) levels drop, making you feel drained. Some people find it helpful to eat four or five smaller meals throughout the day instead of fewer big meals.

- **Drink enough water.** Since our bodies are more than two-thirds H_2O, we need at least 64 ounces of water a day.

- **Take a walk.** If you're feeling drained in the middle of the day, it helps to move around. Do sit-ups or jumping jacks. Go outside for a brisk walk or ride your bike.

Chapter 13

Physical Activity and Teens

Chapter Contents

Section 13.1—Physical Activity Facts 134

Section 13.2—Importance of Physical Activity 136

Section 13.3—Physical Activity Guidelines for
             Children and Adolescents 138

Section 13.1

Physical Activity Facts

This section includes text excerpted from "Healthy
Schools—Physical Activity Facts," Centers for Disease
Control and Prevention (CDC), June 28, 2017.

Regular physical activity in childhood and adolescence is important
for promoting lifelong health and well-being and preventing various
health conditions. The *United States Physical Activity Guidelines for
Americans* recommend that children and adolescents aged 6 to 17 years
should have 60 minutes (1 hour) or more of physical activity each day.
Unfortunately, many children and adolescents do not meet the recommendations set forth in the *Physical Activity Guidelines for Americans.*

Benefits of Physical Activity

Regular physical activity can help children and adolescents improve
cardiorespiratory fitness, build strong bones and muscles, control
weight, reduce symptoms of anxiety and depression, and reduce the
risk of developing health conditions such as:

- Heart disease
- Cancer
- Type 2 diabetes
- High blood pressure
- Osteoporosis
- Obesity

Consequences of Physical Inactivity

Physical inactivity can:

- Lead to energy imbalance (e.g., expend less energy through
  physical activity than consumed through diet) and can increase
  the risk of becoming overweight or obese.

- Increase the risk of factors that cause cardiovascular disease, including hyperlipidemia (e.g., high cholesterol and triglyceride levels), high blood pressure, obesity, and insulin resistance and glucose intolerance.

- Increase the risk for developing type 2 diabetes.

- Increase the risk for developing breast, colon, endometrial, and lung cancers.

- Lead to low bone density, which in turn, leads to osteoporosis.

Physical Activity and Academic Achievement

- Students who are physically active tend to have better grades, school attendance, cognitive performance (e.g., memory), and classroom behaviors (e.g., on-task behavior).

- Higher physical activity and physical fitness levels are associated with improved cognitive performance (e.g., concentration, memory) among students.

Physical Activity Behaviors of Young People

- Only 21 percent of 6 to 19-year old children and adolescents in the Unites States attained 60 or more minutes of moderate to vigorous physical activity on at least 5 days per week.

- Only 27.1 percent of high school students participate in at least 60 minutes per day of physical activity on all 7 days of the week.

- In 2015, 53.4 percent of high school students participated in muscle strengthening exercises (e.g., push-ups, sit-ups, weight-lifting) on 3 or more days during the week.

- In 2015, 51.6 percent of high school students attended physical education classes in an average week, and only 29.8 percent of high school students attended physical education classes daily.

Recommendations for Physical Activity

- The U.S. Department of Health and Human Services (HHS) provides guidance on healthy physical activity habits. The national recommendation is that children and adolescents aged 6 to 17 years should have 60 minutes (1 hour) or more of physical activity each day.

This includes:

- **Aerobic:** Most of the 60 or more minutes a day should be either moderate- or vigorous-intensity aerobic physical activity and should include vigorous-intensity physical activity at least 3 days a week.

- **Muscle-strengthening:** As part of their 60 or more minutes of daily physical activity, children and adolescents should include muscle-strengthening physical activity on at least 3 days of the week.

- **Bone-strengthening:** As part of their 60 or more minutes of daily physical activity, children and adolescents should include bone-strengthening physical activity on at least 3 days of the week.

These *Guidelines* also encourage children and adolescents to participate in physical activities that are appropriate for their age, that are enjoyable, and that offer variety.

- The national recommendation for schools is to have a comprehensive approach for addressing physical education and physical activity in schools. This approach is called Comprehensive School Physical Activity Programs.

Section 13.2

Importance of Physical Activity

This section includes text excerpted from "Importance of Physical Activity," U.S. Department of Health and Human Services (HHS), January 2017.

Physical activity provides long-term health benefits for everyone! By being active, you will burn calories that you store from eating throughout the day and—it can be as easy as walking the dog or as rigorous as running a marathon. Providing opportunities for children to be active early on puts them on a path to better physical and mental health. It's never too late to jumpstart a healthy lifestyle.

Physical Activity and Obesity

Physical activity, along with proper nutrition, is beneficial to people of all ages, backgrounds, and abilities. And it is important that everyone gets active: over the last 20 years, there's been a significant increase in obesity in the United States. About one-third of U.S. adults (33.8%) are obese and approximately 17 percent (or 12.5 million) of children and adolescents (aged 2–19 years) are obese.

The health implications of obesity in America are startling:

- If things remain as they are today, one-third of all children born in the year 2000 or later may suffer from diabetes at some point in their lives, while many others are likely to face chronic health problems such as heart disease, high blood pressure, cancer, diabetes, and asthma.

- Studies indicate that overweight youth may never achieve a healthy weight, and up to 70 percent of obese teens may become obese adults.

- Even more worrisome, the cumulative effect could be that children born in the year 2000 or later may not outlive their parents.

The impact of obesity doesn't end there. Obesity has personal financial and national economic implications as well. Those who are obese have medical costs that are $1,429 more than those of normal weight on average (roughly 42% higher). And annual direct costs of childhood obesity are $14.3 billion.

By incorporating physical activity into your daily life—30 minutes for adults and 60 minutes for children—as well as healthy eating, you will experience positive health benefits and be on the path for a better future.

The Impact of Physical Activity on Your Health

Regular physical activity can produce long-term health benefits. It can help:

- Prevent chronic diseases such as heart disease, cancer, and stroke (the three leading health-related causes of death)

- Control weight

- Make your muscles stronger

- Reduce fat

- Promote strong bone, muscle, and joint development
- Condition heart and lungs
- Build overall strength and endurance
- Improve sleep
- Decrease potential of becoming depressed
- Increase your energy and self-esteem
- Relieve stress
- Increase your chances of living longer

When you are not physically active, you are more at risk for:

- High blood pressure
- High blood cholesterol
- Stroke
- Type 2 diabetes
- Heart disease
- Cancer

Section 13.3

Physical Activity Guidelines for Children and Adolescents

This section includes text excerpted from "2008 Physical Activity Guidelines for Americans," Office of Disease Prevention and Health Promotion (ODPHP), U.S. Department of Health and Human Services (HHS), October 7, 2008. Reviewed November 2017.

Regular physical activity in children and adolescents promotes health and fitness. Compared to those who are inactive, physically active youth have higher levels of cardiorespiratory fitness and stronger muscles. They also typically have lower body fatness. Their bones are stronger, and they may have reduced symptoms of anxiety and depression. Youth who are regularly active also have a better chance of a healthy adulthood. Children and adolescents don't usually develop chronic diseases, such as heart disease, hypertension, type 2 diabetes, or osteoporosis. However, risk factors for these diseases can begin to develop early in life. Regular physical activity makes it less likely that these risk factors will develop and more likely that children will remain healthy as adults. Youth can achieve substantial health benefits by doing moderate- and vigorous-intensity physical activity for periods of time that add up to 60 minutes (1 hour) or more each day. This activity should include aerobic activity as well as age-appropriate muscle- and bone strengthening activities. Although current science is not complete, it appears that, as with adults, the total amount of physical activity is more important for achieving health benefits than is any one component (frequency, intensity, or duration) or specific mix of activities (aerobic, muscle-strengthening, bone strengthening). Even so, bone-strengthening activities remain especially important for children and young adolescents because the greatest gains in bone mass occur during the years just before and during puberty. In addition, the majority of peak bone mass is obtained by the end of adolescence.

This section provides physical activity guidance for children and adolescents aged 6 to 17, and focuses on physical activity beyond baseline activity.

Parents and other adults who work with or care for youth should be familiar with the *Guidelines* in this section. These adults should be aware that, as children become adolescents, they typically reduce their physical activity. Adults play an important role in providing age-appropriate opportunities for physical activity. In doing so, they help lay an important foundation for life-long, health-promoting physical activity. Adults need to encourage active play in children and encourage sustained and structured activity as children grow older.

Explaining the Guidelines

Types of Activity

The *Guidelines* for children and adolescents focus on three types of activity: aerobic, muscle-strengthening, and bone-strengthening. Each type has important health benefits.

- **Aerobic activities** are those in which young people rhythmically move their large muscles. Running, hopping, skipping, jumping rope, swimming, dancing, and bicycling are all examples of aerobic activities. Aerobic activities increase cardiorespiratory fitness. Children often do activities in short bursts, which may not technically be aerobic activities. However, this document will also use the term aerobic to refer to these brief activities.

- **Muscle-strengthening activities** make muscles do more work than usual during activities of daily life. This is called "overload," and it strengthens the muscles. Muscle-strengthening activities can be unstructured and part of play, such as playing on playground equipment, climbing trees, and playing tug-of-war. Or these activities can be structured, such as lifting weights or working with resistance bands.

- **Bone-strengthening activities** produce a force on the bones that promotes bone growth and strength. This force is commonly produced by impact with the ground. Running, jumping rope, basketball, tennis, and hopscotch are all examples of bone-strengthening activities. As these examples illustrate, bone-strengthening activities can also be aerobic and muscle-strengthening.

How Age Influences Physical Activity in Children and Adolescents

Children and adolescents should meet the *Guidelines* by doing activity that is appropriate for their age. Their natural patterns of movement differ from those of adults. For example, children are naturally active in an intermittent way, particularly when they do unstructured active play. During recess and in their free play and games, children use basic aerobic and bone-strengthening activities, such as running, hopping, skipping, and jumping, to develop movement patterns and skills. They alternate brief periods of moderate- and vigorous-intensity activity with brief periods of rest. Any episode of moderate- or vigorous intensity physical activity, however brief, counts toward the *Guidelines*. Children also commonly increase muscle strength through unstructured activities that involve lifting or moving their body weight or working against resistance. Children don't usually do or need formal muscle-strengthening programs, such as lifting weights.

Meeting the Guidelines

American youth vary in their physical activity participation. Some don't participate at all, others participate in enough activity to meet the *Guidelines*, and some exceed the *Guidelines*.

Children and adolescents can meet the *Physical Activity Guidelines* and become regularly physically active in many ways. One practical strategy to promote activity in youth is to replace inactivity with activity whenever possible. For example, where appropriate and safe, young people should walk or bicycle to school instead of riding in a car. Rather than just watching sporting events on television, young people should participate in age appropriate sports or games.

- **Children and adolescents who do not meet the** *Guidelines* should slowly increase their activity in small steps and in ways that they enjoy. A gradual increase in the number of days and the time spent being active will help reduce the risk of injury.

- **Children and adolescents who meet the** *Guidelines* should continue being active on a daily basis and, if appropriate, become even more active. Evidence suggests that even more than 60 minutes of activity every day may provide additional health benefits.

- **Children and adolescents who exceed the** *Guidelines* should maintain their activity level and vary the kinds of activities they do to reduce the risk of overtraining or injury.

Children and adolescents with disabilities are more likely to be inactive than those without disabilities. Youth with disabilities should work with their healthcare provider to understand the types and amounts of physical activity appropriate for them. When possible, children and adolescents with disabilities should meet the *Guidelines*. When young people are not able to participate in appropriate physical activities to meet the *Guidelines*, they should be as active as possible and avoid being inactive.

Chapter 14

Weight Management in Teens

Chapter Contents

Section 14.1—Understanding Your Teen's Body
          Mass Index Measurement 144

Section 14.2—Helping Your Overweight Child........................ 148

Section 14.3—Tips to Help Teens to Lose Weight.................... 153

Section 14.1

Understanding Your Teen's Body Mass Index Measurement

This section includes text excerpted from "Healthy Weight—About Child and Teen BMI," Centers for Disease Control and Prevention (CDC), May 15, 2015.

What Is Body Mass Index (BMI)?

BMI is a person's weight in kilograms divided by the square of height in meters. For children and teens, BMI is age and sex specific and is often referred to as BMI for age. In children, a high amount of body fat can lead to weight related diseases and other health issues and being underweight can also put one at risk for health issues.

A high BMI can be an indicator of high body fatness. BMI does not measure body fat directly, but research has shown that BMI is correlated with more direct measures of body fat, such as skinfold thickness measurements, bioelectrical impedance, densitometry (underwater weighing), dual energy X-ray absorptiometry (DXA), and other methods. BMI can be considered an alternative to direct measures of body fat. In general, BMI is an inexpensive and easy to perform method of screening for weight categories that may lead to health problems.

How Is BMI Calculated for Children and Teens?

Calculating BMI using the BMI Percentile Calculator involves the following steps:

- Measure height and weight.

- Use the Child and Teen BMI Calculator (nccd.cdc.gov/dnpabmi/Calculator.aspx) to calculate BMI. This calculator provides BMI and the corresponding BMI-for-age percentile on a Centers for Disease Control and Prevention (CDC) BMI-for-age growth chart. Use this calculator for children and teens, aged 2 through 19 years old. The BMI number is calculated using standard formulas.

What Is a BMI Percentile and How Is It Interpreted?

After BMI is calculated for children and teens, it is expressed as a percentile which can be obtained from either a graph or a percentile calculator. These percentiles express a child's BMI relative to children in the United States who participated in national surveys that were conducted from 1963–65 to 1988–1944. Because weight and height change during growth and development, as does their relation to body fatness, a child's BMI must be interpreted relative to other children of the same sex and age.

The BMI for age percentile growth charts are the most commonly used indicator to measure the size and growth patterns of children and teens in the United States. BMI for age weight status categories and the corresponding percentiles were based on expert committee recommendations and are shown in the following table.

Table 14.1. Body Mass Index Calculation

Weight Status Category	Percentile Range
Underweight	Less than the 5th percentile
Normal or Healthy Weight	5th percentile to less than the 85th percentile
Overweight	85th to less than the 95th percentile
Obese	Equal to or greater than the 95th percentile

How Is BMI Used with Children and Teens?

For children and teens, BMI is not a diagnostic tool and is used to screen for potential weight and health related issues. For example, a child may have a high BMI for their age and sex, but to determine if excess fat is a problem, a healthcare provider would need to perform further assessments. These assessments might include skinfold thickness measurements, evaluations of diet, physical activity, family history, and other appropriate health screenings. The American Academy of Pediatrics (AAP) recommends the use of BMI to screen for overweight and obesity in children beginning at 2 years old. For children under the age of 2 years old, consult the World Health Organization (WHO) standards.

Is BMI Interpreted the Same Way for Children and Teens as It Is for Adults?

BMI is interpreted differently for children and teens even though it is calculated as weight (÷) height. Because there are changes in weight and height with age, as well as their relation to body fatness, BMI levels among children and teens need to be expressed relative to other children of the same sex and age. These percentiles are calculated from the CDC growth charts, which were based on national survey data collected from 1963–65 to 1988–1994.

Obesity is defined as a BMI at or above the 95th percentile for children and teens of the same age and sex. For example, a 10 year old boy of average height (56 inches) who weighs 102 pounds would have a BMI of 22.9 kg/m2. This would place the boy in the 95th percentile for BMI, and he would be considered to have obesity. This means that the child's BMI is greater than the BMI of 95 percent of 10 year old boys in the reference population.

Why Can't Healthy Weight Ranges Be Provided for Children and Teens?

Normal or healthy weight status is based on BMI between the 5th and 85th percentile on the CDC growth chart. It is difficult to provide healthy weight ranges for children and teens because the interpretation of BMI depends on weight, height, age, and sex.

What Are the BMI Trends for Children and Teens in the United States?

The prevalence of children and teens who measure in the 95th percentile or greater on the CDC growth charts has greatly increased over the past 40 years. However, this trend has leveled off and has even declined in certain age groups.

How Can I Tell If My Child Is Overweight or Obese?

CDC and AAP recommend the use of BMI to screen for overweight and obesity in children and teens age 2 through 19 years. For children under the age of 2 years old, consult the WHO standards. Although BMI is used to screen for overweight and obesity in children and teens, BMI is not a diagnostic tool. To determine whether the child has excess fat, further assessment by a trained health professional would be needed.

Can I Determine If My Child or Teen Is Obese by Using an Adult BMI Calculator?

In general, it's not possible to do this. The adult calculator provides only the BMI value (weight/height) and not the BMI percentile that is needed to interpret BMI among children and teens. It is not appropriate to use the BMI categories for adults to interpret the BMI of children and teens.

However, if a child or teen has a BMI of ≥ 30 kg/m2 the child is almost certainly obese. A BMI of 30 kg/m2 is approximately the 95th percentile among 17-year old girls and 18-year old boys.

My Two Children Have the Same BMI Values, but One Is Considered Obese and the Other Is Not. Why Is That?

The interpretation of BMI varies by age and sex. So if the children are not the same age and the same sex, the interpretation of BMI has different meanings. For children of different age and sex, the same BMI could represent different BMI percentiles and possibly different weight status categories.

What Are the Health Consequences of Obesity during Childhood?

Health Risks Now

Childhood obesity can have a harmful effect on the body in a variety of ways.

- High blood pressure and high cholesterol, which are risk factors for cardiovascular disease (CVD). In one study, 70 percent of obese children had at least one CVD risk factor, and 39 percent had two or more.

- Increased risk of impaired glucose tolerance, insulin resistance and type 2 diabetes.

- Breathing problems, such as sleep apnea, and asthma.

- Joint problems and musculoskeletal discomfort.

- Fatty liver disease, gallstones, and gastro-esophageal reflux (i.e., heartburn).

- Psychological stress such as depression, behavioral problems, and issues in school.

- Low self-esteem and low self-reported quality of life.

- Impaired social, physical, and emotional functioning.

Health Risks Later

Obese children are more likely to become obese adults. Adult obesity is associated with a number of serious health conditions including heart disease, diabetes, and some cancers.

- If children are overweight,

- obesity in adulthood is likely to be more severe.

Section 14.2

Helping Your Overweight Child

This section includes text excerpted from "Weight
Management—Helping Your Child Who Is Overweight,"
National Institute of Diabetes and Digestive and Kidney
Diseases (NIDDK), September 2016.

As a parent or other caregiver, you can do a lot to help your child reach and maintain a healthy weight. Staying active and consuming healthy foods and beverages are important for your child's well-being. You can take an active role in helping your child—and your whole family—learn habits that may improve health.

How Can I Tell If My Child Is Overweight?

Being able to tell whether a child is overweight is not always easy. Children grow at different rates and at different times. Also, the amount of a child's body fat changes with age and differs between girls and boys.

One way to tell if your child is overweight is to calculate his or her body mass index (BMI). BMI is a measure of body weight relative to height. The BMI calculator uses a formula that produces a score often used to tell whether a person is underweight, a normal weight, overweight, or obese. The BMI of children is age and sex specific and known as the "BMI for age."

BMI for age uses growth charts created by the Centers for Disease Control and Prevention (CDC). Doctors use these charts to track a child's growth. The charts use a number called a percentile to show how your child's BMI compares with the BMI of other children. The main BMI categories for children and teens are:

- **healthy weight:** 5th to 84th percentile

- **overweight:** 85th to 94th percentile

- **obese:** 95th percentile or higher

Why Should I Be Concerned?

You should be concerned if your child has extra weight because weighing too much may increase the chances that your child will develop health problems now or later in life.

In the short-run, for example, he or she may have breathing problems or joint pain, making it hard to keep up with friends. Some children may develop health problems, such as type 2 diabetes, high blood pressure, and high cholesterol. Some children also may experience teasing, bullying, depression, or low self-esteem.

Children who are overweight are at higher risk of entering adulthood with too much weight. The chances of developing health problems such as heart disease and certain types of cancer are higher among adults with too much weight.

BMI is a screening tool and does not directly measure body fat or an individual child's risk of health problems. If you are concerned about your child's weight, talk with your child's doctor or other healthcare professional. He or she can check your child's overall health and growth over time and tell you if weight management may be helpful. Many children who are still growing in length don't need to lose weight; they may need to decrease the amount of weight they gain while they grow taller. Don't put your child on a weight loss diet unless your child's doctor tells you to.

How Can I Help My Child Develop Healthy Habits?

You can play an important role in helping your child build healthy eating, drinking, physical activity, and sleep habits. For instance, teach your child about balancing the amount of food and beverages he or she eats and drinks with his or her amount of daily physical activity. Take your child grocery shopping and let him or her choose healthy foods and drinks, and help plan and prepare healthy meals and snacks. The *2015 U.S. Dietary Guidelines* explain the types of foods and beverages to include in a healthy eating plan.

Here are some other ways to help your child develop healthy habits:

- Be a good role model. Consume healthy foods and drinks, and choose active pastimes. Children are good learners, and they often copy what they see.

- Talk with your child about what it means to be healthy and how to make healthy decisions.

  - Discuss how physical activities and certain foods and drinks may help their bodies get strong and stay healthy.

    - Children should get at least an hour of physical activity daily and should limit their screen time (computers, television, and mobile devices) outside of schoolwork to no more than 2 hours each day.

  - Chat about how to make healthy choices about food, drinks, and activities at school, at friends' houses, and at other places outside your home.

- Involve the whole family in building healthy eating, drinking, and physical activity habits. Everyone benefits, and your child who is overweight won't feel singled out.

- Make sure you child gets enough sleep. While research about the relationship between sleep and weight is ongoing, some studies link excess weight to not enough sleep in children and adults. How much sleep your child needs depends on his or her age.

What Can I Do to Improve My Child's Eating Habits?

Besides consuming fewer foods, drinks, and snacks that are high in calories, fat, sugar, and salt, you may get your child to eat healthier by offering these options more often:

- Fruits, vegetables, and whole grains such as brown rice.

- Lean meats, poultry, seafood, beans and peas, soy products, and eggs, instead of meat high in fat.

- Fat free or low fat milk and milk products or milk substitutes, such as soy beverages with added calcium and vitamin D, instead of whole milk or cream.

- Fruit and vegetable smoothies made with fat-free or low-fat yogurt, instead of milk shakes or ice cream.

- Water, fat free, or low fat milk, instead of soda and other drinks with added sugars.

You also may help your child eat better by trying to:

- Avoid serving large portions, or the amount of food or drinks your child chooses for a meal or snack. Start with smaller amounts of food and let your child ask for more if he or she is still hungry. If your child chooses food or drinks from a package, container, or can, read the Nutrition Facts Label to see what amount is equal to one serving. Match your child's portion to the serving size listed on the label to avoid extra calories, fat, and sugar.

- Put healthy foods and drinks where they are easy to see and keep high calorie foods and drinks out of sight—or don't buy them at all.

- Eat fast food less often. If you do visit a fast food restaurant, encourage your child to choose healthier options, such as sliced fruit instead of fries. Also, introduce your child to different foods, such as hummus with veggies.

- Try to sit down to family meals as often as possible, and have fewer meals "on the run."

- Discourage eating in front of the television, computer, or other electronic device.

To help your child develop a healthy attitude toward food and eating:

- Don't make your child clean his or her plate.

- Offer rewards other than food or drinks when encouraging your child to practice healthy habits. Promising dessert for eating vegetables sends a message that vegetables are less valuable than dessert.

Healthy Snack Ideas

To help your child eat less candy, cookies, and other unhealthy snacks, try these healthier snack options instead:

- Air popped popcorn without butter

- fresh, frozen, or fruit canned in natural juices, plain or with fat-free or low fat yogurt

- fresh vegetables, such as baby carrots, cucumbers, zucchini, or cherry tomatoes

- Low sugar, whole grain cereal with fat-free or low-fat milk, or a milk substitute with added calcium and vitamin D

How Can I Help My Child Be More Active?

Try to make physical activity fun for your child. Children need about 60 minutes of physical activity a day, although the activity doesn't have to be all at once. Several short 10 or even 5 minute spurts of activity throughout the day are just as good. If your child is not used to being active, encourage him or her to start out slowly and build up to 60 minutes a day.

To encourage daily physical activity:

- Let your child choose a favorite activity to do regularly, such as climbing a jungle gym at the playground or joining a sports team or dance class.

- Help your child find simple, fun activities to do at home or on his or her own, such as playing tag, jumping rope, playing catch, shooting baskets, or riding a bike (wear a helmet).

- Limit time with the computer, television, cell phone, and other devices to two hours a day.

- Let your child and other family members plan active outings, such as a walk or hike to a favorite spot.

Where Can I Go for Help?

If you have tried to change your family's eating, drinking, physical activity, and sleep habits and your child has not reached a healthy weight, ask your child's healthcare professional about other options. He or she may be able to recommend a plan for healthy eating and physical activity, or refer you to a weight management specialist, registered dietitian, or program. Your local hospital, a community health clinic, or health department also may offer weight-management programs for children and teens or information about where you can enroll in one.

What Should I Look for in a Weight Management Program?

When choosing a weight management program for your child, look for a program that:

- includes a variety of healthcare providers on staff, such as doctors, psychologists and registered dietitians.

- evaluates your child's weight, growth, and health before enrollment and throughout the program.

- adapts to your child's specific age and abilities. Programs for elementary school aged children should be different from those for teens.

- helps your family keep healthy eating, drinking, and physical activity habits after the program ends.

How Else Can I Help My Child?

You can help your child by being positive and supportive throughout any process or program you choose to help him or her achieve a healthy weight. Help your child set specific goals and track progress. Reward successes with praise and hugs.

Tell your child that he or she is loved, special, and important. Children's feelings about themselves are often based on how they think their parents and other caregivers feel about them.

Listen to your child's concerns about his or her weight. He or she needs support, understanding, and encouragement from caring adults.

Section 14.3

Tips to Help Teens to Lose Weight

This section includes text excerpted from "If You Need to Lose Weight," girlshealth.gov, Office on Women's Health (OWH), January 13, 2014. Reviewed November 2017.

Lots of people need to lose some weight. If your doctor tells you that you are overweight or obese, it's important that you try to lose weight. You can ask your doctor and perhaps a dietitian about ways to lose weight. It can be a bit harder for some people to lose weight because of their genes or because of things around them, such as the food choices in their house. But with the right support and a good plan, you can get to a healthy weight.

Great Ways to Lose Weight

You don't need a special diet like a low carb or high protein diet to lose weight. The best way to lose weight is to get the right mix of nutrients and energy your body needs. Here are some tips for losing weight in a healthy way:

- **Follow a food guide.** It can be hard to know which foods to choose. Our MyPlate guide can be a big help. It will encourage you to eat whole grains, vegetables, and fruits. These foods are full of fiber, which can help you feel full. And keeping a record can help.

- **Cut back on fats.** You need some fat, but even small amounts of fats have lots of calories. Read labels to see how much fat a food has. And try to cut back on fried foods and on meats that are high in fat, such as burgers.

- **Eat fewer sweets and unhealthy snacks.** Candy, cookies, and cakes often have a lot of sugar and fat and not many nutrients. Learn about treats that are delicious and nutritious.

- **Avoid sugary drinks.** Try not to drink a lot of sugary sodas, energy drinks, and sports drinks. They can add a lot of calories. (There are about 10 packets of sugar in 12 ounces of soda.) Also try not to drink a lot of fruit juice. Water is a great choice instead. Add a piece of lemon or a splash of juice for more flavor.

- **Get enough sleep at night.** Many teens stay up too late. Staying up late often increases night time snacking and low energy the next morning (which you might be tempted to beat with some extra food).

- **Limit fast food meals.** Studies show that the more fast food you eat each week, the greater the risk of gaining extra weight. So try to limit fast food meals to once a week or less.

- **Tackle hunger with fiber and protein.** Don't wait until you are so hungry that it gets hard to make smart food choices. Instead, when you start to feel hungry, eat a small snack that combines a protein with a food that's high in fiber, such as a whole grain cracker with low-fat cheese. These are filling but not packed with calories.

- **Be aware of how much you are eating.** If you're not sure how much is considered one serving, you can learn how to read labels. You also may eat less if you use a smaller plate. Try not to eat straight from a big package of food—it's easy to lose track that way. And if you're at a restaurant, see if you can take home some leftovers.

- **Think about why you are eating.** Sometimes we eat to fill needs other than hunger, such as being bored, stressed, or lonely. If you do that, see if you can think of some other ways to meet those needs. Consider calling a friend or listening to some great music. And if think you may be having emotional problems, talk to an adult you trust.

- **Get moving.** One great way to lose weight is by being physically active. You should aim for a total of 60 minutes of moderate or vigorous physical activity each day. If you haven't been active in a while, start slowly.

- **Cut down on sitting around.** This means less TV, Internet, and other forms of screen time. Instead, aim for your "hour a day of active play."

How Not to Lose Weight

It can be tempting to look for a quick fix if you need to lose weight. Remember, though, that if something sounds too good to be true, it probably is. Keep these tips in mind:

- **Avoid fad diets.** Fad diets often allow only a few types of food. That means you are not getting all the nutrients you need. And these diets may cause you to lose weight for a short-time, but then you likely will gain it back quickly.

- **Avoid weight loss pills and other quick loss products.** Most weight loss pills, drinks, supplements, and other products you can buy without a prescription have not been shown to work. And they can actually be very dangerous. If you are thinking about taking weight loss pills or similar products, talk to your doctor first.

- **Don't eat too little.** Your body needs fuel to grow and be healthy. If you eat fewer than 1,600 calories each day, you may not get the nutrients you need. And don't skip breakfast. Some research suggests that teens who skip breakfast are more likely to be overweight.

- **Don't try to get rid of food you eat.** Some people think they can lose weight by making themselves vomit or taking laxatives (pills that make you go to the bathroom). These are very dangerous steps and signs of eating disorders. Your body is too precious to treat this way, so get help if you think you may have an eating disorder.

- **Don't expect to lose weight quickly.** Losing about one to two pounds a week is a healthy rate of weight loss. If you are taking extreme steps to lose weight faster, you will probably gain most or all of it back.

Chapter 15

Body Image in Youth

Chapter Contents

Section 15.1—For Teens: Developing Body Image
    and Self-Esteem 158

Section 15.2—Why Do Teens Get Cosmetic Surgery? 162

Section 15.1

For Teens: Developing Body Image and Self-Esteem

This section contains text excerpted from the following sources: Text in this section begins with excerpts from "Having Body Image Issues," girlshealth.gov, Office on Women's Health (OWH), January 7, 2015; Text under the heading "What Is Self-Esteem?" is excerpted from "Self-Esteem and Self-Confidence," girlshealth.gov, Office on Women's Health (OWH), January 7, 2015.

Do you wish you could lose weight, get taller, or develop faster? It's pretty common to worry a little about how your body looks, especially when it's changing. You can learn about body image and ways to take control of yours.

What Is Body Image?

Body image is how you think and feel about your body. It includes whether you think you look good to other people.

Body image is affected by a lot of things, including messages you get from your friends, family, and the world around you. Images we see in the media definitely affect our body image even though a lot of media images are changed or aren't realistic.

Why Does Body Image Matter?

Your body image can affect how you feel about yourself overall. For example, if you are unhappy with your looks, your self-esteem may start to go down. Sometimes, having body image issues or low self-esteem may lead to depression, eating disorders, or obesity.

How Can I Deal with Body Image Issues?

Everyone has something they would like to change about their bodies. But you'll be happier if you focus on the things you like about your body—and your whole self. Need some help? Check out some tips:

- **List your great traits.** If you start to criticize your body, tell yourself to stop. Instead, think about what you like about yourself, both inside and out. The "What's unique about me?" log can get you started.

- **Know your power.** Hey, your body is not just a place to hang your clothes! It can do some truly amazing things. Focus on how strong and healthy your body can be.

- **Treat your body well.** Eat right, sleep tight, and get moving. You'll look and feel your best—and you'll be pretty proud of yourself too.

- **Give your body a treat.** Take a nice bubble bath, do some stretching, or just curl up on a comfy couch. Do something soothing.

- **Mind your media.** Try not to let models and actresses affect how you think you should look. They get lots of help from makeup artists, personal trainers, and photo fixers. And advertisers often use a focus on thinness to get people to buy stuff. Don't let them mess with your mind!

- **Let yourself shine.** A lot of how we look comes from how we carry ourselves. Feeling proud, walking tall, and smiling big can boost your beauty—and your mood.

- **Find fab friends.** Your best bet is to hang out with people who accept you for you! And work with your friends to support each other.

If you can't seem to accept how you look, talk to an adult you trust. You can get help feeling better about your body.

Stressing about Body Changes

During puberty and your teen years, your body changes a lot. All those changes can be hard to handle. They might make you worry about what other people think of how you look and about whether your body is normal. If you have these kinds of concerns, you are not alone.

Here are some common thoughts about changing bodies.

- Why am I taller than most of the boys my age?

- Why haven't I grown?

- Am I too skinny?

- Am I too fat?

- Will others like me now that I am changing?

- Are my breasts too small?

- Are my breasts too large?

- Why do I have acne?

- Do my clothes look right on my body?

- Are my hips getting bigger?

- If you are stressed about your body, you may feel better if you understand why you are changing so fast—or not changing as fast as your friends.

During puberty, you get taller and see other changes in your body, such as wider hips and thighs. Your body will also start to have more fat compared to muscle than before. Each young woman changes at her own pace, and all of these changes are normal.

What Are Serious Body Image Problems?

If how your body looks bothers you a lot and you can't stop thinking about it, you could have body dysmorphic disorder, or BDD.

People with BDD think they look ugly even if they have a small flaw or none at all. They may spend many hours a day looking at flaws and trying to hide them. They also may ask friends to reassure them about their looks or want to have a lot of cosmetic surgery. If you or a friend may have BDD, talk to an adult you trust, such as a parent or guardian, school counselor, teacher, doctor, or nurse. BDD is an illness, and you can get help.

What Is Self-Esteem?

Self-esteem has to do with the **value** and **respect** you have for yourself. Simply put, it's your opinion of yourself.

If you have healthy self-esteem, you feel good about yourself and are proud of what you can do. Having healthy self-esteem can help you feel positive overall. And it can make you brave enough to tackle some serious challenges, like trying out for a school play or standing up to a bully.

If you have low self-esteem, you may not think very highly of yourself. Of course, it's normal to feel down about yourself sometimes.

But if you feel bad about yourself more often than good, you may have low self-esteem. You can read about rating your self-esteem.

How Can Low Self-Esteem Hurt?

Low self-esteem may stop you from doing things you want to do or from speaking up for yourself. Low self-esteem may even lead you to try to feel better in unhealthy ways, like using drugs or alcohol. Also, some people may start to feel so sad or hopeless about themselves that they develop mental health problems like depression and eating disorders.

A lot of things can affect self-esteem. These include how others treat you, your background and culture, and experiences at school. For example, being put down by your boyfriend, classmates, or family or being bullied can affect how you see yourself. But one of the biggest influences on your self-esteem is ... you!

Rate Your Self-Esteem and Self-Confidence

If you have healthy self-esteem and self-confidence, you probably will agree with some or most of the following statements:

- I feel good about who I am.

- I am proud of what I can do, but don't need to show off.

- I know there are some things that I'm good at and some things I need to improve.

- I feel it is okay if I win or if I lose.

- I usually think, "I can do this," before I do something.

- I am eager to learn new things.

- I can handle criticism.

- I like to try to do things without help, but I don't mind asking for help if I need it.

- I like myself.

If some of the items on this checklist are true for you, congrats! You're on the right track. And if your self-esteem ever slips, you can try these steps.

If you have low self-esteem and self-confidence, you probably will agree with some or most of the following statements:

1. I can't do anything well.

2. I have no friends.

3. I do not like to try new things.

4. I get really upset about making mistakes.

5. I'm not as nice, pretty, or smart as the other girls in my class.

6. I don't like it when people say nice things about me.

7. I get very upset when people criticize me.

8. I feel better if I put other people down.

9. I don't know what I'm good at.

10. I usually think, "I can't do this," before I do something.

11. I don't like myself.

12. If many of the items on this list apply to you, try some ways to raise your self-esteem. It's no fun to be hard on yourself, and you can work to stop.

Remember, everyone brings something unique to the world.

Section 15.2

Why Do Teens Get Cosmetic Surgery?

This section includes text excerpted from "Cosmetic Surgery," girlshealth.gov, Office on Women's Health (OWH), April 15, 2014. Reviewed November 2017.

Teens might have cosmetic surgery for a number of reasons, including to remove acne scars, change their noses, and make their breasts smaller or bigger. But if there's something you don't like about your body, your best bet is to try to work on how you feel about it. Your attitude can make a big difference. Try to focus on what you like about yourself. And remember that you've got lots more to offer the world than just how you look.

What Are the Risks of Cosmetic Surgery?

People who have cosmetic surgery face many of the same risks as anyone having surgery. These include:

- Infection

- Not healing well

- Damage to nerves

- Bleeding

- Not being happy with the results

- Risks from anesthesia, such as lung problems

You face additional concerns if you're considering surgery to make your breasts bigger through breast implants. (Keep in mind that you usually can't have this surgery until you're 18.)

For one, these surgeries usually need to be done over at some point. Also, breast implant risks include dimples and wrinkles that won't go away, pain, and an implant breaking. There are other possible problems, too, including that you might not be able to breastfeed when you have a baby and it could be harder to see signs of breast cancer in a mammogram (breast X-ray).

What Else Do I Need to Know about Cosmetic Surgery?

Here are a few key points to keep in mind if you are thinking about plastic surgery:

- Talk to your parents or guardians about any surgery and any concerns you have about how your body looks.

- Don't rely on surgery to change your life in a huge way.

- Make sure any doctor you consider is qualified for the surgery you're considering and is certified by the American Board of Plastic Surgery.

- Some doctors won't perform certain procedures if they don't think you're old enough. For example, it is usually not a good idea to have cosmetic surgery while your body is still growing.

- Health insurance usually does not cover the cost of plastic surgery.

What If I Feel Unhappy about My Body?

Most people want to look good, and in your teen years you've got lots going on with your body. How you feel about how you look is called body image, and it can affect how you feel about yourself overall.

It's not always easy to have a positive body image, but you can work on it. One way is to ignore magazines and TV shows that say you need to look a certain way. Try to hang out with people who have healthy attitudes about how they look and who support and accept you. And remember to focus on what you like about yourself—inside and out.

If how parts of your body look bothers you a huge amount and you can't stop thinking about them, you could have body dysmorphic disorder (BDD). People with BDD spend a lot of time and energy looking at their flaws and trying to hide them. They also may ask friends to reassure them about their looks and sometimes want a lot of cosmetic surgery. BDD is an illness, and you can get help. If you or a friend may have BDD, talk to an adult you trust, such as your parent or guardian, school counselor, doctor, or nurse.

Chapter 16

Sleep and Adolescents

Chapter Contents

Section 16.1—Sleep Deprivation among Teens........................ 166

Section 16.2—Sleep-Smart Tips for Teens 169

Section 16.1

Sleep Deprivation among Teens

This section contains text excerpted from the following sources: Text
in this section begins with excerpts from "Most U.S. Middle and High
Schools Start the School Day Too Early," Centers for Disease Control
and Prevention (CDC), August 6, 2015; Text under the heading
"Teen Sleep Habits" is excerpted from "Teen Sleep Habits—What
Should You Do?" Centers for Disease Control and Prevention (CDC),
October 13, 2011. Reviewed November 2017.

Fewer than 1 in 5 middle and high schools in the United States
began the school day at the recommended 8:30 AM start time or
later during the 2011–2012 school year, according to data published
today in the Centers for Disease Control and Prevention's (CDC)
Morbidity and Mortality Weekly Report. Too-early start times can
keep students from getting the sleep they need for health, safety,
and academic success, according to the American Academy of Pediatrics (AAP).

CDC and U.S. Department of Education (ED) researchers reviewed
data from the 2011–2012 Schools and Staffing Survey of nearly 40,000
public middle, high, and combined schools to determine school start
times.

Schools that have a start time of 8:30 AM or later allow adolescent
students the opportunity to get the recommended amount of sleep
on school nights: about 8.5 to 9.5 hours. Insufficient sleep is common
among high school students and is associated with several health
risks such as being overweight, drinking alcohol, smoking tobacco, and
using drugs—as well as poor academic performance. The proportion
of high school students who fail to get sufficient sleep (2 out of 3) has
remained steady since 2007, according to the 2013 Youth Risk Behavior Surveillance Report (YRBSS).

"Getting enough sleep is important for students' health, safety, and
academic performance," said Anne Wheaton, Ph.D., lead author and
epidemiologist in CDC's Division of Population Health (DPH). "Early
school start times, however, are preventing many adolescents from
getting the sleep they need."

Key Findings

- 42 states reported that 75–100 percent of the public schools in their respective states started before 8:30 AM.

- The average start time was 8:03 AM.

- The percentage of schools with start times of 8:30 AM or later varied greatly by state. No schools in Hawaii, Mississippi, and Wyoming started at 8:30 AM or later; more than 75 percent of schools in Alaska and North Dakota started at 8:30 AM or later.

- Louisiana had the earliest average school start time (7:40 AM), while Alaska had the latest (8:33 AM).

In 2014, the American Academy of Pediatrics (AAP) issued a policy statement urging middle and high schools to modify start times to no earlier than 8:30 AM to aid students in getting sufficient sleep to improve their overall health. School start time policies are not determined at the federal or state level, but at the district or individual school level. Future studies may determine whether this recommendation results in later school start times.

The authors report that delayed school start times do not replace the need for other interventions that can improve sleep among adolescents. Parents can help their children practice good sleep habits. For example, a consistent bedtime and rise time, including on weekends, is recommended for everyone, including children, adolescents, and adults. Healthcare providers who treat adolescents should educate teens and parents about the importance of adequate sleep in maintaining health and well-being.

Teen Sleep Habits

Almost 70 percent of high school students are not getting the recommended hours of sleep on school nights, according to a study by the Centers for Disease Control and Prevention (CDC). Researchers found insufficient sleep (< 8 hours on an average school night) to be associated with a number of unhealthy activities, such as:

- Drinking soda or pop 1 or more times per day (not including diet soda or diet pop)

- Not participating in 60 minutes of physical activity on 5 or more of the past 7 days

- Using computers 3 or more hours each day

- Being in a physical fight 1 or more times
- Cigarette use
- Alcohol use
- Marijuana use
- Current sexual activity
- Feeling sad or hopeless
- Seriously considering attempting suicide

Adolescents not getting sufficient sleep each night may be due to changes in the sleep/wake-cycle as well as everyday activities, such as employment, recreational activities, academic pressures, early school start times, and access to technology.

The National Sleep Foundation (NSF) recommends that teenagers receive between 8.5 hours and 9.25 hours each night.

The following sleep health tips are recommended by the National Sleep Foundation:

- Go to bed at the same time each night and rise at the same time each morning.

- Make sure your bedroom is a quiet, dark, and relaxing environment, which is neither too hot or too cold.

- Make sure your bed is comfortable and use it only for sleeping and not for other activities, such as reading, watching TV, or listening to music. Remove all TVs, computers, and other "gadgets" from the bedroom.

- Avoid large meals a few hours before bedtime.

If your sleep problems persist or if they interfere with how you feel or function during the day, you should seek the assistance of a physician or other health professional. Before visiting your physician, consider keeping a diary of your sleep habits for about ten days to discuss at the visit.

Include the following in your sleep diary, when you:

- Go to bed
- Go to sleep
- Wake up
- Get out of bed

- Take naps
- Exercise
- Consume alcohol and how much
- Consume caffeinated beverages and how much

Section 16.2

Sleep-Smart Tips for Teens

This section contains text excerpted from the following sources: Text under the heading "Get Adequate Sleep" is excerpted from "College Health and Safety," Centers for Disease Control and Prevention (CDC), August 9, 2016; Text beginning with the heading "How Much Is Enough?" is excerpted from "Body—Getting Enough Sleep," girlshealth.gov, Office on Women's Health (OWH), May 27, 2014. Reviewed November 2017.

Get Adequate Sleep

It's a challenge in college to pull late-nighters studying and still get enough sleep to function.

Adolescents should get 8 to 10 hours of sleep a day, although individual needs vary. Lack of sleep can be a risk factor for many chronic diseases and conditions, such as diabetes, cardiovascular diseases, obesity, and depression. Students who work or study long hours may not get enough sleep at night. As a result, they may be sleepy and sluggish during the day and have trouble concentrating, participating in class, taking tests, or making decisions. Sleepiness can also cause car and machinery-related crashes, which cause significant rates of injury and disability each year. Driving while sleepy can be as dangerous as driving while intoxicated. Both are preventable!

How Much Is Enough?

Experts say most teens need a little more than nine hours of sleep each night. Only a tiny number get that much, though. Here are some ways to see if you are getting enough sleep:

- Do you have trouble getting up in the morning?

- Do you have trouble focusing?

- Do you sometimes fall asleep during class?

If you answered yes to these questions, try using the tips above for getting better sleep.

Also keep in mind that good sleep isn't just about the number of hours you're in bed. If you wake up a lot in the night, snore, or have headaches, you may not be getting enough quality sleep to keep you fresh and healthy.

Getting Enough Sleep

What's up with sleep? It may seem like a waste of time when you've got so much going on. But sleep can help you do better in school, stress less, and generally be more pleasant to have around. Sound good? Now consider some possible effects of not getting enough sleep:

- Feeling angry or depressed

- Having trouble learning, remembering, and thinking clearly

- Having more accidents, including when driving or using machines

- Getting sick more often

- Feeling less motivated

- Possibly gaining weight

- Having lower self-esteem

Tips for Better Sleep

- **Go to bed and wake up at the same time every day**—even on the weekends!

- **Exercise regularly.** Don't exercise at the expense of sleep, though.

- **Don't eat a lot close to bedtime.** Food can give you a burst of energy.

- **Avoid bright lights right before bed**, including the ones that come from the TV or the computer. Sleep in a dark room. Darkness tells your body it's time for sleep.

- **Sleep in a slightly cool room.** If you can't control the temperature, try using fewer blankets or dressing lightly.

- **Follow a bedtime routine.** If you do the same things each night before bed, your body will know it's time for sleep. Take a warm bath or shower. Or drink a glass of milk.

- **Wake up to bright light.** Light tells your body it's time to get up.

- **Listen to your body.** If you're feeling tired, go to sleep. If you can't fall asleep within 20 minutes of going to bed, get up and do something else until you feel sleepy.

- **Avoid caffeine.** That means cutting back on coffee, soda, chocolate, and energy drinks—or at least trying not to have any in the afternoon.

- **Don't nap for longer than an hour** or take naps too close to bedtime.

- **Don't stay up all night studying.** Try doing some each night instead. If you pull an all-nighter, you may be too tired to do well on your test.

- **Set aside time to relax for about an hour before bed.** If your tasks have you worried, write them down to get them off your mind.

- **Remove computers, phones, and other gadgets.** Put your cell phone out of your room so you won't be tempted to use it, and so texts and calls won't wake you.

If these tips don't help, tell your parents or guardians. You also might talk to your doctor or nurse.

Part Three

Puberty, Sexuality, and Reproductive Health

Chapter 17

Overview of Reproductive and Sexual Health Trends in Teens

Sexual Activity

Many young people engage in sexual risk behaviors that can result in unintended health outcomes. For example, among U.S. high school students surveyed in 2015.

- 41 percent had ever had sexual intercourse.

This chapter contains text excerpted from the following sources: Text under the heading "Sexual Activity" is excerpted from "Sexual Risk Behaviors: HIV, STD, and Teen Pregnancy Prevention," Centers for Disease Control and Prevention (CDC), August 4, 2017; Text under the heading "Contraceptive Use" is excerpted from "Sexual Activity, Contraceptive Use, and Childbearing of Teenagers Aged 15–19 in the United States," Centers for Disease Control and Prevention (CDC), November 6, 2015; Text under the heading "Sexually Transmitted Diseases" is excerpted from "STDs in Adolescents and Young Adults," Centers for Disease Control and Prevention (CDC), October 17, 2016; Text under the heading "Pregnancy" is excerpted from "Teen Pregnancy—About Teen Pregnancy," Centers for Disease Control and Prevention (CDC), May 4, 2017; Text beginning with the heading "Childbearing" is excerpted from "Trends in Teen Pregnancy and Childbearing," Office of Adolescent Health (OAH), U.S. Department of Health and Human Services (HHS), June 2, 2016.

- 30 percent had had sexual intercourse during the previous 3 months, and, of these

  - 43 percent did not use a condom the last time they had sex.

  - 14 percent did not use any method to prevent pregnancy.

  - 21 percent had drunk alcohol or used drugs before last sexual intercourse.

- Only 10 percent of all students have ever been tested for human immunodeficiency virus (HIV).

Sexual risk behaviors place teens at risk for HIV infection, other sexually transmitted diseases (STDs), and unintended pregnancy:

- Young people (aged 13–24) accounted for an estimated 22 percent of all new HIV diagnoses in the United States in 2015.

- Among young people (aged 13–24) diagnosed with HIV in 2015, 81 percent were gay and bisexual males.

- Half of the nearly 20 million new STDs reported each year were among young people, between the ages of 15 to 24.

- Nearly 230,000 babies were born to teen girls aged 15–19 years in 2015.

Contraceptive Use

- In 2011–2013, 79 percent of female teenagers and 84 percent of male teenagers used a method of contraception the first time they had sexual intercourse. The percentages have not changed over time.

- A higher percentage of female teenagers who had first sexual intercourse at ages 18 or 19 used a method of contraception (93%) compared with those who were 17 and under at first sexual intercourse (77%).

- Almost all male teenagers who had first sexual intercourse at ages 18 or 19 used a method of contraception (99%) compared with those who were 17 and under at first sexual intercourse (82%).

Sexually Transmitted Diseases

Incidence and prevalence estimates suggest that young people aged 15–24 years acquire half of all new STDs and that 1 in 4 sexually active adolescent females has an STD, such as chlamydia or human papillomavirus (HPV). Compared with older adults, sexually active adolescents aged 15–19 years and young adults aged 20–24 years are at higher risk of acquiring STDs for a combination of behavioral, biological, and cultural reasons.

Chlamydia

- In 2015, there were 981,359 reported cases of chlamydial infection among persons aged 15–24 years, representing 64.3 percent of all reported chlamydia cases. Among those aged 15–19 years, the rate of reported cases of chlamydia increased 2.5 percent during 2014–2015 (1,811.9 to 1,857.8 cases per 100,000 population).

- In 2015, the rate of reported chlamydia cases among women aged 15–19 years was 2,994.4 cases per 100,000 females, a 1.5 percent increase from the 2014 rate of 2949.3 cases per 100,000 females.

- In 2015, the rate of reported chlamydia cases among men aged 15–19 years was 767.6 cases per 100,000 males. During 2014–2015, the rate of reported chlamydia cases for men in this age group increased 6.3 percent.

Gonorrhea

During 2014–2015, the rate of reported gonorrhea cases increased 5.2 percent for persons aged 15–19 years. Among women aged 15–24 years, the rate was 496.7 cases per 100,000 females. Rates varied by state, with the majority of states with the highest reported case rates in the South. Among men aged 15–24 years, the overall rate was 398.2 cases per 100,000 males. Rates varied by state, with the majority of states having the highest reported case rates in the South.

- In 2015, women aged 15–19 years had the second highest rate of reported gonorrhea cases (442.2 cases per 100,000 females) compared with other women. During 2014–2015, the rate of reported gonorrhea for women in this age group increased 3.0 percent.

- In 2015, the rate of reported gonorrhea cases among men aged 15–19 years was 244.8 cases per 100,000 males. During 2014–2015, the rate of reported gonorrhea for men in this age group increased 10.1 percent.

Primary and Secondary Syphilis

During 2014–2015, the rate of reported primary and secondary (P&S) syphilis cases increased 10.2 percent among persons aged 15–19 years.

- The rate of reported P&S syphilis cases among women aged 15–19 years decreased each year during 2009–2013 (from 3.3 to 1.9 cases per 100,000 females). However, the rate increased in 2014 and again in 2015.

- In 2015, the rate of reported P&S syphilis among men aged 15–19 years was 8.0 cases per 100,000 males. The P&S syphilis rate among men in this age group has increased each year since 2011. During 2014–2015, the rate increased 12.7 percent.

Pregnancy

- In 2015, a total of 229,715 babies were born to women aged 15–19 years, for a birth rate of 22.3 per 1,000 women in this age group.

- Birth rates fell 9 percent for women aged 15–17 years and 7 percent for women aged 18–19 years.

Although reasons for the declines are not totally clear, evidence suggests these declines are due to more teens abstaining from sexual activity, and more teens who are sexually active using birth control than in previous years. Still, the U.S. teen pregnancy rate is substantially higher than in other western industrialized nations, and racial/ethnic and geographic disparities in teen birth rates persist.

Childbearing

- In 2014, there were 24.2 births for every 1,000 adolescent females ages 15–19, or 249,078 babies born to females in this age group.

- Nearly 89 percent of these births occurred outside of marriage.

- The 2014 teen birth rate indicates a decline of nine percent from 2013 when the birth rate was 26.5 per 1,000.

Abortion

The national teen pregnancy rate has declined almost continuously over the last two decades. The teen pregnancy rate includes pregnancies that end in a live birth, as well as those that end in abortion or miscarriage (fetal loss).* Between 1990 and 2010 (the most recent year for which data are available), the teen pregnancy rate declined by 51 percent—from 116.9 to 57.4 pregnancies per 1,000 teen girls. According to recent national data, this decline is due to the combination of an increased percentage of adolescents who are waiting to have sexual intercourse and the increased use of contraceptives by teens.

About 77 percent of teen pregnancies are unplanned. In other words, they are unwanted or occurred "too soon," according to a national survey of adolescents.6 In 2010, the majority of pregnancies to adolescent females ages 15–19 in the United States—an estimated 60 percent—ended in a live birth; 15 percent ended in a miscarriage; and 30 percent ended in an abortion. The rate of abortions among adolescents is the lowest since abortion was legalized in 1973 and 66 percent lower than its peak in 1988.

* *The teen pregnancy rate is the sum all live births, abortions and miscarriages (or fetal losses) per 1,000 adolescent females ages 15–19 in a given year.*

Chapter 18

Male Reproductive System and Puberty

The Male Reproductive System

The external parts of the male reproductive system consist of the penis, scrotum, and testicles.

The internal organs, or accessory glands, include the epididymis, vas deferens, seminal vesicles, urethra, prostate gland, bulbourethral glands, and the ejaculatory duct.

External Organs

Penis

The penis is the male organ used during intercourse. It consists of two main parts, the shaft and the glans. The glans is a cone-shaped structure situated at the end of the penis and is covered by foreskin, which is a thin, loose layer of skin, which is sometimes removed by a medical procedure called circumcision. Circumcision is done for many reasons; for hygiene; social, religious or cultural reasons. The tip of

This chapter contains text excerpted from the following sources: Text beginning with the heading "The Male Reproductive System" is © 2015 Omnigraphics. Reviewed November 2017; Text beginning with the heading "What Is Puberty?" is excerpted from "BAM! Body and Mind—Body Smarts—Questions Answered," Centers for Disease Control and Prevention (CDC), May 9, 2015.

the penis contains the opening of the urethra, a tube that transports urine and semen. Inside, the penis consists of sponge-like tissues which absorb blood and makes the penis become erect for intercourse.

Scrotum

The scrotum is a bag-like structure that can be found behind the penis. It contains the testicles, which produce sperm, the male gamete, and sex hormones. The scrotum protects the testicles and adjusts the body temperature to ensure the survival of sperm. The scrotum contains special muscles in its wall which helps it to contract and relax according to the body temperature necessary for the proper functioning of the sperm.

Testicles

Also called testes, the testicles are two oval organs inside the scrotum. Testicles produce hormones including testosterone, and create sperm. The sperm are produced by seminiferous tubules inside the testes.

Accessory Glands

Urethra

The urethra is a long tube that carries urine from the urinary bladder. In boys, it also brings semen out of the body, during ejaculation. During sexual intercourse, when the penis becomes erect, urine is blocked and only the semen is allowed to come out of the urethra.

Epididymis

One of the accessory organs of the male reproductive system, the epididymis is found inside the body. Before transporting the sperm to vas deferens, epididymis matures the sperm cells.

Vas Deferens

The vas deferens is a long muscular tube connecting the epididymis and the pelvic area. The vas deferens is the duct system that carries semen—the sperm nourishing fluid—to the urethra.

Other accessory glands of the male reproductive system include the ejaculatory ducts which empty semen into the urethra; the seminal vesicles responsible for producing the majority of the fluid found in semen; the prostate gland which produces fluids that nourish and protect the sperm, and the bulbourethral or Cowper's glands which produce pre-ejaculate to provide lubrication for semen to pass through the urethra.

What Does the Male Reproductive System Do?

All of the organs that make up the male reproductive system are designed to work in harmony to generate and release sperm into the female's vagina during sexual intercourse. Once released into the vagina if a healthy sperm meets a mature egg conception can begin. In addition, the male reproductive system produces hormones that play a vital role in ensuring that a boy will develop into a sexually mature man who is capable of reproducing.

References

1. Dr. David T. Derrer, MD. "The Male Reproductive System," WebMD, February 27, 2014.

2. "Male Reproductive System," The Nemours Foundation/KidsHealth, 2015.

3. "Male Reproductive System," PubMed Health Glossary, n.d.

4. "Bulbourethral Glands," Human Anatomy, 2012.

5. "The Male Reproductive System," The Cleveland Clinic Foundation, 2013.

What Is Puberty?

Puberty is a time in your life when your body makes changes that cause you to develop into an adult. These changes affect both how you look like growing taller and developing more muscle. They also affect how you feel—one minute you want to be treated like an adult, at other times you want to be treated like a kid.

What Causes These Changes?

Hormones in your body increase, and these make the changes of puberty happen. For girls, these hormones are estrogen and progesterone. For boys it's testosterone. Much of what happens to your body is controlled by your hormones and the "genetic map" that your body is following. Of course, no one can control these two things.

When Does Puberty Happen?

Puberty starts and ends at different times for everyone. Girls develop more and change between the ages of 9 and 13. For boys, puberty typically starts a little later, when they are between 10 and 15 years old. This explains why many girls are taller and more mature than boys for a few years until the boys catch up. Just remember, everyone develops at a different rate and African American kids tend to develop earlier.

How Much Will I Grow in Puberty?

During puberty, you may experience a "growth spurt," or period of fast growth. Most girls start their growth spurt between ages 9 and 11, reaching their full height between the ages of 15 and 18. Some girls grow as much as 4 inches per year. Boys typically begin their growth spurt later than girls, between ages 13 and 14. But it lasts longer—until about age 20 or 21. On an average, boys grow about 3 1/2 inches per year during puberty.

There is no way to know for sure how much you will grow. Your body is following a genetic map, which helps determine how you will look as an adult. Things like height, body type, and facial features are determined by your genes. Your special pattern of genes comes to you from members of your family. But, you might ask your parents about what puberty was like for them, and that can help you understand what you should expect.

What Is That Smell?

During puberty, both boys and girls sweat glands are more active. Kids will also sweat more during puberty. A lot of kids notice that they have a new smell under their arms and elsewhere on their bodies when they hit puberty, and believe me, it's not a pretty one. That smell is body odor (you may have heard people call it B.O. for short), and everyone gets it. The hormones become more active, affect the glands in your skin, and the glands make chemicals that smell bad.

So what can you do to feel less stinky? Well, keeping clean can stop you from smelling. You might want to take a shower every day, either in the morning before school or at night before bed. Showering after you've been playing sports or exercising is a really good idea. Another way to cut down on body odor is to use deodorant. If you use a deodorant with antiperspirant, it will cut down on sweat as well.

Does Everyone Get Pimples during Puberty?

About 85–90 percent of all kids—boys and girls—have acne during puberty, and you can count on a zit attack when you want to look your best. The hormonal changes that are happening inside your body cause the oil glands to become more active. It doesn't mean that you are dirty, it just means that what is happening on the inside has put your oil glands into high gear and can cause acne or pimples. You may notice pimples on your face, your upper back, or your upper chest. Pimples usually start around the beginning of puberty and can hang around for a few years as your body changes.

No One Understands Me. I Am Not in Control. Why Do I Feel This Way?

Just as suddenly as your body starts changing, your mind is also making changes. The same hormones that cause changes in your appearance can also affect your emotions, making you feel like no one understands what you're experiencing. You may feel like your emotions are all over the place. One minute you're happy and bouncing off the walls, the next minute you're losing your temper, or bawling your eyes out.

What's going on? Confusion and mixed-up feelings are normal. The different hormones in your body can send your emotions on a roller-coaster ride. Puberty makes almost everyone feel that way. Make no mistake—your body has taken control and you are along for the ride. These changes in emotions are normal and once you've gone through puberty, the emotional roller coaster should slow down. Just keep your cool. It'll gradually become easier as you get used to the new you.

In the meantime, you can control other things that affect how you look, how you feel, and how healthy you are. Taking charge of your health can help you to feel good, and in control during the changes of puberty.

Chapter 19

Male Reproductive Concerns

Chapter Contents

Section 19.1—Erectile Dysfunction... 188

Section 19.2—Disorders of the Scrotum and
Testicles 197

Section 19.3—Testicular Cancer and
Self-Examination.................................... 200

Section 19.4—Gynecomastia (Male Breast
Development)... 206

Section 19.1

Erectile Dysfunction

This section includes text excerpted from "Erectile
Dysfunction (ED)," National Institute of Diabetes and
Digestive and Kidney Diseases (NIDDK), July 2017.

What Is Erectile Dysfunction?

Erectile dysfunction (ED) is a condition in which you are unable to
get or keep an erection firm enough for satisfactory sexual intercourse.
ED can be a short-term or long-term problem. You have ED when you:

• can get an erection sometimes, but not every time you want to
have sex

• can get an erection, but it does not last long enough for fulfilling
or satisfactory sex

• are unable to get an erection at any time

Healthcare professionals, such as primary care providers and urologists, often can treat ED. Although ED is very common, it is not a normal part of aging. Talk with a healthcare professional if you have any
ED symptoms. ED could be a sign of a more serious health problem.

You may find it embarrassing and difficult to talk with a healthcare
professional about ED. However, remember that a healthy sex life
can improve your quality of life and is part of a healthy life overall.
Healthcare professionals, especially urologists, are trained to speak
to people about many kinds of sexual problems.

How Common Is Erectile Dysfunction?

ED is very common. It affects about 30 million men in the United
States.

Who Is More Likely to Develop Erectile Dysfunction?

You are more likely to develop ED if you:

• are older

- have certain diseases or conditions

- take certain medicines

- have certain psychological or emotional issues

- have certain health-related factors or behaviors, such as over-weight or smoking

What Are the Complications of Erectile Dysfunction?

Complications of ED may include:

- an unfulfilled sex life

- a loss of intimacy between you and a partner, resulting in a strained relationship

- depression, anxiety, and low self-esteem

- being unable to get a partner pregnant

Depression, anxiety, and low self-esteem can also contribute to ED, creating a cycle of health problems.

What Are the Symptoms of Erectile Dysfunction?

Symptoms of ED include:

- being able to get an erection sometimes, but not every time you want to have sex

- being able to get an erection, but not having it last long enough for sex

- being unable to get an erection at any time

ED is often a symptom of another health problem or health-related factor.

What Causes Erectile Dysfunction?

Many different factors affecting your vascular system, nervous system, and endocrine system can cause or contribute to ED.

Although you are more likely to develop ED as you age, aging does not cause ED. ED can be treated at any age.

Certain Diseases and Conditions

The following diseases and conditions can lead to ED:

- type 2 diabetes
- heart and blood vessel disease
- atherosclerosis
- high blood pressure
- chronic kidney disease
- multiple sclerosis
- Peyronie disease
- injury from treatments for prostate cancer, including radiation therapy and prostate surgery
- injury to the penis, spinal cord, prostate, bladder, or pelvis
- surgery for bladder cancer

Men who have diabetes are two to three times more likely to develop ED than men who do not have diabetes.

Taking Certain Medicines

ED can be a side effect of many common medicines, such as:

- blood pressure medicines
- antiandrogens—medicines used for prostate cancer therapy
- antidepressants
- tranquilizers, or prescription sedatives—medicines that make you calmer or sleepy
- appetite suppressants, or medicines that make you less hungry
- ulcer medicines

Certain Psychological or Emotional Issues

Psychological or emotional factors may make ED worse. You may develop ED if you have one or more of the following:

- fear of sexual failure
- anxiety

- depression
- guilt about sexual performance or certain sexual activities
- low self-esteem
- stress—about sexual performance, or stress in your life in general

Certain Health-Related Factors and Behaviors

The following health-related factors and behaviors may contribute to ED:

- smoking
- drinking too much alcohol
- using illegal drugs
- being overweight
- not being physically active

How Do Doctors Diagnose Erectile Dysfunction?

A doctor, such as a urologist, diagnoses erectile dysfunction (ED) with a medical and sexual history, and a mental health and physical exam. You may find it difficult to talk with a healthcare professional about ED. However, remember that a healthy sex life is part of a healthy life. The more your doctor knows about you, the more likely he or she can help treat your condition.

Medical and Sexual History

Taking a medical and sexual history is one of the first things a doctor will do to help diagnose ED. He or she will ask you to provide information, such as:

- how you would rate your confidence that you can get and keep an erection
- how often your penis is firm enough for intercourse when you have erections from sexual stimulation
- how often you are able to maintain an erection during sexual intercourse
- how often you find sexual intercourse satisfying

- if you have an erection when you wake up in the morning

- how you would rate your level of sexual desire

- how often you're able to climax, or orgasm, and ejaculate

- any surgeries or treatments that may have damaged your nerves or blood vessels near the penis

- any prescription or over-the-counter (OTC) medicines you take

- if you use illegal drugs, drink alcohol, or smoke

This information will help your doctor understand your ED problem. The medical history can reveal diseases and treatments that lead to ED. Reviewing your sexual activity can help your doctor diagnose problems with sexual desire, erection, climax, or ejaculation.

Mental Health and Physical Exam

A healthcare professional may ask you some personal questions and use a questionnaire to help diagnose any psychological or emotional issues that may be leading to ED. The healthcare professional may also ask your sexual partner questions about your relationship and how it may affect your ED.

He or she also will perform a physical exam to help diagnose the causes of ED. During the physical exam, a healthcare professional most often checks your

- penis to find out if it's sensitive to touch. If the penis lacks sensitivity, a problem in the nervous system may be the cause.

- penis's appearance for the source of the problem. For example, Peyronie disease causes the penis to bend or curve when erect.

- body for extra hair or breast enlargement, which can point to hormonal problems.

- blood pressure.

- pulse in your wrist and ankles to see if you have a problem with circulation.

Lab Tests

Blood tests can uncover possible causes of ED, such as diabetes, atherosclerosis, chronic kidney disease, and hormonal problems.

Imaging Tests

A technician most often performs a Doppler ultrasound in a doctor's office or an outpatient center. The ultrasound can detect poor blood flow through your penis. The technician passes a handheld device lightly over your penis to measure blood flow. Color images on a computer screen show the speed and direction blood is flowing through a blood vessel. A radiologist or urologist interprets the images. During this exam, a healthcare professional may inject medicine into your penis to create an erection.

Other Tests

- Nocturnal erection test
- Injection test

How Can I Treat Erectile Dysfunction?

You can work with a healthcare professional to treat an underlying cause of your erectile dysfunction (ED). Choosing an ED treatment is a personal decision. However, you also may benefit from talking with your partner about which treatment is best for you as a couple.

Lifestyle Changes

Your healthcare professional may suggest that you make lifestyle changes to help reduce or improve ED. You can:

- quit smoking
- limit or stop drinking alcohol
- increase physical activity and maintain a healthy body weight
- stop illegal drug use

You can seek help from a health professional if you have trouble making these changes on your own.

Go to Counseling

Talk with your doctor about going to a counselor if psychological or emotional issues are affecting your ED. A counselor can teach you how to lower your anxiety or stress related to sex. Your counselor may suggest that you bring your partner to counseling sessions to learn how to support you. As you work on relieving your anxiety or stress, a doctor can focus on treating the physical causes of ED.

How Do Doctors Treat Erectile Dysfunction?

Change Your Medicines

If a medicine you need for another health condition is causing ED, your doctor may suggest a different dose or different medicine. Never stop taking a medicine without speaking with your doctor first.

Prescribe Medicines You Take by Mouth

A healthcare professional may prescribe you an oral medicine, or medicine you take by mouth, such as one of the following, to help you get and maintain an erection:

- sildenafil (Viagra)

- vardenafil (Levitra, Staxyn)

- tadalafil (Cialis)

- avanafil (Stendra)

All of these medicines work by relaxing smooth muscles and increasing blood flow in the penis during sexual stimulation. You should not take any of these medicines to treat ED if you are taking nitrates to treat a heart condition. Nitrates widen and relax your blood vessels. The combination can lead to a sudden drop in blood pressure, which may cause you to become faint or dizzy, or fall, leading to possible injuries.

Also talk to your healthcare professional if you are taking alpha blockers to treat prostate enlargement. The combination of alpha blockers and ED medicines also could cause a sudden drop in blood pressure.

A healthcare professional may prescribe testosterone if you have low levels of this hormone in your blood. Although taking testosterone may help your ED, it is often unhelpful if your ED is caused by circulatory or nerve problems. Taking testosterone also may lead to side effects, including a high red blood cell count and problems urinating.

Testosterone treatment also has not been proven to help ED associated with age-related or late-onset hypogonadism. Do not take testosterone therapy that hasn't been prescribed by your doctor. Testosterone therapy can affect how your other medicines work and can cause serious side effects.

Prescribe Injectable Medicines and Suppositories

Many men get stronger erections by injecting a medicine called alprostadil into the penis, causing it to become filled with blood. Oral medicines can improve your response to sexual stimulation, but they do not trigger an automatic erection like injectable medicines do.

Instead of injecting a medicine, some men insert a suppository of alprostadil into the urethra. A suppository is a solid piece of medicine that you insert into your body where it dissolves. A healthcare professional will prescribe a prefilled applicator for you to insert the pellet about an inch into your urethra. An erection will begin within 8 to 10 minutes and may last 30 to 60 minutes.

Discuss Alternative Medicines

Some men say certain alternative medicines taken by mouth can help them get and maintain an erection. However, not all "natural" medicines or supplements are safe. Combinations of certain prescribed and alternative medicines could cause major health problems. To help ensure coordinated and safe care, discuss your use of alternative medicines, including use of vitamin and mineral supplements, with a healthcare professional. Also, never order a medicine online without talking with your doctor.

What Steps Can I Take to Prevent Erectile Dysfunction?

You can help prevent many of the causes of erectile dysfunction (ED).

Quit Smoking

If you smoke, get help quitting. Smoking is linked to heart and blood vessel disease, which can lead to ED. Even when heart and blood vessel disease and other possible causes of ED are taken into account, smoking still increases the chances that you will have ED.

Follow a Healthy Eating Plan

To help maintain erectile function, choose whole-grain foods, low-fat dairy foods, fruits and vegetables, and lean meats. Avoid foods high in fat, especially saturated fat, and sodium. Follow a healthy eating plan to help aim for a healthy weight, and control your blood pressure and diabetes. Controlling your blood pressure and diabetes may help prevent ED.

Also, avoid drinking too much alcohol. If you are having trouble cutting out alcohol, see a counselor who has expert knowledge in treating people who drink too much.

Maintain a Healthy Weight to Prevent Diabetes and High Blood Pressure

Maintaining a healthy weight also can help delay the start of diabetes and keep your blood pressure down. Talk with your doctor about how to prevent diabetes—or manage the disease if you already have it. Get regular checkups to measure your blood pressure.

If you need to lose weight, talk with your healthcare provider about how to lose weight safely. Ask for a referral to a dietitian who can help you plan healthy meals to lose weight. Losing weight may help reduce inflammation, increase testosterone levels, and increase self-esteem, all of which may help prevent ED. If you are at a healthy weight for your height, maintain that weight through healthy eating and physical activity.

Be Physically Active

Physical activity increases blood flow through your body, including the penis. Talk with a healthcare professional before starting new activities. Beginners should start slow, with easier activities such as walking at a normal pace or gardening. You can gradually work up to harder activities, such as walking briskly or swimming. Aim for at least 30 minutes of activity most days of the week.

Avoid Using Illegal Drugs

Using illegal drugs may prevent you from getting or keeping an erection. For instance, some illegal drugs may prevent you from becoming aroused or feeling other sensations. Using illegal drugs may mask other psychological, emotional, or physical factors that may be causing your ED. Talk with your healthcare provider if you think you need help with drug abuse.

Section 19.2

Disorders of the Scrotum and Testicles

This section contains text excerpted from the following sources:
Text under the heading "Epididymitis" is excerpted from
"Epididymitis," Centers for Disease Control and Prevention
(CDC), June 4, 2015; Text under the heading is "Hydrocele," © 2017
Omnigraphics. Reviewed November 2017; Text under the heading
is "Spermatocele," © 2017 Omnigraphics. Reviewed November
2017; Text under the heading "Inguinal Hernia" is excerpted from
"Inguinal Hernia," National Institute of Diabetes and Digestive and
Kidney Diseases (NIDDK), June 2014. Reviewed November 2017;
Text under the heading "Perineal Injury in Males" is excerpted
from "Perineal Injury in Males," National Institute of Diabetes and
Digestive and Kidney Diseases (NIDDK), March 2014.
Reviewed November 2017.

Epididymitis

Acute epididymitis is a clinical syndrome consisting of pain, swelling, and inflammation of the epididymis that lasts <6 weeks. Sometimes the testis is also involved—a condition referred to as epididymo-orchitis. A high index of suspicion for spermatic cord (testicular) torsion must be maintained in men who present with a sudden onset of symptoms associated with epididymitis, as this condition is a surgical emergency.

Among sexually active men aged <35 years, acute epididymitis is most frequently caused by *C. trachomatis* or *N. gonorrhoeae*. Acute epididymitis caused by sexually transmitted enteric organisms (e.g., *Escherichia coli*) also occurs among men who are the insertive partner during anal intercourse. Sexually transmitted acute epididymitis usually is accompanied by urethritis, which frequently is asymptomatic. Other nonsexually transmitted infectious causes of acute epididymitis (e.g., Fournier's gangrene) are uncommon and should be managed in consultation with a urologist.

In men aged ≥35 years who do not report insertive anal intercourse, sexually transmitted acute epididymitis is less common. In this group, the epididymis usually becomes infected in the setting of bacteruria secondary to bladder outlet obstruction (e.g., benign prostatic hyperplasia). In older men, nonsexually transmitted acute epididymitis is also associated with prostate biopsy, urinary tract instrumentation or surgery, systemic disease, and/or immunosuppression.

Chronic epididymitis is characterized by a ≥6 week history of symptoms of discomfort and/or pain in the scrotum, testicle, or epididymis. Chronic infectious epididymitis is most frequently seen in conditions associated with a granulomatous reaction; *Mycobacterium tuberculosis* (TB) is the most common granulomatous disease affecting the epididymis and should be suspected, especially in men with a known history of or recent exposure to TB. The differential diagnosis of chronic noninfectious epididymitis, sometimes termed "orchalgia/epididymalgia" is broad (i.e., trauma, cancer, autoimmune, and idiopathic conditions); men with this diagnosis should be referred to a urologist for clinical management.

Hydrocele

A hydrocele is a generally harmless, painless buildup of fluid around one or both testicles that causes swelling in the scrotum.

Hydroceles can be described as primary or secondary. A primary hydrocele, also called an idiopathic hydrocele, often occurs as a result of an imbalance between the secretion and absorption of fluids in the membranes covering the testes. A secondary hydrocele may follow trauma, infection, or neoplasms.

Common in newborns, congenital hydroceles may form a few weeks prior to birth when the testes descend from the abdomen into the scrotum, surrounded by a fluid-filled sac. Normally, this sac closes and the fluid is absorbed. In some newborns, however, the sac fails to close, which causes a route to the abdominal cavity to remain open. This is called a communicating hydrocele, since it allows the passage of fluid between the abdomen and scrotum. A noncommunicating hydrocele, on the other hand, develops when the sac closes but traps some fluid in the scrotum. Congenital hydroceles are found in about 10 percent of newborns and may regress spontaneously within the first two years of life.

Hydroceles may also affect adolescents and adults, most often men over 40. In these cases, the hydrocele may be caused by a condition in which the passage from abdomen to scrotum either hasn't closed all the way or has reopened. Other causes of hydroceles in adults include injury to the scrotum or inflammation resulting from an infection.

Spermatocele

A spermatocele—often called a spermatic cyst—is a benign fluid-filled mass within the scrotum. The cyst is an accumulation of fluid and sperm cells that typically arises from the caput (head) of the epididymis, a tightly coiled tube located above each testicle that collects and transports sperm. Spermatoceles are common and generally do not require treatment. However, discomfort, pain, or a bothersome enlargement may require surgical intervention.

Spermatoceles are usually asymptomatic, do not affect fertility, and are most often discovered during self-examination or in an imaging test carried out for other conditions.

Inguinal Hernia

An inguinal hernia happens when contents of the abdomen—usually fat or part of the small intestine—bulge through a weak area in the lower abdominal wall. The abdomen is the area between the chest and the hips. The area of the lower abdominal wall is also called the inguinal or groin region.

Two types of inguinal hernias are

- indirect inguinal hernias, which are caused by a defect in the abdominal wall that is congenital, or present at birth

- direct inguinal hernias, which usually occur only in male adults and are caused by a weakness in the muscles of the abdominal wall that develops over time

Inguinal hernias occur at the inguinal canal in the groin region. The inguinal canal is a passage through the lower abdominal wall. People have two inguinal canals—one on each side of the lower abdomen. In males, the spermatic cords pass through the inguinal canals and connect to the testicles in the scrotum—the sac around the testicles. The spermatic cords contain blood vessels, nerves, and a duct, called the spermatic duct, that carries sperm from the testicles to the penis. In females, the round ligaments, which support the uterus, pass through the inguinal canals.

Perineal Injury in Males

Perineal injury is an injury to the perineum, the part of the body between the anus and the genitals, or sex organs. In males, the perineum is the area between the anus and the scrotum, the external pouch of skin that holds the testicles. Injuries to the perineum can happen suddenly, as in an accident, or gradually, as the result of an activity that persistently puts pressure on the perineum. Sudden damage to the perineum is called an acute injury, while gradual damage is called a chronic injury.

The perineum is important because it contains blood vessels and nerves that supply the urinary tract and genitals with blood and nerve signals.

Section 19.3

Testicular Cancer and Self-Examination

This section contains text excerpted from the following sources:
Text in this section begins with excerpts from "Testicular Cancer
Treatment (PDQ®)–Patient Version," National Cancer Institute
(NCI), July 7, 2016; Text beginning with the heading "Testicular Self-
Examination" is © 2017 Omnigraphics.
Reviewed November 2017.

Although testicular cancer has a relatively low rate of occurrence, accounting for just one percent of malignancies in all men, it is the most common neoplasm, or abnormal growth, in adolescent males and young men under 35 years of age. Testicular cancer is easily diagnosable and can be successfully treated, with a high survival rate of more than ten years in nearly 90 percent of patients. As with most types of cancer, the prognosis is particularly good with early detection. While significant advances have been made in developing treatments for testicular cancer in the last few decades, the benefits of early detection through self-examination have not received much attention, often resulting in delays before medical attention is sought.

In the absence of a standard or routine screening for testicular cancer, the condition is most often detected either by a doctor during a routine physical examination, or by an individual during the course of a self-exam. The outlook for testicular cancer depends on whether or not the disease has metastasized to lymph nodes, tissues, and organs, and this underscores the importance of early detection by testicular self-examination (TSE). Early detection involves the diagnosis of testicular cancer through Stages 1 and 2. Stage 1 refers to a "localized" tumor restricted to the primary site, the testes. Stage 2 is the term for a "regional" tumor, one that has spread to other areas. An early diagnosis resulting from a self-exam can greatly enhance treatment outcomes and also reduce the side effects commonly associated with chemotherapy, radiation, and surgery.

Testicular Cancer

Testicular cancer is a disease in which malignant (cancer) cells form in the tissues of one or both testicles. The testicles are 2 egg shaped glands located inside the scrotum (a sac of loose skin that lies directly below the penis). The testicles are held within the scrotum by the spermatic cord, which also contains the vas deferens and vessels and nerves of the testicles.

The testicles are the male sex glands and produce testosterone and sperm. Germ cells within the testicles produce immature sperm that travel through a network of tubules (tiny tubes) and larger tubes into the epididymis (a long coiled tube next to the testicles) where the sperm mature and are stored.

Almost all testicular cancers start in the germ cells. The two main types of testicular germ cell tumors are seminomas and nonseminomas. These 2 types grow and spread differently and are treated differently. Nonseminomas tend to grow and spread more quickly than seminomas. Seminomas are more sensitive to radiation. A testicular tumor that contains both seminoma and nonseminoma cells is treated as a nonseminoma. Testicular cancer is the most common cancer in men 20 to 35 years old.

Health History and the Risk of Testicular Cancer

Health history can affect the risk of testicular cancer. Anything that increases the chance of getting a disease is called a risk factor. Having a risk factor does not mean that you will get cancer; not having risk factors doesn't mean that you will not get cancer. Talk with your doctor if you think you may be at risk. Risk factors for testicular cancer include:

• Having had an undescended testicle.

• Having had abnormal development of the testicles.

• Having a personal history of testicular cancer.

- Having a family history of testicular cancer (especially in a father or brother).

- Being white.

Signs and Symptoms of Testicular Cancer

Signs and symptoms of testicular cancer include swelling or discomfort in the scrotum. These and other signs and symptoms may be caused by testicular cancer or by other conditions. Check with your doctor if you have any of the following:

- A painless lump or swelling in either testicle.

- A change in how the testicle feels.

- A dull ache in the lower abdomen or the groin.

- A sudden buildup of fluid in the scrotum.

- Pain or discomfort in a testicle or in the scrotum.

Tests for Diagnosing Testicular Cancer

Tests that examine the testicles and blood are used to detect and diagnose testicular cancer. The following tests and procedures may be used:

- **Physical exam and history:** An exam of the body to check general signs of health, including checking for signs of disease, such as lumps or anything else that seems unusual. The testicles will be examined to check for lumps, swelling, or pain. A history of the patient's health habits and past illnesses and treatments will also be taken.

- **Ultrasound exam:** A procedure in which high energy sound waves (ultrasound) are bounced off internal tissues or organs and make echoes. The echoes form a picture of body tissues called a sonogram.

- **Serum tumor marker test:** A procedure in which a sample of blood is examined to measure the amounts of certain substances released into the blood by organs, tissues, or tumor cells in the body. Certain substances are linked to specific types of cancer when found in increased levels in the blood. These are called tumor markers. The following tumor markers are used to detect testicular cancer:

- Alpha fetoprotein (AFP).

- Beta human chorionic gonadotropin (β-hCG).

Tumor marker levels are measured before inguinal orchiectomy and biopsy, to help diagnose testicular cancer.

- **Inguinal orchiectomy:** A procedure to remove the entire testicle through an incision in the groin. A tissue sample from the testicle is then viewed under a microscope to check for cancer cells. (The surgeon does not cut through the scrotum into the testicle to remove a sample of tissue for biopsy, because if cancer is present, this procedure could cause it to spread into the scrotum and lymph nodes. It's important to choose a surgeon who has experience with this kind of surgery.) If cancer is found, the cell type (seminoma or nonseminoma) is determined in order to help plan treatment.

Prognosis and Treatment Options

The prognosis and treatment options depend on the following:

- Stage of the cancer (whether it is in or near the testicle or has spread to other places in the body, and blood levels of AFP, β-hCG, and lactate dehydrogenase (LDH).

- Type of cancer.

- Size of the tumor.

- Number and size of retroperitoneal lymph nodes.

Testicular cancer can usually be cured in patients who receive adjuvant chemotherapy or radiation therapy after their primary treatment.

Treatment for Testicular Cancer Can Cause Infertility

Certain treatments for testicular cancer can cause infertility that may be permanent. Patients who may wish to have children should consider sperm banking before having treatment. Sperm banking is the process of freezing sperm and storing it for later use.

Testicular Self-Examination

Although testicular cancer has a relatively low rate of occurrence, accounting for just one percent of malignancies in all men, it is the most common neoplasm, or abnormal growth, in adolescent males and young men under 35 years of age. Testicular cancer is easily diagnosable and can be successfully treated, with a high survival rate of more than ten years in nearly 90 percent of patients. As with most types of cancer, the prognosis is particularly good with early detection. While significant advances have been made in developing treatments for testicular cancer in the last few decades, the benefits of early detection through self-examination have not received much attention, often resulting in delays before medical attention is sought.

Importance of Testicular Self-Examination (TSE)

In the absence of a standard or routine screening for testicular cancer, the condition is most often detected either by a doctor during a routine physical examination, or by an individual during the course of a self-exam. The outlook for testicular cancer depends on whether or not the disease has metastasized to lymph nodes, tissues, and organs, and this underscores the importance of early detection by TSE. Early detection involves the diagnosis of testicular cancer through Stages 1 and 2. Stage 1 refers to a "localized" tumor restricted to the primary site, the testes. Stage 2 is the term for a "regional" tumor, one that has spread to other areas. An early diagnosis resulting from a self-exam can greatly enhance treatment outcomes and also reduce the side effects commonly associated with chemotherapy, radiation, and surgery.

How to Perform a Self-Exam

It is important to perform a self-examination every month. This allows you to familiarize yourself with the size, shape, and consistency of your testes and sensitize you to any abnormality in the future. This also helps you to distinguish the epididymis—a highly coiled duct behind the testis for the temporary storage of sperm—from an abnormal lump or growth. Further, it is quite normal for most men to have testicular asymmetry. Differently sized testes with one hanging lower than the other is a normal anatomical feature and should not be construed as a sign of abnormality.

The ideal time to perform a self-exam is right after a warm shower when the scrotum is relaxed and can be easily drawn back to examine the testicles.

TSE is a simple procedure that takes no more than a couple of minutes:

- Hold the penis away from the scrotum to enable close examination of the testes.

- Hold the testicles between your thumb and fingers and roll gently.

- Feel each testicle for any painless lump, usually grain or pea-sized, in the front or sides, taking care not to confuse a lump with supporting tissues and blood vessels.

- If you detect any thickening, discomfort, or pain in the testicles or groin, contact your healthcare professional immediately.

Studies show that men often delay seeking medical attention because early symptoms are typically mild, and many men tend to believe that a lump is benign or harmless and may go away on its own. Concerns about loss of sexuality, or sterility, may also get in the way of seeking professional help when an abnormality is detected.

While the majority of scrotal and testicular irregularities may not be associated with malignancy, it is important for all men—especially those who carry a high risk for testicular tumors—to perform regular self-exams. A family history of testicular cancer and previous history of malignant tumors in one or both of the testes are regarded as high-risk factors, as are conditions such as cryptorchidism, a common birth defect associated with undescended testes.

References

1. "How to Perform a Testicular Self-Examination," The Nemours Foundation, 2012.

2. "Testicular Examination and Testicular Self-Examination (TSE)," Healthwise, Incorporated, June 4, 2014.

3. "SEER Stat Fact Sheets: Testis Cancer," National Institutes of Health (NIH), April 2016.

Section 19.4

Gynecomastia (Male Breast Development)

"Gynecomastia (Male Breast Development),"
© 2017 Omnigraphics. Reviewed November 2017.

What Is Gynecomastia?

Gynecomastia is the enlargement of male breast tissue, most often due to an imbalance of the hormones estrogen and testosterone. The condition can affect one or both breasts and can make the breast tender. It is usually not permanent or dangerous; however, affected males can experience a considerable amount of social embarrassment and psychological distress. Pseudogynecomastia (false gynecomastia) can sometimes be confused with gynecomastia; but the former is caused by an excessive amount of fat tissue on the chest, while the latter is an above-average growth of the breast tissue itself.

Prevalence

Gynecomastia can occur at any stage of a man's life, depending on the degree of hormonal change. Newborn babies often have this condition for a short time immediately after birth when the mother's estrogen remains in their bloodstreams. In infants, it usually disappears within the first year of life. Teenage boys may experience gynecomastia during puberty starting from as early as age 10, with aggressive growth between the ages 13 and 14, and slowly regressing in the later teen years. Statistically, only about 4 percent of males between the ages 10 and 19 are found to have gynecomastia. The condition is most prevalent among older adults, aged 50 to 80. One in every four men in this age group is affected, and in these cases, there may be other medical problems associated with the condition.

Causes and Risk Factors

The exact cause of gynecomastia is unclear; however, in most cases it is thought to be the result of an imbalance between estrogen and testosterone. These hormones are responsible for the development and control of sex characteristics in both males and females. In general, testosterone helps create typically male characteristics, such as facial hair, muscle mass, body hair, and a deep voice. Estrogen aids in the development of what are commonly regarded as feminine characteristics, including breast development. Since men have both hormones in their systems, if an imbalance favors estrogen, gynecomastia can result.

Some other causes and risk factors of gynecomastia include:

- Medication, such as antibiotics, anti-anxiety drugs, anabolic steroids, heart medications, anti-androgens, tricyclic antidepressants, gastric motility medications, and ulcer medications.

- Cancer and AIDS treatments.

- The use of substance like alcohol, heroin, methadone, marijuana, and amphetamines.

- A variety of physical conditions, including hypogonadism, tumors, kidney failure, liver failure, cirrhosis, malnutrition, and starvation.

- The use of tea tree oil or lavender oil, herbal products that contain natural estrogen.

- Obesity or lack of proper diet and nutrition.

Diagnosis

To begin evaluating a patient for gynecomastia, a healthcare provider will ask for a medical history, including such information as the symptoms being experienced, how long they have persisted, if tenderness is present around the breast area, type of medication being taken, general health condition, drug history, and family health history. The healthcare provider will then perform a careful examination of the breast tissue, genitals, and abdomen.

Tests a doctor may order to help confirm a diagnosis of gynecomastia include:

- computerized tomography (CT) scans

- blood tests

- mammograms

- magnetic resonance imaging (MRI) scans

- tissue biopsies

- testicular ultrasounds

Treatment

In young patients, treatment is often not necessary, since in such cases, gynecomastia usually resolves on its own. For older individuals, a number of treatment methods can be recommended by healthcare providers. For example, medications may be prescribed to help restore hormone balance. Certain medications, such as tamoxifen, aromatase inhibitors (Arimidex), and raloxifene (Evista)--while not specifically approved for the treatment of gynecomastia--may help in some cases. If any health condition is causing the gynecomastia, it will need to be addressed through specific treatment. If gynecomastia has been resulted from the use of certain drugs, doctors may prescribe a different medication that may help improve the condition.

In rare cases, surgery may be an option if medication and other treatment prove ineffective. Surgical options include liposuction, a procedure that removes the breast fat but not the breast gland tissue, and mastectomy, a procedure that removes the breast gland tissue.

In order to make good decisions and ensure the best possible outcome, before beginning any treatment, the patient should ask the following questions of the healthcare provider:

- Is the breast enlargement likely to resolve on its own?

- What types of treatments are available?

- How long will treatment last?

- Are there any health conditions that are triggering the gynecomastia?

- Should I avoid any particular substance or medication to improve the condition?

- Should I be tested for breast cancer?

- If breasts are hurting, what can I do to stop the pain?

Treatment options also include getting psychological counseling, as well as help and support from family. The condition can cause stress and embarrassment, and so counseling, group therapy, and help explaining the condition to family and friends can have a major impact on the recovery process.

References

1. Booth, Stephanie. "Enlarged Breasts in Men: Causes and Treatments," WebMD, December 13, 2015.

2. "Enlarged Breasts in Men (Gynecomastia)," Mayo Clinic, August 29, 2017.

3. "Gynecomastia," Cleveland Clinic, n.d.

4. "Gynecomastia," Familydoctor.org, March 2014.

5. Lemaine, Valerie, M.D., Cenk Cayci, M.D., Patricia S. Simmons, M.D., and Paul Petty, M.D. "Gynecomastia in Adolescent Males," National Library of Medicine (NLM), February 27, 2013.

Chapter 20

Female Reproductive System and Puberty

How the Female Reproductive System Works

The female reproductive system is all the parts of your body that help you reproduce, or have babies. And it is quite amazing! Consider these two fabulous facts:

- Your body likely has hundreds of thousands of eggs that could grow into a baby. And you have them from the time you're born.

- Right inside you is a perfect place for those eggs to meet with sperm and grow a whole human being!

What's Inside the Female Reproductive System?

The ovaries are two small organs. Before puberty, it's as if the ovaries are asleep. During puberty, they "wake up." The ovaries start making more estrogen and other hormones, which cause body changes.

This chapter contains text excerpted from the following sources: Text beginning with the heading "How the Female Reproductive System Works" is excerpted from "How the Female Reproductive System Works," girlshealth.gov, Office on Women's Health (OWH), May 23, 2014. Reviewed November 2017; Text beginning with the heading "What Is Puberty?" is excerpted from "Body," girlshealth.gov, Office on Women's Health (OWH), May 23, 2014. Reviewed November 2017.

One important body change is that these hormones cause you to start getting your period, which is called menstruating.

Once a month, the ovaries release one egg (ovum). This is called ovulation.

The fallopian tubes connect the ovaries to the uterus. The released egg moves along a fallopian tube.

The uterus—or womb—is where a baby would grow. It takes several days for the egg to get to the uterus.

As the egg travels, estrogen makes the lining of the uterus (called the endometrium) thick with blood and fluid. This makes the uterus a good place for a baby to grow. You can get pregnant if you have sex with a male without birth control and his sperm joins the egg (called fertilization) on its way to your uterus.

If the egg doesn't get fertilized, it will be shed along with the lining of your uterus during your next period. But don't look for the egg—it's too small to see!

The blood and fluid that leave your body during your period passes through your cervix and vagina.

The cervix is the narrow entryway in between the vagina and uterus. The cervix is flexible so it can expand to let a baby pass through during childbirth.

The vagina is like a tube that can grow wider to deliver a baby that has finished growing inside the uterus.

The hymen covers the opening of the vagina. It is a thin piece of tissue that has one or more holes in it. Sometimes a hymen may be stretched or torn when you use a tampon or during a first sexual experience. If it does tear, it may bleed a little bit.

What's Outside the Vagina?

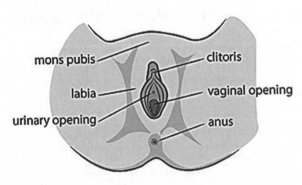

Figure 20.1. *Outside the Vagina*

The vulva covers the entrance to the vagina. The vulva has five parts: mons pubis, labia, clitoris, urinary opening, and vaginal opening. The mons pubis is the mound of tissue and skin above your legs, in the middle. This area becomes covered with hair when you go through puberty. The labia are the two sets of skin folds (often called lips) on either side of the opening of the vagina. The labia majora are the outer lips, and the labia minora are the inner lips. It is normal for the labia to look different from each other. The clitoris is a small, sensitive bump at the bottom of the mons pubis that is covered by the labia minora. The urinary opening, below the clitoris, is where your urine (pee) leaves the body. The vaginal opening is the entry to the vagina and is found below the urinary opening.

What Is Puberty?

Puberty is when you start making the change from being a child to being an adult. And it's when your body develops the ability to have a baby. It all happens thanks to changing hormones, or natural body chemicals.

With everything that's changing, life can feel a little overwhelming. But you can feel more in control if you take good care of your body. Knowing what to expect can help, too, so keep reading. (And don't forget that puberty also involves changes you can't see—like changes to your self-esteem and your feelings.

Timing and Stages of Puberty

Adolescence and puberty can be so confusing! Here's some info on what to expect and when:

- Puberty in girls usually starts between the ages of 8 and 13 and ends by around 14. For boys, puberty usually starts between 10 and 14, and ends by around 15 or 16.

- For girls, one of the first signs of puberty usually is their breasts starting to grow.

- Getting your period (menstruation) usually happens later, around two years after breast growth starts.

- In between, you'll probably start to see more hair in places like under your arms and in your pubic area.

- Puberty involves big changes to your shape, including getting taller (which stops when puberty ends).

Of course, it can be hard to have your body change at a slower or faster rate than your friends' bodies. If how fast or slow your body is changing is upsetting you, talk to an adult you trust.

If you're developing slower or faster than you think you should, your body may just be changing at its own natural rate. It's a good idea to let your doctor know if you start puberty before age 8. Also let your doctor know if you don't have any signs of puberty by the time you're 14. Your doctor can check whether a medical problem is involved.

Changes to Your Shape

How your body looks changes a lot during puberty. For one, usually between the ages of 9 and 13, girls grow much faster than they had been growing. This process, called a growth spurt, happens later for boys. That explains why you may be taller than the boys in your grade for a while.

You likely will also see lots of other changes in your body during puberty.

Changes in Your Body during Puberty

These are some of the changes you can expect during puberty:

- A curvier shape
- Wider hips, thighs, and bottom
- Normal weight gain as your body structure grows
- Stretch marks, or little scars, where your skin was pulled from growing fast (but that usually fade over time)

You'll also see more body hair, changes to your breasts, and possibly some acne. We've got lots of helpful tips on each of those topics, too!

Keep in mind that these changes all are common and normal! And make sure to take good care of your great, growing body. With everything that's going on, it's important to eat well, stay fit, and get enough sleep.

Your Feelings about Your Changing Body

During puberty your body may seem very different from what you're used to, and you might feel uncomfortable or shy about it. Remember that everyone goes through these changes—it's just part of life—and every girl grows at her own pace.

During puberty, it's common to struggle with body image, or how you feel about your body. This can be especially hard when models in magazines have bodies that seem "perfect." But a lot of what you see in magazines and online is either fake or unhealthy.

If you think you or a friend may have a problem with body image or an eating disorder, talk to a parent, a doctor, or another adult you trust. Help is available, and it's important to get treated. You can get better!

Remember, measure yourself by your great traits and loving heart—not by the size and shape of your body!

Changes to Your Breasts

It's natural for girls to wonder about their breasts: Are they too big? Too small? If your breasts are large, they may get you unwanted attention. If they're small, you may worry that they'll never grow. Remember that your breasts don't need to look like your friend's breasts or a magazine model's breasts. The world would be boring if everyone looked the same!

What Happens to Breasts during Puberty?

Throughout puberty, you will experience changes in your breasts. The first change is developing a very small bump under the nipple. Early on, you may also notice that your breasts feel a little itchy or achy. Later on, they also may feel tender or sore during your period.

Keep in mind that it is very common for your two breasts to be different sizes, especially as they first start to grow. Other people can't tell that your breasts are different sizes. Give your body time to grow at its own rate and in its own way. Vitamins, herbal teas, and creams—even exercises—won't change the size of your breasts.

What about Lumps and Other Changes?

Most of the changes your breasts will go through are normal. Let your doctor know if you find a lump or have a pain that you are not sure about. Although lumps are common in young women, keep in mind that it is very rare for the lumps to be cancer.

Should I Wear a Bra?

Wearing a bra can help support and protect your breasts. If you find that exercise is not as comfortable when your breasts start to grow, try wearing a sports bra with a snug fit for support.

Are you having a hard time finding a bra that fits well? Often, you can get help in a department store or special bra store. There are certain steps people there can take for measuring your body to get a good fit.

Body Hair

Even before you get your first period, you will likely see new hair growing in your pubic area, under your arms, and on your legs. The hair may start out light and there won't be a lot of it, but then it will grow darker and thicker as you go through the stages of puberty. Hair in the pubic area starts near the opening and spreads up in a V shape over time.

Body hair is normal, and some people think it looks cool. Lots of women and girls remove body hair from places such as their legs and underarms, although there is no real health reason to do so.

If you are thinking about removing hair for the first time, it makes sense to talk to your parents or guardians. They may have an opinion about how old you should be to start removing hair or advice on ways to do it.

Tips for Removing Pubic Hair

In recent years, more girls and women have also begun removing all or some of the hair around their vagina. There is no need to remove the hair to keep the area clean. The decision to remove pubic hair often is based just on trends, which change over time.

If you're thinking about removing pubic hair, keep a few facts in mind:

- Your pubic hair helps protect the sensitive lips around the opening to your vagina from painful rubbing by your underwear.

- The pubic area is very sensitive. It can easily get irritated or infected when removing hair.

- Waxing works by pulling out the hair, which can hurt.

- If you shave, you can give yourself a painful cut.

- As shaved hair grows back, it can feel itchy and uncomfortable.

- If you decide to use a hair-removal cream, make sure it says it's gentle enough for the pubic area.

- Don't put on any product that could sting, like aftershave lotion. To help avoid irritation, don't use products with added dyes or fragrances.

If you have more questions about taking care of this sensitive area, talk with an adult you trust.

Changes in Your Mind

During puberty, changes don't happen only to your body—changes happen in your mind, too.

- You are able to understand more complex matters.
- You are starting to make more of your own moral choices.
- You know more about who you are, and what your likes and dislikes are.
- You may have some new, strong emotions.

The teen years can seem like an emotional roller coaster, with worries about your changing looks, the demands of school, and pressure to fit in. You might feel alone on this ride, but everyone struggles with it. And some of your experiences have to do with the physical changes of this age, including shifts in your hormones and a brain that's developing just like your body is.

Chapter 21

Menstruation and the Menstrual Cycle

The menstrual cycle is the hormonal process a woman's body goes through each month to prepare for a possible pregnancy. Regular menstrual periods in the years between puberty and menopause are usually a sign that your body is working normally. Irregular or heavy, painful periods are not normal. Many women also get premenstrual syndrome (PMS) symptoms. You can take steps at home and talk to your doctor or nurse about ways to treat your period problems and PMS.

What Is Menstruation?

Menstruation is a woman's monthly bleeding, often called your "period." When you menstruate, your body discards the monthly buildup of the lining of your uterus (womb). Menstrual blood and tissue flow from your uterus through the small opening in your cervix and pass out of your body through your vagina.

During the monthly menstrual cycle, the uterus lining builds up to prepare for pregnancy. If you do not get pregnant, estrogen and progesterone hormone levels begin falling. Very low levels of estrogen and progesterone tell your body to begin menstruation.

This chapter includes text excerpted from "Menstrual Cycle," Office on Women's Health (OWH), U.S. Department of Health and Human Services (HHS), June 12, 2017.

What Is the Menstrual Cycle?

The menstrual cycle is the monthly hormonal cycle a female's body goes through to prepare for pregnancy. Your menstrual cycle is counted from the first day of your period up to the first day of your next period. Your hormone levels (estrogen and progesterone) usually change throughout the menstrual cycle and can cause menstrual symptoms.

How Long Is a Typical Menstrual Cycle?

The typical menstrual cycle is 28 days long, but each woman is different. Also, a woman's menstrual cycle length might be different from month-to-month. Your periods are still "regular" if they usually come every 24 to 38 days. This means that the time from the first day of your last period up to the start of your next period is at least 24 days but not more than 38 days.

Some women's periods are so regular that they can predict the day and time that their periods will start. Other women are regular but can only predict the start of their period within a few days.

What Is Ovulation?

Ovulation is when the ovary releases an egg so it can be fertilized by a sperm in order to make a baby. A woman is most likely to get pregnant if she has sex without birth control in the three days before and up to the day of ovulation (since the sperm are already in place and ready to fertilize the egg as soon as it is released). A man's sperm can live for 3 to 5 days in a woman's reproductive organs, but a woman's egg lives for just 12 to 24 hours after ovulation.

Each woman's cycle length may be different, and the time between ovulation and when the next period starts can be anywhere from one week (7 days) to more than 2 weeks (19 days).

At different times in a woman's life, ovulation may or may not happen:

- Women who are pregnant do not ovulate.

- Women who are breastfeeding may or may not ovulate. Women who are breastfeeding should talk to their doctor about birth control methods if they do not want to get pregnant.

- During perimenopause, the transition to menopause, you may not ovulate every month.

- After menopause you do not ovulate.

How Do I Know If I'm Ovulating?

A few days before you ovulate, your vaginal mucus or discharge changes and becomes more slippery and clear. This type of mucus helps sperm move up into your uterus and into the fallopian tubes where it can fertilize an egg. Some women feel minor cramping on one side of their pelvic area when they ovulate. Some women have other signs of ovulation.

Luteinizing hormone (LH) is a hormone released by your brain that tells the ovary to release an egg (called ovulation). LH levels begin to surge upward about 36 hours before ovulation, so some women and their doctors test for LH levels. LH levels peak about 12 hours before ovulation. Women who are tracking ovulation to become pregnant will notice a slight rise in their basal temperature (your temperature after sleeping before you get out of bed) around ovulation.

How Does My Menstrual Cycle Change as I Get Older?

Your cycles may change in different ways as you get older. Often, periods are heavier when you are younger (in your teens) and usually get lighter in your 20s and 30s. This is normal.

- **For a few years after your first period**, menstrual cycles longer than 38 days are common. Girls usually get more regular cycles within three years of starting their periods. If longer or irregular cycles last beyond that, see your doctor or nurse to rule out a health problem, such as polycystic ovary syndrome (PCOS).

- **In your 20s and 30s**, your cycles are usually regular and can last anywhere from 24 to 38 days.

- **In your 40s**, as your body starts the transition to menopause, your cycles might become irregular. Your menstrual periods might stop for a month or a few months and then start again. They also might be shorter or last longer than usual, or be lighter or heavier than normal.

Talk to your doctor or nurse if you have menstrual cycles that are longer than 38 days or shorter than 24 days, or if you are worried about your menstrual cycle.

Why Should I Keep Track of My Menstrual Cycle?

If your periods are regular, tracking them will help you know when you ovulate, when you are most likely to get pregnant, and when to expect your next period to start.

If your periods are not regular, tracking them can help you share any problems with your doctor or nurse.

If you have period pain or bleeding that causes you to miss school or work, tracking these period symptoms will help you and your doctor or nurse find treatments that work for you. Severe pain or bleeding that causes you to miss regular activities is not normal and can be treated.

How Can I Keep Track of My Menstrual Cycle?

You can keep track of your menstrual cycle by marking the day you start your period on a calendar. After a few months, you can begin to see if your periods are regular or if your cycles are different each month.

You may want to track:

- **Premenstrual syndrome (PMS) symptoms:** Did you have cramping, headaches, moodiness, forgetfulness, bloating, or breast tenderness?

- **When your bleeding begins:** Was it earlier or later than expected?

- **How heavy the bleeding was on your heaviest days:** Was the bleeding heavier or lighter than usual? How many pads or tampons did you use?

- **Period symptoms:** Did you have pain or bleeding on any days that caused you to miss work or school?

- **How many days your period lasted:** Was your period shorter or longer than the month before?

You can also download apps (sometimes for free) for your phone to track your periods. Some include features to track your PMS symptoms, energy and activity levels, and more.

When Does a Girl Usually Get Her First Period?

The average age for a girl in the United States to get her first period is 12. This does not mean that all girls start at the same age.

A girl may start her period anytime between 8 and 15. The first period normally starts about two years after breasts first start to develop and pubic hair begins to grow. The age at which a girl's mother started her period can help predict when a girl may start her period.

A girl should see her doctor if:

- She starts her period before age 8.

- She has not had her first period by age 15.

- She has not had her first period within three years of breast growth.

How Long Does a Woman Usually Have Periods?

On average, women get a period for about 40 years of their life. Most women have regular periods until perimenopause, the time when your body begins the change to menopause. Perimenopause, or transition to menopause, may take a few years. During this time, your period may not come regularly. Menopause happens when you have not had a period for 12 months in a row. For most women, this happens between the ages of 45 and 55. The average age of menopause in the U.S. is 52.

Periods also stop during pregnancy and may not come back right away if you breastfeed.

But if you don't have a period for 90 days (three months), and you are not pregnant or breastfeeding, talk to your doctor or nurse. Your doctor will check for pregnancy or a health problem that can cause periods to stop or become irregular.

What Is a Normal Amount of Bleeding during My Period?

The average woman loses about two to three tablespoons of blood during her period.8 Your periods may be lighter or heavier than the average amount. What is normal for you may not be the same for someone else. Also, the flow may be lighter or heavier from month to month.

Your periods may also change as you get older. Some women have heavy bleeding during perimenopause, the transition to menopause. Symptoms of heavy menstrual bleeding may include:

- Bleeding through one or more pads or tampons every one to two hours

- Passing blood clots larger than the size of quarters

- Bleeding that often lasts longer than eight days

How Often Should I Change My Pad, Tampon, Menstrual Cup, Sponge, or Period Panties?

Follow the instructions that came with your period product. Try to change or rinse your feminine hygiene product before it becomes soaked through or full.

- Most women change their **pads** every few hours.

- A **tampon** should not be worn for more than 8 hours because of the risk of toxic shock syndrome (TSS)

- **Menstrual cups and sponges** may only need to be rinsed once or twice a day.

- **Period panties** (underwear with washable menstrual pads sewn in) can usually last about a day, depending on the style and your flow.

Use a product appropriate in size and absorbency for your menstrual bleeding. The amount of menstrual blood usually changes during a period. Some women use different products on different days of their period, depending on how heavy or light the bleeding is.

You could be at risk for TSS if you use more absorbent tampons than you need for your bleeding or if you do not change your tampon often enough (at least every four to eight hours). Menstrual cups, cervical caps, sponges, or diaphragms (anything inserted into your vagina) may also increase your risk for TSS if they are left in place for too long (usually 24 hours). Remove sponges within 30 hours and cervical caps within 48 hours.

If you have any symptoms of TSS, take out the tampon, menstrual cup, sponge, or diaphragm, and call 911 or go to the hospital right away.

Symptoms of TSS include:

- Sudden high fever
- Muscle aches
- Vomiting
- Nausea
- Diarrhea
- Rash
- Kidney or other organ failure

How Does the Menstrual Cycle Affect Other Health Problems?

The changing hormone levels throughout the menstrual cycle can also affect other health problems:

- **Depression and anxiety disorders.** These conditions often overlap with premenstrual syndrome (PMS). Depression and anxiety symptoms are similar to PMS and may get worse before or during your period.

- **Asthma.** Your asthma symptoms may be worse during some parts of your cycle.

- **Irritable bowel syndrome (IBS).** IBS causes cramping, bloating, and gas. Your IBS symptoms may get worse right before your period.

- **Bladder pain syndrome.** Women with bladder pain syndrome are more likely to have painful cramps during PMS.

Chapter 22

Female Reproductive Health Concerns

Chapter Contents

Section 22.1—Why See a Gynecologist? 228

Section 22.2—Premenstrual Syndrome (PMS) 231

Section 22.3—Menstrual Irregularities 237

Section 22.4—Vaginal Yeast Infections 240

Section 22.5—Vaginal Discharge Concerns 245

Section 22.1

Why See a Gynecologist?

This section includes text excerpted from "Why See a
Gynecologist?" girlshealth.gov, Office on Women's
Health (OWH), April 15, 2014. Reviewed November 2017.

Going to see a gynecologist—a doctor who focuses on women's reproductive health—means you're taking responsibility for your body in
new ways. It can be very exciting to know you're making sure all is
going well with puberty, your reproductive system, and more.

Keep in mind that other doctors also can help with gynecological
issues. For example, an adolescent medicine specialist, family doctor,
or pediatrician can answer questions and may be able to examine your
vagina, too.

Of course, it can be stressful to deal with a whole new type of doctor's visit, but learning more can help you know what to expect.

Why See a Gynecologist?

Seeing a gynecologist can:

- Help you understand your body and how to care for it

- Give you and the doctor a sense of what is normal for you so
  you can notice any problem changes, like signs of a vaginal
  infection

- Let the doctor find problems early so they can be treated

- Explain what a normal vaginal discharge should look like and
  what could be a sign of a problem

- Teach you how to protect yourself if you have sex

Your gynecologist can answer any questions you have about the
many changes that may be happening to your body. It's great to build
a relationship with your gynecologist over the years so he or she understands your health and what matters to you.

When Do I Need to Go?

The American College of Obstetricians and Gynecologists (ACOG) recommends that teenage girls start seeing a gynecologist between the ages of 13 and 15.

If you don't go at that time, you should make sure to visit a gynecologist, adolescent health specialist, or other health professional who can take care of women's reproductive health if:

- You have ever had sex (vaginal, oral, or anal) or intimate sexual contact

- It has been three months or more since your last period and you haven't gotten it again

- You have stomach pain, fever, and fluid coming from your vagina that is yellow, gray, or green with a strong smell—all of which are possible signs of a serious condition called pelvic inflammatory disease (PID) that needs immediate treatment

- You are having problems with your period, like a lot of pain, bleeding heavily, or bleeding for longer than usual, or it has stopped coming regularly

- You have not gotten your period by the age of 15 or within three years of when your breasts started to grow

- You've had your period for two years and it's still not regular or comes more than once a month

- You are having sex and missed your period

What Will Happen at the Visit?

It's understandable if you're nervous about your first visit. Keep in mind that part of the time will be spent just talking. Your doctor may ask questions about you and your family to learn if you have a history of illnesses. And you can ask the doctor any questions you might have. Don't worry—your doctor probably has already heard every question imaginable! You can talk about any concerns you have, including:

- Cramps and questions about periods

- Acne

- Weight issues

- Feeling depressed

- Sexually transmitted diseases or STDs (also known as sexually transmitted infections or STIs)

- Drinking, using drugs, or smoking

Stay Safe

If you are sexually active, tell your doctor. You likely will need to be tested for STDs like human immunodeficiency virus (HIV) and chlamydia. STDs are common among young people. Plus, you can have an STD without having any symptoms. Don't let any possible embarrassment put your health—or your life—at risk.

During your visit, your doctor will probably go through some of the usual items on a doctor's checkup checklist, like weighing you and measuring your blood pressure. He or she also may check the outside of your genitals and do a breast exam. It's common for young women to have some lumpiness in their breasts, but your doctor may want to make sure you don't have problem lumps or pain.

You may have heard of Pap tests and pelvic exams and wonder if you need them. Most likely you won't need either of these until you're 21. If you are sexually active or have symptoms like an unusual vaginal fluid or a history of problems, there's a chance your doctor may choose to do one or both of these. It's helpful, then, to know what to expect.

A pelvic exam usually involves the doctor examining the outside of your genital area (the vulva). It may also involve the doctor using a tool called a speculum to look inside your vagina and check to make sure your cervix is healthy. Frequently, he or she also will feel inside to make sure organs like your ovaries and uterus feel okay. You probably will feel pressure, but it shouldn't hurt. Try to relax—breathing deeply can help.

A Pap test is done by gently taking some cells from your cervix. These cells are checked for changes that could be cancer or that could turn into cancer.

If you haven't already had the human papillomavirus (HPV) vaccine, ask your doctor about it. It helps guard against the human papillomavirus, which can cause genital warts and is the major cause of cervical cancer.

You have options to make your visit more comfortable:

- During the exam, if the doctor is a man, a female nurse or assistant should also be in the room. You can also ask if you can see a female doctor.

- You can ask to have your mom, sister, or a friend stay in the room with you during the visit if that would help.

- You can ask questions about what's going to happen so you know what to expect.

- You can ask the doctor about keeping things you discuss private. Taking care of your health is a huge sign that you are growing up. Be proud of yourself for learning information that can protect your health.

Section 22.2

Premenstrual Syndrome (PMS)

This section includes text excerpted from "Premenstrual Syndrome (PMS)," Office on Women's Health (OWH), U.S. Department of Health and Human Services (HHS), June 12, 2017.

Premenstrual syndrome (PMS) is a combination of physical and emotional symptoms that many women get after ovulation and before the start of their menstrual period. Researchers think that PMS happens in the days after ovulation because estrogen and progesterone levels begin falling dramatically if you are not pregnant. PMS symptoms go away within a few days after a woman's period starts as hormone levels begin rising again.

Some women get their periods without any signs of PMS or only very mild symptoms. For others, PMS symptoms may be so severe that it makes it hard to do everyday activities like go to work or school. Severe PMS symptoms may be a sign of premenstrual dysphoric disorder (PMDD). PMS goes away when you no longer get a period, such as after menopause. After pregnancy, PMS might come back, but you might have different PMS symptoms.

Who Gets PMS?

As many as three in four women say they get PMS symptoms at some point in their lifetime. For most women, PMS symptoms are mild.

Less than 5 percent of women of childbearing age get a more severe form of PMS, called premenstrual dysphoric disorder (PMDD).

PMS may happen more often in women who:

- Have high levels of stress

- Have a family history of depression

- Have a personal history of either postpartum depression or depression

Does PMS Change with Age?

Yes. PMS symptoms may get worse as you reach your late 30s or 40s and approach menopause and are in the transition to menopause, called perimenopause.

This is especially true for women whose moods are sensitive to changing hormone levels during the menstrual cycle. In the years leading up to menopause, your hormone levels also go up and down in an unpredictable way as your body slowly transitions to menopause. You may get the same mood changes, or they may get worse.

PMS stops after menopause when you no longer get a period.

What Are the Symptoms of PMS?

PMS symptoms are different for every woman. You may get physical symptoms, such as bloating or gassiness, or emotional symptoms, such as sadness, or both. Your symptoms may also change throughout your life.

Physical symptoms of PMS can include:

- Swollen or tender breasts

- Constipation or diarrhea

- Bloating or a gassy feeling

- Cramping

- Headache or backache

- Clumsiness

- Lower tolerance for noise or light

Emotional or mental symptoms of PMS include:

- Irritability or hostile behavior
- Feeling tired
- Sleep problems (sleeping too much or too little)
- Appetite changes or food cravings
- Trouble with concentration or memory
- Tension or anxiety
- Depression, feelings of sadness, or crying spells
- Mood swings
- Less interest in sex

Talk to your doctor or nurse if your symptoms bother you or affect your daily life.

What Causes PMS?

Researchers do not know exactly what causes PMS. Changes in hormone levels during the menstrual cycle may play a role. These changing hormone levels may affect some women more than others.

How Is PMS Diagnosed?

There is no single test for PMS. Your doctor will talk with you about your symptoms, including when they happen and how much they affect your life.

You probably have PMS if you have symptoms that:

- Happen in the five days before your period for at least three menstrual cycles in a row
- End within four days after your period starts
- Keep you from enjoying or doing some of your normal activities

Keep track of which PMS symptoms you have and how severe they are for a few months. Write down your symptoms each day on a calendar or with an app on your phone. Take this information with you when you see your doctor.

How Does PMS Affect Other Health Problems?

About half of women who need relief from PMS also have another health problem, which may get worse in the time before their menstrual period. These health problems share many symptoms with PMS and include:

- **Depression and anxiety disorders.** These are the most common conditions that overlap with PMS. Depression and anxiety symptoms are similar to PMS and may get worse before or during your period.

- **Myalgic encephalomyelitis/chronic fatigue syndrome (ME/CFS).** Some women report that their symptoms often get worse right before their period. Research shows that women with ME/CFS may also be more likely to have heavy menstrual bleeding and early or premature menopause.

- **Irritable bowel syndrome (IBS).** IBS causes cramping, bloating, and gas. Your IBS symptoms may get worse right before your period.

- **Bladder pain syndrome.** Women with bladder pain syndrome are more likely to have painful cramps during PMS.

PMS may also worsen some health problems, such as asthma, allergies, and migraines.

What Can I Do at Home to Relieve PMS Symptoms?

These tips will help you be healthier in general, and may relieve some of your PMS symptoms.

- **Get regular aerobic physical activity throughout the month.** Exercise can help with symptoms such as depression, difficulty concentrating, and fatigue.

- **Choose healthy foods most of the time.** Avoiding foods and drinks with caffeine, salt, and sugar in the two weeks before your period may lessen many PMS symptoms.

- **Get enough sleep.** Try to get about eight hours of sleep each night. Lack of sleep is linked to depression and anxiety and can make PMS symptoms such as moodiness worse.

- **Find healthy ways to cope with stress.** Talk to your friends or write in a journal. Some women also find yoga, massage, or meditation helpful.

- **Don't smoke.** In one large study, women who smoked reported more PMS symptoms and worse PMS symptoms than women who did not smoke.

What Medicines Can Treat PMS Symptoms?

Over-the-counter (OTC) and prescription medicines can help treat some PMS symptoms. Over-the-counter pain relievers you can buy in most stores may help lessen physical symptoms, such as cramps, headaches, backaches, and breast tenderness. These include:

- Ibuprofen
- Naproxen
- Aspirin

Some women find that taking an over-the-counter pain reliever right before their period starts lessens the amount of pain and bleeding they have during their period.

Prescription medicines may help if over-the-counter pain medicines don't work:

- **Hormonal birth control** may help with the physical symptoms of PMS, but it may make other symptoms worse. You may need to try several different types of birth control before you find one that helps your symptoms.

- **Antidepressants** can help relieve emotional symptoms of PMS for some women when other medicines don't help. Selective serotonin reuptake inhibitors, or SSRIs, are the most common type of antidepressant used to treat PMS.

- **Diuretics** ("water pills") may reduce symptoms of bloating and breast tenderness.

- **Antianxiety medicine** may help reduce feelings of anxiousness.

All medicines have risks. Talk to your doctor or nurse about the benefits and risks.

Should I Take Vitamins or Minerals to Treat PMS Symptoms?

Maybe. Studies show that certain vitamins and minerals may help relieve some PMS symptoms. The U.S. Food and Drug Administration

(FDA) does not regulate vitamins or mineral and herbal supplements in the same way they regulate medicines. Talk to your doctor before taking any supplement.

Studies have found benefits for:

- **Calcium.** Studies show that calcium can help reduce some PMS symptoms, such as fatigue, cravings, and depression. Calcium is found in foods such as milk, cheese, and yogurt. Some foods, such as orange juice, cereal, and bread, have calcium added (fortified). You can also take a calcium supplement.

- **Vitamin B6.** Vitamin B6 may help with PMS symptoms, including moodiness, irritability, forgetfulness, bloating, and anxiety. Vitamin B6 can be found in foods such as fish, poultry, potatoes, fruit (except for citrus fruits), and fortified cereals. You can also take it as a dietary supplement.

Studies have found mixed results for:

- **Magnesium.** Magnesium may help relieve some PMS symptoms, including migraines. If you get menstrual migraines, talk to your doctor about whether you need more magnesium. Magnesium is found in green, leafy vegetables such as spinach, as well as in nuts, whole grains, and fortified cereals. You can also take a supplement.

- **Polyunsaturated fatty acids (omega-3 and omega-6).** Studies show that taking a supplement with 1 to 2 grams of polyunsaturated fatty acids may help reduce cramps and other PMS symptoms. Good sources of polyunsaturated fatty acids include flaxseed, nuts, fish, and green leafy vegetables.

What Complementary or Alternative Medicines May Help Relieve PMS Symptoms?

Some women report relief from their PMS symptoms with yoga or meditation. Others say herbal supplements help relieve symptoms. Talk with your doctor or nurse before taking any of these supplements. They may interact with other medicines you take, making your other medicine not work or cause dangerous side effects. The U.S. Food and Drug Administration (FDA) does not regulate herbal supplements at the same level that it regulates medicines.

Some research studies show relief from PMS symptoms with these herbal supplements, but other studies do not. Many herbal supplements should not be used with other medicines. Some herbal supplements women use to ease PMS symptoms include:

- **Black cohosh.** The underground stems and root of black cohosh are used fresh or dried to make tea, capsules, pills, or liquid extracts. Black cohosh is most often used to help treat menopausal symptoms, and some women use it to help relieve PMS symptoms.

- **Chasteberry.** Dried ripe chasteberry is used to prepare liquid extracts or pills that some women take to relieve PMS symptoms. Women taking hormonal birth control or hormone therapy for menopause symptoms should not take chasteberry.

- **Evening primrose oil.** The oil is taken from the plant's seeds and put into capsules. Some women report that the pill helps relieve PMS symptoms, but the research results are mixed.

Section 22.3

Menstrual Irregularities

This section includes text excerpted from "Irregularities,"
Eunice Kennedy Shriver National Institute of Child Health and
Human Development (NICHD), June 5, 2017.

What Are Menstrual Irregularities?

For most women, a normal menstrual cycle ranges from 21 to 35 days. However, 14 percent to 25 percent of women have irregular menstrual cycles, meaning the cycles are shorter or longer than normal; are heavier or lighter than normal; or are experienced with other problems, like abdominal cramps. Irregular cycles can be ovulatory, meaning that ovulation occurs, or anovulatory, meaning ovulation does not occur.

The most common menstrual irregularities include:

- **Amenorrhea or absent menstrual periods:** When a woman does not get her period by age 16, or when she stops getting her period for at least 3 months and is not pregnant.

- **Oligomenorrhea or infrequent menstrual periods:** Periods that occur more than 35 days apart.

- **Menorrhagia or heavy menstrual periods:** Also called excessive bleeding. Although anovulatory bleeding and menorrhagia are sometimes grouped together, they do not have the same cause and require different diagnostic testing.

- **Prolonged menstrual bleeding:** Bleeding that exceeds 8 days in duration on a regular basis.

- **Dysmenorrhea:** Painful periods that may include severe menstrual cramps.

Additional menstrual irregularities include:

- **Polymenorrhea:** Frequent menstrual periods occurring less than 21 days apart

- **Irregular menstrual periods** with a cycle-to-cycle variation of more than 20 days

- **Shortened menstrual bleeding** of less than 2 days in duration

- **Intermenstrual bleeding:** Episodes of bleeding that occur between periods, also known as spotting

What Causes Menstrual Irregularities?

Menstrual irregularities can have a variety of causes, including pregnancy, hormonal imbalances, infections, diseases, trauma, and certain medications.

Causes of irregular periods (generally light) include:

- Perimenopause (generally in the late 40s and early 50s)

- Primary ovarian insufficiency (POI)

- Eating disorders (anorexia nervosa or bulimia)

- Excessive exercise

- Thyroid dysfunction (too much or too little thyroid hormone)

- Elevated levels of the hormone prolactin, which is made by the pituitary gland to help the body produce milk

- Uncontrolled diabetes

- Cushing's syndrome (elevated levels of the hormone cortisol, used in the body's response to stress)
- Late-onset congenital adrenal hyperplasia (problem with the adrenal gland)
- Hormonal birth control (birth control pills, injections, or implants)
- Hormone-containing intrauterine devices (IUDs)
- Scarring within the uterine cavity (Asherman syndrome)
- Medications, such as those to treat epilepsy or mental health problems

Common causes of heavy or prolonged menstrual bleeding include:

- Adolescence (during which cycles may not be associated with ovulation)
- Polycystic ovary syndrome (PCOS) (bleeding irregular but heavy)
- Uterine fibroids (benign growths of uterine muscle)
- Endometrial polyps (benign overgrowth of the lining of the uterus)
- Adenomyosis (the presence of uterine lining in the wall of the uterus)
- Nonhormonal IUDs
- Bleeding disorders, such as leukemia, platelet disorders, clotting factor deficiencies, or (less common) von Willebrand disease
- Pregnancy complications (miscarriage)

Common causes of dysmenorrhea (menstrual pain) include:

- Endometriosis (uterine lining grows outside the uterus)
- Uterine abnormalities (fibroids or adenomyosis)
- IUDs
- Pelvic scarring due to STIs, such as chlamydia or gonorrhea
- Heavy menstrual flow

Section 22.4

Vaginal Yeast Infections

This section includes text excerpted from "Vaginal Yeast Infections," Office on Women's Health (OWH), U.S. Department of Health and Human Services (HHS), August 3, 2017.

A vaginal yeast infection is an infection of the vagina that causes itching and burning of the vulva, the area around the vagina. Vaginal yeast infections are caused by an overgrowth of the fungus *Candida*.

Who Gets Vaginal Yeast Infections?

Women and girls of all ages can get vaginal yeast infections. Three out of four women will have a yeast infection at some point in their life. Almost half of women have two or more infections.

Vaginal yeast infections are rare before puberty and after menopause.

Are Some Women More at Risk for Yeast Infections?

Yes. Your risk for yeast infections is higher if:

- You are pregnant
- You have diabetes and your blood sugar is not under control
- You use a type of hormonal birth control that has higher doses of estrogen
- You douche or use vaginal sprays
- You recently took antibiotics such as amoxicillin or steroid medicines
- You have a weakened immune system, such as from human immunodeficiency virus (HIV)

What Are the Symptoms of Vaginal Yeast Infections?

The most common symptom of a vaginal yeast infection is extreme itchiness in and around the vagina.

Other signs and symptoms include:

- Burning, redness, and swelling of the vagina and the vulva
- Pain when urinating
- Pain during sex
- Soreness
- A thick, white vaginal discharge that looks like cottage cheese and does not have a bad smell

You may have only a few of these symptoms. They may be mild or severe.

What Causes Yeast Infections?

Yeast infections are caused by overgrowth of the microscopic fungus *Candida*. Your vagina may have small amounts of yeast at any given time without causing any symptoms. But when too much yeast grows, you can get an infection.

Can I Get a Yeast Infection from Having Sex?

Yes. A yeast infection is not considered an sexually transmitted infection (STI), because you can get a yeast infection without having sex. But you can get a yeast infection from your sexual partner. Condoms and dental dams may help prevent getting or passing yeast infections through vaginal, oral, or anal sex.

Should I Call My Doctor or Nurse If I Think I Have a Yeast Infection?

Yes. Seeing your doctor or nurse is the only way to know for sure if you have a yeast infection and not a more serious type of infection.

The signs and symptoms of a yeast infection are a lot like symptoms of other more serious infections, such as STIs and bacterial vaginosis (BV). If left untreated, STIs and BV raise your risk of getting other STIs, including HIV, and can lead to problems getting pregnant. BV can also lead to problems during pregnancy, such as premature delivery.

How Is a Yeast Infection Diagnosed?

Your doctor will do a pelvic exam to look for swelling and discharge. Your doctor may also use a cotton swab to take a sample of the discharge from your vagina. A lab technician will look at the sample under a microscope to see whether there is an overgrowth of the fungus *Candida* that causes a yeast infection.

How Is a Yeast Infection Treated?

Yeast infections are usually treated with antifungal medicine. See your doctor or nurse to make sure that you have a vaginal yeast infection and not another type of infection.

You can then buy antifungal medicine for yeast infections at a store, without a prescription. Antifungal medicines come in the form of creams, tablets, ointments, or suppositories that you insert into your vagina. You can apply treatment in one dose or daily for up to seven days, depending on the brand you choose.

Your doctor or nurse can also give you a single dose of antifungal medicine taken by mouth, such as fluconazole. If you get more than four vaginal yeast infections a year, or if your yeast infection doesn't go away after using over-the-counter (OTC) treatment, you may need to take regular doses of antifungal medicine for up to six months.

Is It Safe to Use Over-the-Counter (OTC) Medicines for Yeast Infections?

Yes, but always talk with your doctor or nurse before treating yourself for a vaginal yeast infection. This is because:

- **You may be trying to treat an infection that is not a yeast infection.** Studies show that two out of three women who buy yeast infection medicine don't really have a yeast infection. Instead, they may have an STI or bacterial vaginosis (BV). STIs and BV require different treatments than yeast infections and, if left untreated, can cause serious health problems.

- **Using treatment when you do not actually have a yeast infection can cause your body to become resistant to the yeast infection medicine.** This can make actual yeast infections harder to treat in the future.

- **Some yeast infection medicine may weaken condoms and diaphragms, increasing your chance of getting pregnant or an STI when you have sex.** Talk to your doctor or nurse about what is best for you, and always read and follow the directions on the medicine carefully.

How Do I Treat a Yeast Infection If I'm Pregnant?

During pregnancy, it's safe to treat a yeast infection with vaginal creams or suppositories that contain miconazole or clotrimazole.

Do **not** take the oral fluconazole tablet to treat a yeast infection during pregnancy. It may cause birth defects.

Can I Get a Yeast Infection from Breastfeeding?

Yes. Yeast infections can happen on your nipples or in your breast (commonly called "thrush") from breastfeeding. Yeast thrive on milk and moisture. A yeast infection you get while breastfeeding is different from a vaginal yeast infection. However, it is caused by an overgrowth of the same fungus.

Symptoms of thrush during breastfeeding include:

- Sore nipples that last more than a few days, especially after several weeks of pain-free breastfeeding

- Flaky, shiny, itchy, or cracked nipples

- Deep pink and blistered nipples

- Achy breast

- Shooting pain in the breast during or after feedings

If you have any of these signs or symptoms or think your baby might have thrush in his or her mouth, call your doctor.

If I Have a Yeast Infection, Does My Sexual Partner Need to Be Treated?

Maybe. Yeast infections are not STIs. But it is possible to pass yeast infections to your partner during vaginal, oral, or anal sex.

- **If your partner is a man,** the risk of infection is low. About 15 percent of men get an itchy rash on the penis if they have unprotected sex with a woman who has a yeast infection. If this happens to your partner, he should see a doctor. Men who haven't been circumcised and men with diabetes are at higher risk.

- **If your partner is a woman,** she may be at risk. She should be tested and treated if she has any symptoms.

How Can I Prevent a Yeast Infection?

You can take steps to lower your risk of getting yeast infections:

- Do not douche. Douching removes some of the normal bacteria in the vagina that protects you from infection.

- Do not use scented feminine products, including bubble bath, sprays, pads, and tampons.

- Change tampons, pads, and panty liners often.

- Do not wear tight underwear, pantyhose, pants, or jeans. These can increase body heat and moisture in your genital area.

- Wear underwear with a cotton crotch. Cotton underwear helps keep you dry and doesn't hold in warmth and moisture.

- Change out of wet swimsuits and workout clothes as soon as you can.

- After using the bathroom, always wipe from front to back.

- Avoid hot tubs and very hot baths.

- If you have diabetes, be sure your blood sugar is under control.

Does Yogurt Prevent or Treat Yeast Infections?

Maybe. Studies suggest that eating eight ounces of yogurt with "live cultures" daily or taking *Lactobacillus acidophilus* capsules can help prevent infection.

But, more research still needs to be done to say for sure if yogurt with Lactobacillus or other probiotics can prevent or treat vaginal yeast infections. If you think you have a yeast infection, see your doctor or nurse to make sure before taking any over-the-counter medicine.

What Should I Do If I Get Repeat Yeast Infections?

If you get four or more yeast infections in a year, talk to your doctor or nurse.

About 5 percent of women get four or more vaginal yeast infections in one year. This is called recurrent vulvovaginal candidiasis (RVVC). RVVC is more common in women with diabetes or weak immune systems, such as with HIV, but it can also happen in otherwise healthy women.

Doctors most often treat RVVC with antifungal medicine for up to six months.

Section 22.5

Vaginal Discharge Concerns

This section includes text excerpted from "Douching," Office on Women's Health (OWH), U.S. Department of Health and Human Services (HHS), August 3, 2017.

What Is Douching?

The word "douche" means to wash or soak. Douching is washing or cleaning out the inside of the vagina with water or other mixtures of fluids. Most douches are sold in stores as prepackaged mixes of water and vinegar, baking soda, or iodine. The mixtures usually come in a bottle or bag. You squirt the douche upward through a tube or nozzle into your vagina. The water mixture then comes back out through your vagina.

Douching is different from washing the outside of your vagina during a bath or shower. Rinsing the outside of your vagina with warm water will not harm your vagina. But, douching can lead to many different health problems.

Most doctors recommend that women do not douche.

How Common Is Douching?

In the United States, almost one in five women 15 to 44 years old douche.

More African-American and Hispanic women douche than white women. Douching is also common in teens of all races and ethnicities.

Studies have not found any health benefit to douching. But, studies have found that douching is linked to many health problems.

Why Should Women Not Douche?

Most doctors recommend that women do not douche. Douching can change the necessary balance of vaginal flora (bacteria that live in the vagina) and natural acidity in a healthy vagina.

A healthy vagina has good and harmful bacteria. The balance of bacteria helps maintain an acidic environment. The acidic environment protects the vagina from infections or irritation.

245

Douching can cause an overgrowth of harmful bacteria. This can lead to a yeast infection or bacterial vaginosis. If you already have a vaginal infection, douching can push the bacteria causing the infection up into the uterus, fallopian tubes, and ovaries. This can lead to pelvic inflammatory disease, a serious health problem.

Douching is also linked to other health problems.

What Health Problems Are Linked to Douching?

Health problems linked to douching include:

- **Bacterial vaginosis (BV)**, which is an infection in the vagina. Women who douche often (once a week) are five times more likely to develop BV than women who do not douche.

- **Pelvic inflammatory disease**, an infection in the reproductive organs that is often caused by an STI

- **Problems during pregnancy**, including preterm birth and ectopic pregnancy

- **STIs**, including human immunodeficiency virus (HIV)

- **Vaginal irritation** or dryness

Researchers are studying whether douching causes these problems or whether women at higher risk for these health problems are more likely to douche.

Should I Douche to Get Rid of Vaginal Odor or Other Problems?

No. You should not douche to try to get rid of vaginal odor or other vaginal problems like discharge, pain, itching, or burning.

Douching will only cover up odor for a short time and will make other problems worse. Call your doctor or nurse if you have:

- Vaginal discharge that smells bad

- Vaginal itching and thick, white, or yellowish-green discharge with or without an odor

- Burning, redness, and swelling in or around the vagina

- Pain when urinating

- Pain or discomfort during sex

These may be signs of a vaginal infection, or an STI. Do not douche before seeing your doctor or nurse. This can make it hard for the doctor or nurse to find out what may be wrong.

Should I Douche to Clean inside My Vagina?

No. Doctors recommend that women do not douche. You do not need to douche to clean your vagina. Your body naturally flushes out and cleans your vagina. Any strong odor or irritation usually means something is wrong.

Douching also can raise your chances of a vaginal infection or an STI. If you have questions or concerns, talk to your doctor.

What Is the Best Way to Clean My Vagina?

It is best to let your vagina clean itself. The vagina cleans itself naturally by making mucous. The mucous washes away blood, semen, and vaginal discharge.

If you are worried about vaginal odor, talk to your doctor or nurse. But you should know that even healthy, clean vaginas have a mild odor that changes throughout the day. Physical activity also can give your vagina a stronger, muskier scent, but this is still normal.

Keep your vagina clean and healthy by:

- Washing the outside of your vagina with warm water when you bathe. Some women also use mild soaps. But, if you have sensitive skin or any current vaginal infections, even mild soaps can cause dryness and irritation.

- Avoiding scented tampons, pads, powders, and sprays. These products may increase your chances of getting a vaginal infection.

Can Douching before or after Sex Prevent STIs?

No. Douching before or after sex does not prevent STIs. In fact, douching removes some of the normal bacteria in the vagina that protect you from infection. This can actually increase your risk of getting STIs, including HIV, the virus that causes Acquired Immune Deficiency Syndrome (AIDS).

Should I Douche If I Had Sex without Using Protection or If the Condom Broke?

No. Douching removes some of the normal bacteria in the vagina that protect you from infection. This can increase your risk of getting STIs, including HIV. Douching also does not protect against pregnancy.

If you had sex without using protection or if the condom broke during sex, see a doctor right away. You can get medicine to help prevent HIV and unwanted pregnancy.

Should I Douche If I Was Sexually Assaulted?

No, you should not douche, bathe, or shower. As hard as it may be to not wash up, you may wash away important evidence if you do. Douching may also increase your risk of getting STIs, including HIV. Go to the nearest hospital emergency room as soon as possible. The National Sexual Assault Hotline at 800-656-HOPE (800-656-4673) can help you find a hospital able to collect evidence of sexual assault. Your doctor or nurse can help you get medicine to help prevent HIV and unwanted pregnancy.

Can Douching after Sex Prevent Pregnancy?

No. Douching **does not** prevent pregnancy. It should never be used for birth control. If you had sex without using birth control or if your birth control method did not work correctly (failed), you can use emergency contraception to keep from getting pregnant.

If you need birth control, talk to your doctor or nurse about which type of birth control method is best for you.

How Does Douching Affect Pregnancy?

Douching can make it harder to get pregnant and can cause problems during pregnancy:

- **Trouble getting pregnant.** Women who douched at least once a month had a harder time getting pregnant than those women who did not douche.

- **Higher risk of ectopic pregnancy.** Douching may increase a woman's chance of damaged fallopian tubes and ectopic pregnancy. Ectopic pregnancy is when the fertilized egg attaches to the inside of the fallopian tube instead of the uterus. If left untreated, ectopic pregnancy can be life-threatening. It can also make it hard for a woman to get pregnant in the future.

- **Higher risk of early childbirth.** Douching raises your risk for premature birth. One study found that women who douched during pregnancy were more likely to deliver their babies early. This raises the risk for health problems for you and your baby.

Chapter 23

Precocious and Delayed Puberty

Chapter Contents

Section 23.1—Precocious Puberty 252

Section 23.2—Delayed Puberty 257

Section 23.1

Precocious Puberty

This section includes text excerpted from "Puberty and Precocious Puberty: Overview," *Eunice Kennedy Shriver* National Institute of Child Health and Human Development (NICHD), December 1, 2012. Reviewed November 2017.

The onset of puberty, the time in life when a person becomes sexually mature, typically occurs between ages 8 and 13 for girls and ages 9 and 14 for boys. Precocious puberty is puberty that begins abnormally early, and delayed puberty is puberty that begins abnormally late. The *Eunice Kennedy Shriver* National Institute of Child Health and Human Development (NICHD) and other National Institutes of Health (NIH) Institutes and federal agencies support and conduct research on the causes of precocious puberty and delayed puberty. They also investigate the biology and chemistry of normal puberty to shed light on the mechanisms responsible for precocious and delayed puberty.

What Are Precocious Puberty?

Precocious Puberty

Precocious puberty is a condition that occurs when sexual maturity begins earlier than normal. Precocious (meaning prematurely developed) puberty begins before age 8 for girls and before age 9 for boys.

Children affected by precocious puberty may experience problems such as:

- Failure to reach their full height because their growth halts too soon.

- Psychological and social problems, such as anxiety over being "different" from their peers. However, many children do not experience major psychological or social problems, particularly when the onset of puberty is only slightly early.

What Are the Symptoms of Precocious Puberty?

Precocious Puberty

The symptoms of precocious puberty are similar to the signs of normal puberty but they manifest earlier—before the age of 8 in girls and before age 9 in boys.

How Many Children Are Affected by/at Risk of Precocious Puberty?

Precocious puberty affects about 1 percent of the U.S. population (roughly 3 million children). Many more girls are affected than boys. One study suggests that African American girls have some early breast development or some early pubic hair more often than white girls or Hispanic girls.

Who Is at Risk?

There is a greater chance of being affected by precocious puberty if a child is:

- Female

- African American

- Obese

What Causes Precocious Puberty?

Precocious Puberty

In approximately 90 percent of girls who experience precocious puberty, no underlying cause can be identified—although heredity and being overweight may contribute in some cases. When a cause cannot be identified, the condition is called idiopathic precocious puberty. In boys with precocious puberty, approximately 50 percent of cases are idiopathic. In the remaining 10 percent of girls and 50 percent of boys with precocious puberty, an underlying cause can be identified.

Sometimes the cause is an abnormality involving the brain. In other children, the signs of puberty occur because of a problem such as a tumor or genetic abnormality in the ovaries, testes, or adrenal glands, causing overproduction of sex hormones.

253

Precocious puberty can be divided into two categories, depending on where in the body the abnormality occurs—central precocious puberty and peripheral precocious puberty.

Central Precocious Puberty

This type of early puberty, also known as gonadotropin-dependent precocious puberty, occurs when the abnormality is located in the brain. The brain signals the pituitary gland to begin puberty at an early age. Central precocious puberty is the most common form of precocious puberty and affects many more girls than boys. The causes of central precocious puberty include:

• Brain tumors

• Prior radiation to the brain

• Prior infection of the brain

• Other brain abnormalities

Often, however, there is no identifiable abnormality in the brain; this is called idiopathic central precocious puberty.

Peripheral Precocious Puberty

This form of early puberty is also called gonadotropin-independent precocious puberty. In peripheral precocious puberty, the abnormality is not in the brain but in the testicles, ovaries, or adrenal glands, causing overproduction of sex hormones, like testosterone and estrogens. Peripheral precocious puberty may be caused by:

• Tumors of the ovary, testis, or adrenal gland

• In boys, tumors that secrete a hormone called hCG, or human chorionic gonadotropin

• Certain rare genetic syndromes, such as McCune-Albright syndrome or familial male precocious puberty

• Severe hypothyroidism, in which the thyroid gland secretes abnormally low levels of hormones

• Disorders of the adrenal gland, such as congenital adrenal hyperplasia

• Exposure of the child to medicines or creams that contain estrogens or androgens

How Do Healthcare Providers Diagnose Precocious Puberty?

To identify whether a child is entering puberty, a pediatrician (a physician specializing in the treatment of children) will carefully examine the following:

- In girls, the growth of pubic hair and breasts
- In boys, the increase in size of the testicles and penis and the growth of pubic hair

The pediatrician will compare what he or she finds against the Tanner scale, a 5-point scale that gauges the extent of puberty development in children.

Precocious Puberty

After giving a child a complete physical examination and analyzing his or her medical history, a healthcare provider may perform tests to diagnose precocious puberty, including:

- A blood test to check the level of hormones, such as the gonadotropins (luteinizing hormone [LH] and follicle-stimulating hormone [FSH]), estradiol, testosterone, dehydroepiandrosterone sulfate (DHEAS), and thyroid hormones
- A gonadotropin-releasing hormone agonist (GnRHa) stimulation test, which can tell whether a child's precocious puberty is gonadotropin-dependent or gonadotropin-independent
- Measuring blood 17-hydroxyprogesterone to test for congenital adrenal hyperplasia
- A "bone age" X-ray to determine if bones are growing at a normal rate

The healthcare provider may also use imaging techniques to rule out a tumor or other organ abnormality as a cause. These imaging methods may include:

- Ultrasound (sonography) to examine the gonads. An ultrasound painlessly creates an image on a computer screen of blood vessels and tissues, allowing a healthcare provider to monitor organs and blood flow in real time
- An MRI (magnetic resonance imaging) scan of the brain and pituitary gland using an instrument that produces detailed images of organs and bodily structures.

What Are Common Treatments for Problems of Puberty?

Precocious Puberty

There are a number of reasons to treat precocious puberty.

Treatment for precocious puberty can help stop puberty until the child is closer to the normal time for sexual development. One reason to consider treating precocious puberty is that rapid growth and bone maturation, caused by precocious puberty, can prevent a child from reaching his or her full height potential. Children grow rapidly in height during puberty and reach their final adult height after puberty. Children who go through puberty too early may not reach their full adult height potential because their growth stops too soon.

Another reason to consider treating precocious puberty is that a young child may not be psychologically ready for the physical and hormonal changes that occur in puberty.

However, not all children with precocious puberty require treatment, particularly if the onset of puberty is only slightly early. The goal of treatment is to prevent the production of sex hormones to prevent the early halt of growth, short stature in adulthood, emotional effects, social problems, and problems with libido (especially in boys).

If precocious puberty is caused by a specific medical problem, treating the underlying problem can often stop the progression of precocious puberty. In addition, precocious puberty can often be stopped by medical treatment to block the hormones that cause puberty. For example, medications called gonadotropin-releasing hormone agonists (GnRHa) are used to treat central precocious puberty. These medications, some of which are injected, suppress production of luteinizing hormone (LH) and follicle-stimulating hormone (FSH).

Section 23.2

Delayed Puberty

This section includes text excerpted from "Puberty and Precocious Puberty: Condition Information," *Eunice Kennedy Shriver* National Institute of Child Health and Human Development (NICHD), December 1, 2012. Reviewed November 2017.

What Is Delayed Puberty?

Delayed puberty is the term for a condition in which the body's timing for sexual maturity is later than the normal range of ages.

Many children with delayed puberty will eventually go through an otherwise normal puberty, just at a late age. Other children have a long-lasting condition known as hypogonadism in which the sex glands (the testes in men and the ovaries in women) produce few or no hormones. For example, hypogonadism can occur in girls with Turner syndrome or in individuals with hypogonadotropic hypogonadism, which occurs when the hypothalamus produces little to no gonadotropin-releasing hormone (GnRH).

What Are the Symptoms of Delayed Puberty?

Delayed puberty is characterized by the lack of onset of puberty within the normal range of ages.

What Causes Delayed Puberty?

Many children with delayed puberty will eventually go through an otherwise normal puberty, just at a late age. Sometimes, this delay occurs because the child is just maturing more slowly than average, a condition called constitutional delay of puberty. This condition often runs in families.

Puberty can be delayed in children who have not gotten proper nutrition due to long-term illnesses. Also, some young girls who undergo intense physical training for a sport, such as running or gymnastics, start puberty later than normal.

In other cases, the delay in puberty is not just due to slow maturation but occurs because the child has a long-term medical condition
known as hypogonadism, in which the sex glands (the testes in men
and the ovaries in women) produce few or no hormones. Hypogonadism can be divided into two categories: secondary hypogonadism and
primary hypogonadism.

- Secondary hypogonadism (also known as central hypogonadism
  or hypogonadotropic hypogonadism), is caused by a problem
  with the pituitary gland or hypothalamus (part of the brain). In
  secondary hypogonadism, the hypothalamus and the pituitary
  gland fail to signal the gonads to properly release sex hormones.
  Causes of secondary hypogonadism include:

  - Kallmann syndrome, a genetic problem that also diminishes
    the sense of smell

  - Isolated hypogonadotropic hypogonadism, a genetic condition
    that only affects sexual development but not the sense of smell

  - Prior radiation, trauma, surgery, or other injury to the brain
    or pituitary

  - Tumors of the brain or pituitary

- In primary hypogonadism, the problem lies in the ovaries or
  testes, which fail to make sex hormones normally. Some causes
  include:

  - Genetic disorders, especially Turner syndrome (in women)
    and Klinefelter syndrome (in men)

  - Certain autoimmune disorders

  - Developmental disorders

  - Radiation or chemotherapy

  - Infection

  - Surgery

How Do Healthcare Providers Diagnose Delayed Puberty?

To identify whether a child is entering puberty, a pediatrician (a
physician specializing in the treatment of children) will carefully examine the following:

- In girls, the growth of pubic hair and breasts

- In boys, the increase in size of the testicles and penis and the growth of pubic hair

The pediatrician will compare what he or she finds against the Tanner scale, a 5-point scale that gauges the extent of puberty development in children.

To diagnose hypogonadotropic hypogonadism, a healthcare provider may prescribe these tests:

- Blood tests to measure hormone levels

- Blood tests to measure if the pituitary gland can correctly respond to GnRH

- An MRI of the brain and pituitary gland

What Are Common Treatments for Problems of Puberty?

With delayed puberty or hypogonadism, treatment varies with the origin of the problem but may involve:

- In males, testosterone injections, skin patches, or gel

- In females, estrogen and/or progesterone given as pills or skin patches

Chapter 24

Teaching Teens about Sexual Activity

Chapter Contents

Section 24.1—Making Healthy Sexual Decisions 262

Section 24.2—Facts on Sex Education in the
  United States.. 266

Section 24.1

Making Healthy Sexual Decisions

This section includes text excerpted from documents
published by two public domain sources. Text under headings
marked 1 are excerpted from "Why Waiting to Have Sex Makes
Sense," girlshealth.gov, Office on Women's Health (OWH),
November 25, 2015; Text under headings marked 2 are excerpted
from "Deciding about Sex," girlshealth.gov, Office on Women's
Health (OWH), November 25, 2015; Text under heading marked 3 is
excerpted from "Sexually Transmitted Diseases (STDs)—How You
Can Prevent Sexually Transmitted Diseases," Centers for Disease
Control and Prevention (CDC), January 21, 2016.

Why Waiting to Have Sex Makes Sense[1]

You may hear so many messages suggesting that it's a good idea to
have sex, from songs on the radio to talk at school. You may also feel
curious about sex or have a strong attraction to someone.

Deciding to have sex is a big deal, though, so think it through. You
could wind up with an unplanned pregnancy. You could also catch
an STD, or sexually transmitted disease (also known as an STI, or
sexually transmitted infection).

Having sex before you're ready can seriously hurt your relationship—and your feelings. Few people regret waiting to have sex, but
many wish they hadn't started early.

Keep in mind that even if you've already had sex, you can still
choose to stop.

Ways to Decide If You're Ready for Sex[2]

If you are deciding about sex, you've got a lot to think about. And it
makes sense to do your thinking in advance—not when you're swept
up in the excitement of the moment.

Think about your values, deepest feelings, and future goals.
Remember that having sex with someone is no guarantee that you'll
stay together. Not even having a baby together guarantees that. And

as much as you care what the other person thinks, it's what you think that really matters!

For teens, not having sex—abstinence—makes good sense. That's partly because your chances of staying safe from unplanned pregnancy and human immunodeficiency virus (HIV) and other STDs are better if you wait. It's also partly because being older can help you handle the strong emotional aspects of sex. Just because your body seems ready doesn't mean that you are!

Questions to Ask Yourself about Sex[2]

Here are some questions you can ask yourself to help decide about sex:

- Do you really feel ready to have sex and not just excited about the idea?

- Do you really trust and feel safe with your partner?

- Are you feeling pressure—from friends, your partner, or even yourself—or is this something that's really right for you?

- Are you doing this because you think everyone else is? (More than half of high schoolers haven't had sex yet.)

- Do you feel really nervous—not just a little worried but really concerned or scared?

- Can you talk to your partner about preventing pregnancy and STDs?

- Do you know what to do help prevent pregnancy and STDs?

- Do you know what you would do if you got pregnant?

- How would you feel if other people found out you had sex?

Unplanned Pregnancy[1]

Three 3 of 10 teen girls in the United States get pregnant before they turn 20. And most teen pregnancies are not planned.

Getting pregnant before you're ready can be a huge shock. The emotional stress and money worries of raising a baby can be a lot even for an older couple. Imagine what your life would be like if you had to get up with a baby in the night and take care of it every day!

Abstinence is the safest way to prevent the challenges that come with teen pregnancy. Check out some of these facts about teen pregnancy:

- Teen mothers are less likely to finish high school.

- Teen moms are more likely to be—and stay—single parents.

- Babies born to teen moms face greater health risks.

- Teen moms face health risks, too, including possibly being obese later in life.

- Teen moms are at a higher risk of being poor.

- Kids of teen moms are more likely to have problems in school and with the police.

If you do get pregnant, remember that you need to take care of yourself. Be sure to see a doctor. Get help from a trusted adult, like your parents, grandparents, or school counselor.

Sexually Transmitted Diseases (STDs)[1]

Sexually transmitted diseases, or STDs (also known as sexually transmitted infections or STIs) are a huge problem among young people.

Consider some reasons that abstinence makes sense in staying safe from STDs:

- One in 4 teen girls has an STD.

- Condoms decrease the risk of STDs, but they are not 100 percent effective. This is especially true for STDs that can spread just by skin-to-skin contact, such as herpes, which has no cure.

- Having an STD increases your chances of getting HIV, too, and there is no cure for HIV.

- Some STDs have no symptoms, so you can't know if your partner is infected. A partner with no symptoms can still give the STD to you, though.

- Some STDs have no symptoms, so you can't know if you have them, but they can cause serious health problems. These problems include trouble getting pregnant when you are ready to have a baby.

What If I Don't Have "Real" Sex?[1]

Different people may have different definitions of abstinence. Some think it means not having sexual intercourse, but others think it means avoiding other sexual acts, too. Experts say complete abstinence—not having vaginal, oral, and anal sex—is safest. Consider these facts:

- Even if you don't have intercourse but semen (cum) gets in your vagina, there's a chance you could get an STD or get pregnant.
- You can get some STDs from oral sex.
- It's easier to get some STDs from anal sex than from vaginal sex.

Avoiding intimate sexual contact, including skin-to-skin genital contact, is the only sure way to prevent all STDs and pregnancy. If you are having sexual contact, though, it's super-smart to use a condom.

Also keep in mind that acts like oral sex are intimate acts. Try to think about whether you want to do something intimate before you do it. Think about having respect for yourself and having the respect of your partner.

Prevention[3]

Abstinence

The most reliable way to avoid infection is to not have sex (i.e., anal, vaginal, or oral).

Vaccination

Vaccines are safe, effective, and recommended ways to prevent hepatitis B and human papilloma virus (HPV). HPV vaccines for males and females can protect against some of the most common types of HPV. It is best to get all three doses (shots) before becoming sexually active. However, HPV vaccines are recommended for all teen girls and women through age 26 and all teen boys and men through age 21, who did not get all three doses of the vaccine when they were younger. You should also get vaccinated for hepatitis B if you were not vaccinated when you were younger.

Reduce Number of Sex Partners

Reducing your number of sex partners can decrease your risk for STDs. It is still important that you and your partner get tested, and that you share your test results with one another.

Mutual Monogamy

Mutual monogamy means that you agree to be sexually active with only one person, who has agreed to be sexually active only with you. Being in a long-term mutually monogamous relationship with an uninfected partner is one of the most reliable ways to avoid STDs. But you must both be certain you are not infected with STDs. It is important to have an open and honest conversation with your partner.

Use Condoms

Correct and consistent use of the male latex condom is highly effective in reducing STD transmission. Use a condom every time you have anal, vaginal, or oral sex.

If you have latex allergies, synthetic nonlatex condoms can be used. But it is important to note that these condoms have higher breakage rates than latex condoms. Natural membrane condoms are not recommended for STD prevention.

Section 24.2

Facts on Sex Education in the United States

This section includes text excerpted from "Educating Teenagers about Sex in the United States," Centers for Disease Control and Prevention (CDC), November 6, 2015.

Key Findings

- Most teenagers received formal sex education before they were 18 (96% of female and 97% of male teenagers).

- Female teenagers were more likely than male teenagers to report first receiving instruction on birth control methods in high school (47% compared with 38%).

- Younger female teenagers were more likely than younger male teenagers to have talked to their parents about sex and birth control.

- Nearly two out of three female teenagers talked to their parents about "how to say no to sex" compared with about two out of five male teenagers.

Sex education in schools and other places, as well as received from parents, provides adolescents with information to make informed choices about sex at a crucial period of their development. Using data from the 2006–2008 National Survey of Family Growth (NSFG), this report examines the percentage of male and female teenagers 15–19 years who received sex education. Teenagers were asked if they received formal instruction on four topics of sex education at school, church, a community center, or some other place before they were 18 years old and the grade they were in when this first occurred. In addition, they were asked if they talked to their parents before they were 18 about topics concerning sex, birth control, sexually transmitted diseases (STDs), and the human immunodeficiency virus (HIV)/ acquired immunodeficiency syndrome (AIDS) prevention.

What Percentage of Teenagers Received Formal Sex Education?

- Most teenagers received formal sex education before they were 18 (96% of female and 97% of male teenagers)

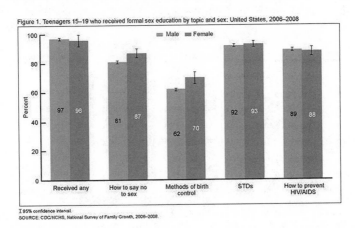

Figure 1. Teenagers 15–19 who received formal sex education by topic and sex: United States, 2006–2008

I 95% confidence interval.
SOURCE: CDC/NCHS, National Survey of Family Growth, 2006–2008.

Figure 24.1. *Teenagers 15–19 Who Received Formal Sex Education by Topic and Sex*

- Ninety-two percent of male and 93 percent of female teenagers reported being taught about STDs and 89 percent of male and

88 percent of female teenagers reported receiving instruction on how to prevent HIV/AIDS.

- A larger percentage of teenagers reported receiving formal sex education on "how to say no to sex" (81% of male and 87% female teenagers) than reported receiving formal sex education on methods of birth control.

- Male teenagers were less likely than female teenagers to have received instructions on methods of birth control (62% of male and 70% female teenagers).

What Grade Are Teenagers in When They First Receive Formal Sex Education?

- Among teenagers who reported receiving formal sex education from a school, church, community center, or some other place, the majority first received instruction on "how to say no to sex," STDs, or how to prevent HIV/AIDS while in middle school (grades 6–8).

- Teenagers who reported first receiving sex education prior to middle school were more likely to report instruction on "how to say no to sex" than other topics. About one in five teenagers reported first receiving instruction on "how to say no to sex" while in first through fifth grade.

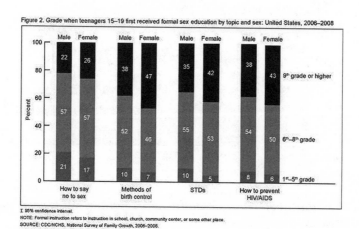

Figure 2. Grade when teenagers 15–19 first received formal sex education by topic and sex: United States, 2006–2008

I 95% confidence interval.
NOTE: Formal instruction refers to instruction in school, church, community center, or some other place.
SOURCE: CDC/NCHS, National Survey of Family Growth, 2006–2008.

Figure 24.2. *Grades When Teenagers 15–19 First Received Formal Sex Education by Topic and Sex*

- Male teenagers were about as likely as female teenagers to report first receiving formal sex education on methods of birth control while in middle school (52% male teenagers compared with 46% female teenagers) and less likely than female teenagers to report first receiving instruction on methods of birth control while in high school (38% males compared with 47% females).

- Female teenagers were equally likely to report first receiving instruction on methods of birth control while in middle school or high school.

Do Teenagers Talk about Sex-Related Topics with Their Parents?

- More than two out of every three male teenagers and almost four out of every five female teenagers talked with a parent about at least one of six sex education topics ("how to say no to sex," methods of birth control, STDs, where to get birth control, how to prevent HIV/AIDS, and how to use a condom).

- Younger teenage (15–17 years old) females were more likely (80%) than younger male teenagers (68%) to have talked to their parents about these topics. On the other hand, there was virtually no difference for older teenage (18–19 years old) males and females in whether they talked to their parents about these topics.

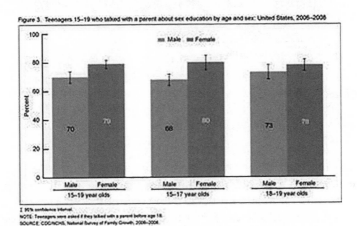

Figure 24.3. *Teenagers 15–19 Who Talked with a Parent about Sex Education by Age and Sex*

Do Male and Female Teenagers Differ in Whether They Talk to Their Parents about Sex and Birth Control?

• Female teenagers were more likely than male teenagers to talk to their parents about "how to say no to sex," methods of birth control, and where to get birth control.

• Nearly two-thirds of female teenagers have talked to their parents about "how to say no to sex" compared with about two out of five male teenagers.

• Male teenagers were more likely than female teenagers to talk to their parents about how to use a condom (38% of males compared with 29% of females).

• Female and male teenagers were equally likely to have talked with their parents about STDs and how to prevent HIV/AIDS.

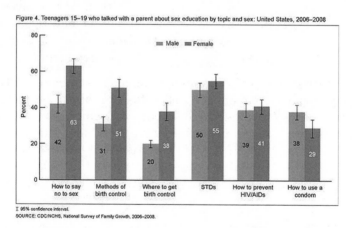

Figure 4. Teenagers 15–19 who talked with a parent about sex education by topic and sex: United States, 2006–2008

Figure 24.4. *Teenagers 15–19 Who Talked with a Parent about Sex Education by Topic and Sex*

Summary

Parental communication about sex education topics with their teenagers is associated with delayed sexual initiation and increased birth control method and condom use among sexually experienced teenagers (1–4). Although the impact of formal sex education on teenagers' behavior is harder to assess and depends on its content, studies show it can be effective at reducing risk behaviors. These data show that the majority of male and female teenagers 15–19 years are receiving formal sex education on "how to say no to sex," methods of birth control, STDs, and how to prevent HIV/AIDS. About one-half of teenagers reported first receiving instruction on "how to say no to sex," STDs, and how to prevent HIV/AIDS while in middle school. Most teenagers have talked to their parents about at least one of the six sex education topics. Female teenagers are more likely than male teenagers to talk to their parents about "how to say no to sex," methods of birth control, and where to get birth control. These findings for 2006–2008 suggest little change since 2002 in receipt of formal sex education or information from parents among teenagers.

Chapter 25

Sexually Transmitted Diseases (STDs) and Their Prevention

Chapter Contents

Section 25.1—Frequently Asked Questions about
STDs and STIs.. 274

Section 25.2—Human Immunodeficiency Virus (HIV)
Testing among Adolescents 279

Section 25.3—Vaccine to Prevent Human
Papillomavirus 281

Section 25.4—Practicing Safer Sex.. 287

Section 25.1

Frequently Asked Questions about STDs and STIs

This section includes text excerpted from "What Are STDs and STIs?" girlshealth.gov, Office on Women's Health (OWH), November 25, 2015.

What's the difference between STDs (sexually transmitted diseases) and STIs (sexually transmitted infections)? They are really the same thing. So why do some doctors use the word "infections" instead of "diseases"? Because the word "diseases" can make people think of having an obvious problem—but many STDs often have no signs or symptoms.

It can be hard to think about illness when you're feeling attracted to someone. But STDs are serious stuff, and you owe it to yourself to know the facts.

STDs spread very easily, and young people have been hit hard by them. In fact, 1 out of 4 teenage girls has an STD.

Untreated STDs can cause some scary health problems. These include problems with your reproductive system, like not being able to have children when you want to. And they include pain, cancer, and permanent damage to your body.

What Are STDs (STIs)?

Sexually transmitted diseases or STDs (also called sexually transmitted infections or STIs) are caused by many different bacteria and viruses—and even tiny insects. You can get an STD by having sexual contact with someone who already has one. That means you can get an STD through sexual intercourse, or by putting your mouth, hands, or genitals on the genitals or on the sores of someone who is infected.

Keep in mind that women who have sex with women also are at risk for some STDs.

Can STDs Be Cured for Good?

Some STDs can be treated and cured and will go away completely. Even if you get treated, though, you can get the STD again if you continue to have sex—especially if you have unprotected sex.

Ask your doctor or nurse about treatment for your partner. Otherwise, you might just keep giving the infection back and forth to each other.

Some STDs can't be cured, but you can get help with the symptoms. A few STDs can put your life in danger if they are not treated.

How Can I Keep from Getting STDs?

The surest way to avoid getting an STD is not to have sexual intercourse or other kinds of intimate sexual contact. Even waiting to have sex until you are older lowers your chances of getting an STD. It's also a good idea to stay away from drugs and alcohol, which can lead to having unsafe sex.

If you do have sex, you'll be safer if:

- Both you and your partner get tested for STDs (and treated if necessary)

- The two of you have sex only with each other

- You always use a latex condom (and use it correctly)

Lots of myths about STDs get passed around. Have you heard that you can prevent STDs by urinating, washing, or douching after sex? Well, unfortunately, none of these methods work. And you should not ever douche. Douching can increase your risk of getting STDs because it washes away bacteria that help prevent infection.

There is no vaccine to prevent most STDs. But there are vaccines that can help prevent two STDs:

- The hepatitis B vaccine can help protect against this dangerous STD, which can damage your liver. Most people get the hepatitis B vaccine as babies, but it's a good idea to ask whether you've already gotten yours.

- The HPV vaccine guards against some forms of human papillomavirus. HPV can cause genital warts and cervical cancer.

How Do You Know If You Have an STD?

The only way to know if you have an STD is to be tested. You may have symptoms from an STD. But lots of infections have no symptoms, especially in the early stages. By the time symptoms do show up, the infection may already have done damage.

If you have symptoms that could be coming from an STD, like stomach pain, see a doctor right away. Also see a doctor if fluid comes out of your vagina that is yellow, gray, or green, or has a strong smell. A clear or whitish fluid could be normal discharge, but if it's new and you have been sexually active, ask your doctor about it.

If you are having sex—or have had sex even once—see your doctor to find out which STD tests you may need.

Do Condoms Protect against STDs?

Latex condoms can lower your chances of getting human immuno-deficiency virus (HIV) and some other STDs a lot. They don't totally remove the risk, though. And they work better at preventing some STDs than others.

Who Can Get an STD?

Here are some key points about who can get an STD:

- Anyone who has sexual contact—including oral sex, anal sex, and contact between genital areas—can get an STD.

- STDs affect women and men of all ages and racial and ethnic backgrounds.

- Teenage girls and young women get STDs more easily than older women do.

- Young women who have sex with women are still at risk for STDs.

- Becoming sexually active at an earlier age and having more partners increase the chances of getting an STD.

- If you have sex with someone who has an STD you can catch it even if that person has no symptoms.

How Can I Get Tested for STDs?

Sometimes people are too scared or embarrassed to ask for STD information or testing. But keep in mind that many STDs are easy to treat—and dangerous if they're not detected and treated.

When you visit your doctor, he or she probably will examine your skin, throat, and genital area for sores, growths, and rashes. He or she also may look inside your vagina and at your cervix.

Your doctor may take a sample to test from:

- Fluid or tissue from your genital, vaginal, or anal areas

- Your blood

- Your urine (pee)

Of course, you may be nervous during these tests, but they usually are painless and quick.

When the doctor gets the results, he or she will let you know if you have an STD and what to do to take care of your health. Sometimes, your doctor may want to treat you even before you get your test results. If so, you should still follow up to get the results and any other care you need.

Are you worried about paying for testing? In the United States, the Affordable Care Act (ACA) requires most health insurance plans to cover the whole cost of STD testing.

Can I Ask the Doctor Personal Questions about Sex and STDs?

Doctors and nurses are there to talk to you about anything you need to protect your health!

If you are worried about your doctor telling your parents or guardians you are having sex, ask about his or her privacy policy before you begin. It's possible your doctor may encourage you to talk to your parents. But in most states, doctors can't share information about your reproductive health (especially about STDs) with anyone else without your permission. They can share the information without your permission only in special situations, such as if they think you have been sexually abused.

If you're having sex, it's very important to see your doctor regularly. You also might suggest that your partner see a doctor,

277

Adolescent Health Sourcebook, Fourth Edition

too. That way, your partner can get any necessary tests and helpful information to stay well, too.

What Should I Do If I Have an STD or Think I May Have an STD?

If you think you have an STD, follow these important steps:

- **Try to talk to your parents/guardians.** If you don't feel like you can do this, talk to someone else you trust, like a nurse or a teacher.

- **Make an appointment right away to see a healthcare provider**, such as a pediatrician, an adolescent medicine specialist, or a gynecologist.

- **Be sure to tell your sexual partner if you think you have an STD.** Both of you should be tested and treated if necessary, or you can pass it back and forth. Remember that your partner can have the STD and not have any symptoms.

- **If you have an STD, follow your doctor's instructions carefully.**

- **Avoid all sexual activity while you are being treated for an STD.**

- **Some STDs like HPV (human papillomavirus) and HIV cannot be cured** and can be passed to someone else, even if you don't have symptoms. Talk with your doctor about ways to help protect your partner.

- For STDs that can be cured, get a follow-up test to make sure that the infection is gone.

- **If you think you might be pregnant, be sure to tell your doctor.** Some medicines aren't safe to take if you are pregnant, so you may need to take a different drug to treat the STD.

What Is Pelvic Inflammatory Disease (PID)?

PID stands for pelvic inflammatory disease. It is a serious infection in your reproductive system that you can get from having some STDs. PID can lead to problems like ongoing pain in your pelvic area and not being able to have a baby when you are ready.

Teen girls (and young women) who have sex are most at risk for PID. This is partly because having a cervix that is still developing

278

increases the chances of getting STDs that can lead to PID. And the more sex partners you have, the greater your chances of getting PID.

If you want to avoid getting STDs, your best bet is not to have sex. Latex condoms can reduce the chance of getting STDs that can lead to PID, but you have to use condoms the right way and every time.

If you are having sex, make sure to see your doctor and get tested for STDs. Treating STDs early can help prevent PID.

Section 25.2

Human Immunodeficiency Virus (HIV) Testing among Adolescents

This section includes text excerpted from "HIV Testing among Adolescents," Centers for Disease Control and Prevention (CDC), July 2014. Reviewed November 2017.

Routine human immunodeficiency virus (HIV) testing for adolescents and adults aged 13–64 years is one of the most important strategies Centers for Disease Control and Prevention (CDC) recommends for reducing the spread of HIV. HIV testing is also an integral part of the National HIV/AIDS (Acquired Immune Deficiency Syndrome) Strategy to prevent the spread of HIV and improve health outcomes for those who are already infected. Because youth spend a significant part of their day in school, education agencies and schools can play key roles in supporting HIV testing.

Why HIV Testing Is Important for Adolescents

Many young people in the United States remain at risk for HIV infection. In 2010,

- Youth aged 13–24 years accounted for 7 percent of the estimated 1.1 million persons living with HIV infection.

- 26 percent (about 1 in 4) of the estimated 47,500 new HIV infections were among youth aged 13–24 years: 57 percent among blacks/African Americans, 20 percent among Hispanics/Latinos, and 20 percent among whites.

Adolescents engage in behaviors that put them at risk for HIV infection. Among U.S. high school students in 2013,

- 47 percent have had sexual intercourse at least once.
- 34 percent are currently sexually active.
- 41 percent of currently sexually active students did not use a condom the last time they had sexual intercourse.
- 15 percent have had four or more sex partners.
- 6 percent had sexual intercourse for the first time before age 13.

Knowing one's HIV status is one of the most important parts of prevention. Studies show that people who know they are infected are far less likely to have unprotected sex than those who do not know. Early diagnosis of HIV infection and linkage to care enable people to start treatment sooner, leading to better health outcomes and longer lives, and reducing the risk of spreading HIV to others.

How Schools and Education Agencies Can Support HIV Testing

Collect and use health risk behavior data. CDC's national Youth Risk Behavior Survey (YRBS), a school-based survey that monitors health risk behaviors among high school students, measures the percentage of students who have been tested for HIV infection. According to the 2013 national YRBS, only 13 percent of 9th–12th grade students had ever been tested for HIV.

Although the national YRBS data are useful for characterizing HIV testing trends nationwide, state and local data are also needed to examine local trends in testing behaviors, identify disparities in testing for certain groups, and determine whether young people at high risk are being tested. Starting in 2015, the state/local standard questionnaire will include a question measuring HIV testing.

Teach students about HIV and other sexually transmitted diseases. Educating students about HIV and other sexually transmitted diseases (STDs) could increase students' likelihood of being tested. According to an analysis of YRBS data, HIV testing was more common among students who had ever been taught in school about AIDS or

HIV infection (13%) than among those who had not (10%). The CDC's *2006 School Health Policies and Programs Study* found that nationwide, in required health education courses, 85 percent of high schools taught students how HIV is spread and 77 percent taught students how HIV is diagnosed and treated. High schools can strengthen their HIV prevention curricula by including information on locations and procedures for obtaining free, or low-cost, confidential HIV testing.

Support student access to HIV counseling and testing services. Schools can play a critical role in facilitating access to HIV testing. A school-based referral program can help connect students to adolescent-friendly community healthcare providers. Some schools may be able to offer onsite testing in conjunction with a school-linked or school-based clinic or in partnership with mobile (e.g., van-based) testing programs.

Promote communication between parents and adolescents. Effective communication between parents and adolescents about HIV is important. Approximately 60 percent of adolescents aged 15–19 years report that they have not had a conversation with their parents about how to prevent HIV infection. Schools can encourage activities shown to promote parent-child communication, such as assigning sex education homework assignments to be completed with a parent or trusted adult, or providing multi-session parent-child sex education programs.

Section 25.3

Vaccine to Prevent Human Papillomavirus

This section includes text excerpted from "HPV Vaccine Information for Young Women," Centers for Disease Control and Prevention (CDC), December 28, 2016.

Vaccines are available to prevent the human papillomavirus (HPV) types that cause most cervical cancers as well as some cancers of the anus, vulva (area around the opening of the vagina),

vagina, and oropharynx (back of throat including base of tongue and tonsils). The vaccine also prevents HPV types that cause most genital warts.

Why Is the HPV Vaccine Important?

Genital HPV is a common virus that is passed from one person to another through direct skin-to-skin contact during sexual activity. Most sexually active people will get HPV at some time in their lives, though most will never even know it. HPV infection is most common in people in their late teens and early 20s.

There are about 40 types of HPV that can infect the genital areas of men and women. Most HPV types cause no symptoms and go away on their own. But some types can cause cervical cancer in women and other less common cancers—like cancers of the anus, penis, vagina, and vulva and oropharynx. Other types of HPV can cause warts in the genital areas of men and women, called genital warts. Genital warts are not life-threatening. But they can cause emotional stress and their treatment can be very uncomfortable. Every year, about 12,000 women are diagnosed with cervical cancer and 4,000 women die from this disease in the U.S. About 1 percent of sexually active adults in the U.S. have visible genital warts at any point in time.

Which Girls/Women Should Receive HPV Vaccination?

HPV vaccination is recommended for 11 and 12 year-old girls. It is also recommended for girls and women age 13 through 26 years of age who have not yet been vaccinated or completed the vaccine series; HPV vaccine can also be given to girls beginning at age 9 years. CDC recommends 11 to 12 year olds get two doses of HPV vaccine to protect against cancers caused by HPV.

Will Sexually Active Females Benefit from the Vaccine?

Ideally females should get the vaccine before they become sexually active and exposed to HPV. Females who are sexually active may also benefit from vaccination, but they may get less benefit. This is because they may have already been exposed to one or more of the HPV types targeted by the vaccines. However, few sexually active young women are infected with all HPV types prevented by the vaccines, so most young women could still get protection by getting vaccinated.

Can Pregnant Women Get the Vaccine?

The vaccine is not recommended for pregnant women. Studies show that the HPV vaccine does not cause problems for babies born to women who were vaccinated while pregnant, but more research is still needed. A pregnant woman should not get any doses of the HPV vaccine until her pregnancy is completed.

Getting the HPV vaccine when pregnant is not a reason to consider ending a pregnancy. If a woman realizes that she got one or more shots of an HPV vaccine while pregnant, she should do two things:

- Wait until after her pregnancy to finish any remaining HPV vaccine doses.

- Call the pregnancy registry [800-986-8999 for Gardasil and Gardasil 9, or 888-825-5249 for Cervarix].

Should Girls and Women Be Screened for Cervical Cancer before Getting Vaccinated?

Girls and women do not need to get an HPV test or Pap test to find out if they should get the vaccine. However it is important that women continue to be screened for cervical cancer, even after getting all recommended shots of the HPV vaccine. This is because the vaccine does not protect against all types of cervical cancer.

How Effective Is the HPV Vaccine?

The HPV vaccine targets the HPV types that most commonly cause cervical cancer and can cause some cancers of the vulva, vagina, anus, and oropharynx. It also protects against the HPV types that cause most genital warts. The HPV vaccine is highly effective in preventing the targeted HPV types, as well as the most common health problems caused by them.

The vaccine is less effective in preventing HPV-related disease in young women who have already been exposed to one or more HPV types. That is because the vaccine prevents HPV before a person is exposed to it. The HPV vaccine does not treat existing HPV infections or HPV-associated diseases.

How Long Does Vaccine Protection Last?

Research suggests that vaccine protection is long-lasting. Current studies have followed vaccinated individuals for ten years, and show that there is no evidence of weakened protection over time.

What Does the Vaccine Not Protect Against?

The vaccine does not protect against all HPV types—so they will not prevent all cases of cervical cancer. Since some cervical cancers will not be prevented by the vaccine, it will be important for women to continue getting screened for cervical cancer. Also, the vaccine does not prevent other sexually transmitted infections (STIs). So it will still be important for sexually active persons to lower their risk for other STIs.

How Safe Is the HPV Vaccine?

The HPV vaccine has been licensed by the U.S. Food and Drug Administration (FDA). The CDC has approved this vaccine as safe and effective. The vaccine was studied in thousands of people around the world, and these studies showed no serious safety concerns. Side effects reported in these studies were mild, including pain where the shot was given, fever, dizziness, and nausea. Vaccine safety continues to be monitored by CDC and the FDA. More than 60 million doses of HPV vaccine have been distributed in the United States as of March 2014.

Fainting, which can occur after any medical procedure, has also been noted after HPV vaccination. Fainting after any vaccination is more common in adolescents. Because fainting can cause falls and injuries, adolescents and adults should be seated or lying down during HPV vaccination. Sitting or lying down for about 15 minutes after a vaccination can help prevent fainting and injuries.

Why Is HPV Vaccination Only Recommended for Women through Age 26?

HPV vaccination is not currently recommended for women over age 26 years. Clinical trials showed that, overall, HPV vaccination offered women limited or no protection against HPV-related diseases. For women over age 26 years, the best way to prevent cervical cancer is to get routine cervical cancer screening, as recommended.

What about Vaccinating Boys and Men?

HPV vaccine is licensed for use in boys and men. It has been found to be safe and effective for males 9–26 years. Advisory Committee on Immunization Practices (ACIP) recommends routine vaccination of boys aged 11 or 12 years with a series of doses. The vaccination series can be started beginning at age 9 years. Vaccination is recommended for males aged 13 through 21 years who have not already been vaccinated or who have not received all recommended doses. The vaccine is most effective when given at younger ages; males aged 22 through 26 years may be vaccinated. CDC recommends 11 to 12 year olds get two doses of HPV vaccine to protect against cancers caused by HPV.

Is HPV Vaccine Covered by Insurance Plans?

Health insurance plans cover the cost of HPV vaccines. If you don't have insurance, the Vaccines for Children (VFC) program may be able to help.

How Can I Get Help Paying for HPV Vaccine?

The Vaccines for Children (VFC) program helps families of eligible children who might not otherwise have access to vaccines. The program provides vaccines at no cost to doctors who serve eligible children. Children younger than 19 years of age are eligible for VFC vaccines if they are Medicaid-eligible, American Indian, or Alaska Native or have no health insurance. "Underinsured" children who have health insurance that does not cover vaccination can receive VFC vaccines through Federally Qualified Health Centers or Rural Health Centers. Parents of uninsured or underinsured children who receive vaccines at no cost through the VFC Program should check with their healthcare providers about possible administration fees that might apply. These fees help providers cover the costs that result from important services like storing the vaccines and paying staff members to give vaccines to patients. However, VFC vaccines cannot be denied to an eligible child if a family can't afford the fee.

What Vaccinated Girls/Women Need to Know: Will Girls/ Women Who Have Been Vaccinated Still Need Cervical Cancer Screening?

Yes, vaccinated women will still need regular cervical cancer screening because the vaccine protects against most but not all HPV types that cause cervical cancer. Also, women who got the vaccine after becoming sexually active may not get the full benefit of the vaccine if they had already been exposed to HPV.

Are There Other Ways to Prevent Cervical Cancer?

Regular cervical cancer screening (Pap and HPV tests) and follow-up can prevent most cases of cervical cancer. The Pap test can detect cell changes in the cervix before they turn into cancer. The HPV test looks for the virus that can cause these cell changes. Screening can detect most, but not all, cervical cancers at an early, treatable stage. Most women diagnosed with cervical cancer in the U.S. have either never been screened, or have not been screened in the last 5 years.

Are There Other Ways to Prevent HPV?

For those who are sexually active, condoms may lower the chances of getting HPV, if used with every sex act, from start to finish. Condoms may also lower the risk of developing HPV-related diseases (genital warts and cervical cancer). But HPV can infect areas that are not covered by a condom—so condoms may not fully protect against HPV.

People can also lower their chances of getting HPV by being in a faithful relationship with one partner; limiting their number of sex partners; and choosing a partner who has had no or few prior sex partners. But even people with only one lifetime sex partner can get HPV. And it may not be possible to determine if a partner who has been sexually active in the past is currently infected. That's why the only sure way to prevent HPV is to avoid all sexual activity.

Section 25.4

Practicing Safer Sex

This section contains text excerpted from the following
sources: Text under the heading "What Is 'Safer Sex'?" is excerpted
from "HIV/AIDS—What Is 'Safer Sex'?" U.S. Department of Veterans
Affairs (VA), July 30, 2015; Text under the heading "Tips for Using
Condoms and Dental Dams" is excerpted from "HIV/AIDS—Tips for
Using Condoms and Dental Dams," U.S. Department of Veterans
Affairs (VA), February 2017.

What Is 'Safer Sex'?

We know a lot about how human immunodeficiency virus (HIV) is
transmitted from person to person. Having safer sex means you take
this into account and avoid risky practices.

There are two reasons to practice safer sex: to protect yourself and
to protect others.

Protecting Yourself

If you have HIV, you need to protect your health. When it comes
to sex, this means practicing safer sex to avoid sexually transmitted
diseases like herpes and hepatitis. HIV makes it harder for your body
to fight off diseases. What might be a small health problem for someone
without HIV could be big health problem for you.

Protecting Your Partner

Taking care of others means making sure that you do not pass along
HIV to them. If your sex partners already have HIV, you should still
avoid infecting them with another sexually transmitted disease you
may be carrying.

Most people would agree that you owe it to your sexual partners
to tell them that you have HIV. This is being honest with them. Even
though it can be very hard to do, in the long run you will probably feel
much better about yourself.

Some people with HIV have found that people who love them think that unsafe sex is a sign of greater love or trust. If someone offers to have unsafe sex with you, it is still up to you to protect them by being safe.

"Being safe" usually means protecting yourself and others by using condoms for the highest-risk sex activities, specifically for anal and vaginal sex. When done correctly, condom use is very effective at preventing HIV transmission. In recent years, "being safe" has come to include two other important strategies for reducing HIV infections; these are HIV treatment for HIV-positive people and PrEP for HIV negatives (see below). Both of these are very effective at reducing the risk of HIV infection. One or more of them is likely to be appropriate for you—be sure to ask your healthcare provider about them.

What about Pre-Exposure Prophylaxis (PrEP)?

Some HIV-negative individuals may, under the supervision of their healthcare providers, take anti-HIV medications every day to prevent themselves from becoming infected. This is called pre-exposure prophylaxis, or PrEP. Usually these are persons who are at relatively high risk of becoming infected with HIV (for example, because they have an HIV-infected partner, they have risky sexual exposures, or they share injection drug equipment). The medication used for PrEP is Truvada, a combination tablet containing tenofovir and emtricitabine. PrEP appears to be very effective if it is taken every day, and is not effective if it is taken irregularly. Your U.S. Department of Veterans Affairs (VA) healthcare provider can tell you more about the potential benefits and shortcomings of PrEP for HIV-negative persons.

Tips for Using Condoms and Dental Dams

Some people think that using a condom makes sex less fun. Other people have become creative and find condoms sexy. Not having to worry about infecting someone will definitely make sex much more enjoyable!

If you are not used to using condoms: practice, practice, practice.

Condom Do's and Don'ts:

- **Shop around:** Use lubricated latex condoms. Always use latex, because lambskin condoms don't block HIV and STDs, and polyurethane condoms break more often than latex (if you are allergic to latex, polyurethane condoms are an option). Shop around and find your favorite brand. Try different sizes and shapes (yes, they come in different sizes and shapes!). There are a lot of choices—one will work for you.

- **Keep it fresh:** Store condoms loosely in a cool, dry place (not your wallet). Make sure your condoms are fresh—check the expiration date. Throw away condoms that have expired, been very hot, or been washed in the washer. If you think the condom might not be good, get a new one. You and your partner are worth it.

- **Take it easy:** Open the package carefully, so that you don't rip the condom. Be careful if you use your teeth. Make sure that the condom package has not been punctured (there should be a pocket of air). Check the condom for damaged packaging and signs of aging such as brittleness, stickiness, and discoloration.

- **Keep it hard:** Put on the condom after the penis is erect and before it touches any part of a partner's body. If a penis is uncircumcised (uncut), the foreskin must be pulled back before putting on the condom.

- **Heads up!** Make sure the condom is right-side out. It's like a sock—there's a right side and a wrong side. Before you put it on the penis, unroll the condom about half an inch to see which direction it is unrolling. Then put it on the head of the penis and hold the tip of the condom between your fingers as you roll it all the way down the shaft of the penis from head to base. This keeps out air bubbles that can cause the condom to break. It also leaves a space for semen to collect after ejaculation.

- **Slippery when wet:** If you use a lubricant (lube), it should be a water-soluble lubricant (for example, ID Glide, K-Y Jelly, Slippery Stuff, Foreplay, Wet, Astroglide) in order to prevent breakdown of the condom. Products such as petroleum jelly, massage oils, butter, Crisco, Vaseline, and hand creams are not considered water-soluble lubricants and should not be used. Put lubricant on after you put on the condom, not before—it could slip off. Add more lube often. Dry condoms break more easily.

- **Come and go:** Withdraw the penis immediately after ejaculation, while the penis is still erect; grasp the rim of the condom between your fingers and slowly withdraw the penis (with the condom still on) so that no semen is spilled.

- **Clean up:** Throw out the used condom right away. Tie it off
to prevent spillage or wrap it in bathroom tissue and put it in
the garbage. Condoms can clog toilets. Use a condom only once.
Never use the same condom for vaginal and anal intercourse.
Never use a condom that has been used by someone else.

Do You Have to Use a Condom for Oral Sex?

It is possible for oral sex to transmit HIV, whether the infected
partner is performing or receiving oral sex. But the risk is very low
compared with unprotected vaginal or anal sex.

If you choose to perform oral sex, and your partner is male, you may:

- use a latex condom on the penis; or

- if you or your partner is allergic to latex, plastic (polyurethane)
condoms can be used.

If you choose to have oral sex, and your partner is female, you may:

- use a latex barrier (such as a natural rubber latex sheet, a dental dam, or a cut-open condom that makes a square) between
your mouth and the vagina. A latex barrier such as a dental dam
reduces the risk of blood or vaginal fluids entering your mouth.
Plastic food wrap also can be used as a barrier.

If you choose to perform oral sex with either a male or female partner and this sex includes oral contact with your partner's anus (ani-
lingus or rimming),

- use a latex barrier (such as a natural rubber latex sheet, a dental dam, or a cut-open condom that makes a square) between
your mouth and the anus. Plastic food wrap also can be used
as a barrier. This barrier is to prevent getting another sexually
transmitted disease or parasites, not HIV.

If you choose to share sex toys, such as dildos or vibrators, with
your partner,

- each partner should use a new condom on the sex toy; and be
sure to clean sex toys between each use.

Internal Condom (Female Condom)

This type of condom was originally designed to be inserted into the
vagina before sex. It also can be used in the anus, by either men or

women, though its effectiveness in preventing HIV transmission via anal sex has not been studied.

The internal condom is a large condom fitted with larger and smaller rings at each end. The rings help keep it inside the vagina during sex; for anal sex, the inner ring usually is removed before it is inserted. It is made of nitrile, so any lubricant can be used without damaging it. It may seem a little awkward at first, but can be a useful alternative to the traditional "male" condom. Female condoms generally cost more than male condoms.

- Store the condom in a cool dry place, not in direct heat or sunlight.

- Throw away any condoms that have expired—the date is printed on individual condom wrappers.

- Check the package for damage and check the condom for signs of aging such as brittleness, stickiness, and discoloration. The internal condom is lubricated, so it will be somewhat wet.

- Before inserting the condom, you can squeeze lubricant into the condom pouch and rub the sides together to spread it around.

- Put the condom in before sex play because pre-ejaculatory fluid, which comes from the penis, may contain HIV. The condom can be inserted up to 8 hours before sex.

- The internal condom has a firm ring at each end of it. To insert the condom in the vagina, squeeze the ring at the closed end between the fingers (like a diaphragm), and push it up into the back of the vagina. The open ring must stay outside the vagina at all times, and it will partly cover the lip area. For use in the anus, most people remove the internal ring before insertion.

- Do not use a male condom with the internal condom.

- Do not use an internal condom with a diaphragm.

- If the penis is inserted outside the condom pouch or if the outer ring (open ring) slips into the vagina, stop and take the condom out. Use a new condom before you start sex again.

- Don't tear the condom with fingernails or jewelry.

- Use a condom only once and properly dispose of it in the trash (not the toilet).

Dental Dams and Plastic Wrap

Even though oral sex is a low-risk sexual practice, you may want to use protection when performing oral sex on someone who has HIV.

Dental dams are small squares of latex that were made originally for use in dental procedures. They are now commonly used as barriers when performing oral sex on women, to keep in vaginal fluids or menstrual blood that could transmit HIV or other STDs.

Some people use plastic wrap instead of a dental dam. It's thinner. Here are some things to remember:

- Before using a dental dam, first check it visually for any holes.

- If the dental dam has cornstarch on it, rinse that off with water (starch in the vagina can lead to an infection).

- Cover the woman's genital area with the dental dam.

- For oral-anal sex, cover the opening of the anus with a new dental dam.

- A new dental dam should be used for each act of oral sex; it should never be reused.

Chapter 26

Understanding Abstinence

Sexual abstinence is defined as refraining from all forms of sexual activity and genital contact such as vaginal, oral, or anal sex.

Protect against Pregnancy

Abstinence is the only 100 percent effective way to protect against pregnancy, ensuring that there is no exchange of bodily fluids (such as vaginal secretions and semen). Abstinence prevents pregnancy by keeping semen away from the vagina so the sperm cells in semen cannot meet with an egg and fertilize it. If you are abstinent 100 percent of the time, pregnancy cannot happen. People sometimes also use abstinence to prevent pregnancy on days they are fertile (most likely to get pregnant), but they may have vaginal sex at other times.

It will be important to discuss with your partner what abstinence means to you, especially if you are developing a new relationship. Someone that cares about you will honor your choices and not push for sexual behavior that makes you uncomfortable.

This chapter contains text excerpted from the following sources: Text in this chapter begins with excerpts from "Abstinence," U.S. Department of Health and Human Services (HHS), August 23, 2017; Text under the heading "Ways to Stick to Abstinence" is excerpted from "Why Waiting to Have Sex Makes Sense," girlshealth.gov, Office on Women's Health (OWH), November 25, 2015.

How Effective Is Abstinence?

When practiced consistently, abstinence provides the most effective protection against unplanned pregnancy and sexually transmitted diseases (STDs) including human immunodeficiency virus (HIV) infection. It is only effective when both partners are completely committed and practice abstinence (no genital contact or sharing semen or vaginal fluid) 100 percent of the time. Abstinence is most effective when both partners talk and agree about their reasons to remain abstinent.

Discuss It with Partner

Abstinence is a personal decision that should be discussed with your partner.

Table 26.1. Advantages and Drawbacks of Abstinence

Advantages of Abstinence	Drawbacks of Abstinence
• Abstinence has no health risks.	• It is sometimes hard to abstain from sex, particularly in the moment. You should always communicate with your partner ahead of time about your decision to be abstinent.
• It is a personal decision, available to anyone at any time.	• There may be pressure from your partner or friends to have sex.
• It is free.	
• You can be abstinent at different times in your life for different reasons that may change over time.	
• You can choose to be abstinent whenever you want, no matter your age, gender, sexual orientation, or previous sexual experience.	

Ways to Stick to Abstinence

It's not always easy to abstain from sex. It can help to make a plan ahead of time and get support from people you trust. You might try talking with your parents/guardians about sex to see if they have advice. You also might keep in mind the reasons you made the choice to be abstinent.

Don't be afraid to take a stand with your partner. If you are close enough with someone to consider having sex, you should be close enough to talk about the decision. If you and your partner can't agree, then you might think about whether you'd be better off with someone whose beliefs are closer to your own.

Your own body may tell you to give up on abstinence. Remember that your body is not in charge! Remind yourself of the possible physical, emotional, and financial costs of having sex before you're really ready.

Consider these tips for staying abstinent:

- **Get involved.** Some people find it helps to get involved in activities that let them focus on something other than sex, like volunteering or joining a sports team.

- **Get together.** When you hang out with your date, it can help to hang out in a group. Also, try not to spend a lot of time in secluded places with no one else around or at someone's house when no adults are home.

- **Get out.** Always take a cell phone and cab or bus money in case you want to get out of an uncomfortable situation.

- **Practice.** Think about how to say "no" ahead of time, so you don't have to come up with replies on the spot.

- **Stay sober.** Drugs and alcohol can make you more likely to do something you otherwise never would.

Chapter 27

Birth Control Methods (Contraception)

Birth control (contraception) is any method, medicine, or device used to prevent pregnancy. Women can choose from many different types of birth control. Some work better than others at preventing pregnancy. The type of birth control you use depends on your health, your desire to have children now or in the future, and your need to prevent sexually transmitted infections (STIs). Your doctor can help you decide which type is best for you right now.

What Is the Best Method of Birth Control?

There is no "best" method of birth control for every woman. The birth control method that is right for you and your partner depends on many things, and may change over time.

Before choosing a birth control method, talk to your doctor or nurse about:

- Whether you want to get pregnant soon, in a few years, or never

- How well each method works to prevent pregnancy

- Possible side effects

This chapter includes text excerpted from "Birth Control Methods," Office on Women's Health (OWH), U.S. Department of Health and Human Services (HHS), October 15, 2015.

- How often you have sex

- The number of sex partners you have

- Your overall health

- How comfortable you are with using the method (For example, can you remember to take a pill every day? Will you have to ask your partner to put on a condom each time?)

Keep in mind that even the most effective birth control methods can fail. But your chances of getting pregnant are lower if you use a more effective method.

What Are the Different Types of Birth Control?

Women can choose from many different types of birth control methods. These include, in order of most effective to least effective at preventing pregnancy:

- **Female and male sterilization** (female tubal ligation or occlusion, male vasectomy)—Birth control that prevents pregnancy for the rest of your life through surgery or a medical procedure.

- *Long-acting* **reversible contraceptives or "LARC" methods** (intrauterine devices, hormonal implants)—Birth control your doctor inserts one time and you do not have to remember to use birth control every day or month. LARCs last for 3 to 10 years, depending on the method.

- *Short-acting* **hormonal methods** (pill, mini pills, patch, shot, vaginal ring)—Birth control your doctor prescribes that you remember to take every day or month. The shot requires you to get a shot from your doctor every 3 months.

- **Barrier methods** (condoms, diaphragms, sponge, cervical cap)—Birth control you use each time you have sex.

- **Natural rhythm methods**—Not using a type of birth control but instead avoiding sex and/or using birth control only on the days when you are most fertile (most likely to get pregnant).

How Can I Compare the Different Types of Birth Control?

Table 27.1. Types of Birth Control

Method	Number of Pregnancies per 100 Women within Their First Year of Typical use1	"Side Effects and Risks* *These Are Not All of the Possible Side Effects and Risks. Talk to Your Doctor or Nurse for More Information."	How Often You Have to Take or Use
Abstinence (no sexual contact)	Unknown (0 for perfect use)	No medical side effects	No action required, but it does take willpower. You may want to have a backup birth control method, such as condoms.
Permanent sterilization surgery for women (tubal ligation, "getting your tubes tied")	Less than 1	• Possible pain during recovery (up to 2 weeks) • Bleeding or other complications from surgery • Less common risk includes ectopic (tubal) pregnancy	No action required after surgery
Permanent sterilization implant for women (Essure®)	Less than 1	• Pain during the insertion of Essure; some pain during recovery • Cramping, vaginal bleeding, back pain during recovery • Implant may move out of place • Less common but serious risk includes ectopic (tubal) pregnancy	No action required after surgery
Permanent sterilization surgery for men (vasectomy)	Less than 1	• Pain during recovery • Complications from surgery	No action required after surgery

299

Table 27.1. Continued

Method	Number of Pregnancies per 100 Women within Their First Year of Typical use1	"Side Effects and Risks* *These Are Not All of the Possible Side Effects and Risks. Talk to Your Doctor or Nurse for More Information."	How Often You Have to Take or Use
Implantable rod (Implanon®, Nexplanon®)	Less than 1	• Headache • Irregular periods • Weight gain • Sore breasts • Less common risk includes difficulty in removing the implant	No action required for up to 3 years before removing or replacing
Copper intrauterine device (IUD) (ParaGard®)	Less than 1	• Cramps for a few days after insertion • Missed periods, bleeding between periods, heavier periods • Less common but serious risks include pelvic inflammatory disease and the IUD being expelled from the uterus or going through the wall of the uterus.	No action required for up to 10 years before removing or replacing
Hormonal intrauterine devices (IUDs) (Liletta, Mirena®, and Skyla®)	Less than 1	• Irregular periods, lighter or missed periods • Ovarian cysts • Less common but serious risks include pelvic inflammatory disease and the IUD being expelled from the uterus or going through the wall of the uterus.	No action required for 3 to 5 years, depending on the brand, before removing or replacing

Table 27.1. Continued

Method	Number of Pregnancies per 100 Women within Their First Year of Typical use1	"Side Effects and Risks* *These Are Not All of the Possible Side Effects and Risks. Talk to Your Doctor or Nurse for More Information."	How Often You Have to Take or Use
Shot/Injection (Depo-Provera®)	6	• Bleeding between periods, missed periods • Weight gain • Changes in mood • Sore breasts • Headaches • Bone loss with long-term use (bone loss may be reversible once you stop using this type of birth control)	Get a new shot every 3 months
Oral contraceptives, combination hormones ("the pill")	9	• Headache • Upset stomach • Sore breasts • Changes in your period • Changes in mood • Weight gain • High blood pressure • Less common but serious risks include blood clots, stroke and heart attack; the risk is higher in smokers and women older than 35	Take at the same time every day

Table 27.1. Continued

Method	Number of Pregnancies per 100 Women within Their First Year of Typical use1	"Side Effects and Risks* *These Are Not All of the Possible Side Effects and Risks. Talk to Your Doctor or Nurse for More Information."	How Often You Have to Take or Use
Oral contraceptives, progestin-only pill ("mini-pill")	9	<ul><li>Spotting or bleeding between periods</li><li>Weight gain</li><li>Sore breasts</li><li>Headache</li><li>Nausea</li></ul>	Take at the same time every day
Skin patch (Xulane®)	9 May be less effective in women weighing 198 pounds or more2	<ul><li>Skin irritation</li><li>Upset stomach</li><li>Changes in your period</li><li>Changes in mood</li><li>Sore breasts</li><li>Headache</li><li>Weight gain</li><li>High blood pressure</li><li>Less common but serious risks include blood clots, stroke and heart attack; the risk is higher in smokers and women older than 35</li></ul>	Wear for 21 days, remove for 7 days, replace with a new patch

Birth Control Methods (Contraception)

Table 27.1. Continued

Method	Number of Pregnancies per 100 Women within Their First Year of Typical use1	"Side Effects and Risks* *These Are Not All of the Possible Side Effects and Risks. Talk to Your Doctor or Nurse for More Information."	How Often You Have to Take or Use
Vaginal ring (NuvaRing®)	9	• Headache • Upset stomach • Sore breasts • Vaginal irritation and discharge • Changes in your period • High blood pressure • Less common but serious risks include blood clots, stroke and heart attack; the risk is higher in smokers and women older than 35	Wear for 21 days, remove for 7 days, replace with a new ring
Diaphragm with spermicide (Koromex®, Ortho-Diaphragm®)	12 If you gain or lose than 15 pounds, or have a baby, have your doctor check you to make sure the diaphragm still fits.	• Irritation • Allergic reactions • Urinary tract infection (UTI) • Vaginal infections • Rarely, toxic shock if left in for more than 24 hours Using a spermicide often might increase your risk of getting HIV	Insert each time you have sex
Sponge with spermicide (Today Sponge®)	12 (among women who have never given birth before) or 24 (among women who have given birth)3	• Irritation • Allergic reactions • Rarely, toxic shock if left in for more than 24 hours • Using a spermicide often might increase your risk of getting HIV	Insert each time you have sex

303

Table 27.1. Continued

Method	Number of Pregnancies per 100 Women within Their First Year of Typical use1	"Side Effects and Risks*****These Are Not All of the Possible Side Effects and Risks. Talk to Your Doctor or Nurse for More Information."	How Often You Have to Take or Use
Cervical cap with spermicide (FemCap®)	233	• Vaginal irritation or odor • Urinary tract infections (UTIs) • Allergic reactions • Rarely, toxic shock if left in for more than 48 hours • Using a spermicide often might increase your risk of getting HIV	Insert each time you have sex
Male condom	18	• Irritation • Condom may tear, break or slip off • Allergic reactions to latex condoms	Use each time you have sex
Female condom	21	• Irritation • Condom may tear or slip out • Allergic reaction	Use each time you have sex
Withdrawal—when a man takes his penis out of a woman's vagina (or "pulls out") before he ejaculates (has an orgasm or "comes")	22	• Sperm can be released before the man pulls out, putting you at risk for pregnancy	Use each time you have sex

Table 27.1. Continued

Method	Number of Pregnancies per 100 Women within Their First Year of Typical use1	"Side Effects and Risks* *These Are Not All of the Possible Side Effects and Risks. Talk to Your Doctor or Nurse for More Information."	How Often You Have to Take or Use
Natural family planning (rhythm method)	24	• Can be hard to know the days you are most fertile (when you need to avoid having sex or use backup birth control)	Depending on method used, takes planning each month
Spermicide alone	28 Works best if used along with a barrier method, such as a diaphragm	• Irritation • Allergic reactions • Urinary tract infection • Frequent use of a spermicide might increase your risk of getting HIV	Use each time you have sex

Which Types of Birth Control Help Prevent Sexually Transmitted Infections (STIs)?

Only two types can protect you from sexually transmitted infections (STIs), including human immunodeficiency virus (HIV): male condoms and female condoms.

While condoms are the best way to prevent STIs if you have sex, they are not the most effective type of birth control. If you have sex, the best way to prevent both STIs and pregnancy is to use what is called "dual protection." Dual protection means you use a condom to prevent STIs each time you have sex, and at the same time, you use a more effective form of birth control, such as an intrauterine device (IUD), implant, or shot.

Which Types of Birth Control Can I Get without a Prescription?

You can buy these types of birth control over the counter at a drugstore or supermarket:

- Male condoms

- Female condoms

- Sponges

- Spermicides

- Emergency contraception (EC) pills. Plan B One-Step® and its generic versions are available in drugstores and some supermarkets to anyone, without a prescription. However you should not use EC as your regular birth control because it does not work as well as regular birth control. EC is meant to be used only when your regular birth control does not work for some unexpected reason.

Which Types of Birth Control Do I Have to See My Doctor to Get?

You need a prescription for these types of birth control:

- Oral contraceptives: the pill and the mini-pill (in some states, birth control pills are now available without a prescription, through the pharmacy)

- Patch

- Vaginal ring

- Diaphragms (your doctor or nurse needs to fit one to the shape of your vagina)

- Shot/injection (you get the shot at your doctor's office or family planning clinic)

- Cervical cap

- Implantable rod (inserted by a doctor in the office or clinic)

- IUD (inserted by a doctor in the office or clinic)

You will need surgery or a medical procedure for:

- Female sterilization (tubal ligation)

- Male sterilization (vasectomy)

- Tubal implant (Essure®)

How Does Birth Control Work?

Birth control works to prevent pregnancy in different ways, depending upon the type of birth control you choose:

Female or male sterilization surgery prevents the sperm from reaching the egg by cutting or damaging the tubes that carry sperm (in men) or eggs (in women).

Long-acting **reversible contraceptives or "LARC" methods** (intrauterine devices, hormonal implants) prevent your ovaries from releasing eggs, prevent sperm from getting to the egg, or make implantation of the egg in the uterus (womb) unlikely.

Short-acting hormonal methods, such as the pill, mini-pill, patch, shot, and vaginal ring, prevent your ovaries from releasing eggs or prevent sperm from getting to the egg.

Barrier methods, such as condoms, diaphragms, sponge, cervical cap, prevent sperm from getting to the egg.

- **Natural rhythm methods** involve avoiding sex or using other forms of birth control on the days when you are most fertile (most likely to get pregnant).

Are Birth Control Pills Safe?

Yes, hormonal birth control methods, such as the pill, are safe for most women. Today's birth control pills have lower doses of hormones than in the past. This has lowered the risk of side effects and serious health problems.

Today's birth control pills can have health benefits for some women, such as a lower risk of some kinds of cancer. Also, different brands and types of birth control pills (and other forms of hormonal birth control) can increase your risk for some health problems and side effects. Side effects can include weight gain, headaches, irregular bleeding, breast tenderness, and mood changes.

Talk to your doctor about whether hormonal birth control is right for you.

Does Birth Control Raise My Risk for Health Problems?

It can, depending on your health and the type of birth control you use. Talk to your doctor to find the birth control method that is right for you.

Different forms of birth control have different health risks and side effects. Some birth control methods that increase your risk for health problems include:

- **Hormonal birth control.** Combination birth control pills (birth control with both estrogen and progesterone) and some other forms of hormonal birth control, such as the vaginal ring or skin patch, may raise your risk for blood clots and high blood pressure. Blood clots and high blood pressure can cause a heart attack or stroke. A blood clot in the legs can also go to your lungs, causing serious damage or even death. These are serious side effects of hormonal birth control, but they are rare.

- **Spermicides (used alone or with the cervical cap, diaphragm or sponge).** Spermicides that have nonoxynol-9 can irritate the vagina. This can raise your risk for getting HIV. Use spermicides with nonoxynol-9 only if you are in a monogamous relationship (you have sex only with each other) with a man you know is HIV-negative. Also, medicines for vaginal yeast infections may make spermicides less effective.

- **Intrauterine devices (IUDs).** IUDs can slightly raise your risk of an ectopic pregnancy. Ectopic pregnancies happen when a fertilized egg implants somewhere outside of the uterus (womb), usually in one of the fallopian tubes. An ectopic pregnancy is a serious medical problem that should be treated as soon as possible. IUDs also have a very rare but serious risk of infection or puncture of the uterus.

What Are the Health Risks for Smokers Who Use Birth Control?

If you smoke and are 35 or older, you should not use hormonal birth control. Smoking tobacco and using hormonal birth control raises your risk for blood clots and high blood pressure. Smoking and high blood pressure are risk factors for a heart attack or stroke. The risk for a heart attack or stroke also goes up as you age.

Can Birth Control Help with My Painful or Heavy Periods?

Maybe. Research shows that hormonal birth control, such as the pill, patch, shot, ring, implantable rod, and hormonal IUD, may help with heavy, painful, or long-term bleeding. These methods can also help you have lighter, shorter periods.

What Are Some Other Benefits of Hormonal Birth Control?

Research shows that other benefits of hormonal birth control may include:

- More regular and lighter periods
- Fewer menstrual cramps
- Less acne
- A lower risk of ovary, endometrial (uterus), and colon cancers, pelvic inflammatory disease (PID), noncancerous ovarian cysts, and iron-deficiency anemia

What Do I Do If I Miss a Day Taking the Pill?

Follow the instructions that came with your birth control about using backup birth control (such as a condom and spermicide). You also can follow these recommendations from the Centers for Disease Control and Prevention (CDC).

If you are late or miss a day taking your pill:

- Take the late or missed pill as soon as possible.
- Continue taking the rest of your pills at your normal time, even if it means taking two pills on the same day.

- You do not need other forms of birth control, such as a condom, unless you need to protect against STIs.

If you miss two or more days in a row:

- Take only the most recent missed pill as soon as possible.

- Continue taking the rest of your pills at your normal time, even if it means taking two pills on the same day.

- Use backup birth control, such as a condom and spermicide, or do not have sex until you have taken a pill for seven days in a row.

- If you missed pills during days in the last week of active pills (days 15–21 for 28-day pill packs), start a new pack the next day. If you are not able to start a new pack right away, use backup birth control or avoid sex until hormone pills from a new pack have been taken for 7 days in a row.

- Consider emergency contraception if you missed pills during the first week and had sex.

Talk to your doctor if you continue to miss taking your birth control pill or find it hard to take the pill at the same time each day. You may want to consider a different type of birth control, such as an IUD, an implant, shot, ring, or patch that you don't have to remember to take every day.

How Effective Is the Withdrawal Method?

Not very! About 22 out of 100 women who use withdrawal as their only form of birth control for a year will get pregnant. See the (Table 27.1) for how this number compares to other methods of birth control.

Withdrawal is when a man takes his penis out of a woman's vagina ("pulls out") before he ejaculates or "comes" (has an orgasm). This lowers the chance of sperm from going to the egg. "Pulling out" can be hard for a man to do. It takes a lot of self-control.

Even if you use withdrawal, sperm can be released before the man pulls out. When a man's penis first becomes erect, some fluid may be on the tip of the penis. This fluid has sperm in it, so you could still get pregnant. Withdrawal also does not protect you from STIs, including HIV.

Does Breastfeeding Prevent Pregnancy?

Breastfeeding can be a short-term method of birth control in very specific situations. The risk of pregnancy is less than 2 in 100 if all three of these describe you:

- You have a baby who is less than 6 months old

  and

- You exclusively breastfeed, meaning that you only feed your baby your breastmilk all of the time (no formula, no breast milk from other people, and no solid food)

  and

- You have not gotten a period after childbirth

Talk to your doctor about birth control if you do not want to get pregnant while nursing.

How Can I Get Free or Low-Cost Birth Control?

Under the Affordable Care Act (ACA) (the healthcare law), most insurance plans cover U.S. Food and Drug Administration (FDA)-approved prescription birth control for women, such as the pill, IUDs, and female sterilization, at no additional cost to you. This also includes birth control counseling.

- If you have insurance, check with your insurance provider to find out what is included in your plan.

- If you have Medicaid, your insurance covers birth control. This includes birth control prescriptions and visits to your doctor related to birth control.

- If you don't have insurance, don't panic. Family planning (reproductive health) clinics may provide some birth control methods for free or at low cost.

Chapter 28

Teen Pregnancy

Chapter Contents

Section 28.1—Statistics on Teen Pregnancy in
the United States 314

Section 28.2—Could I Get Pregnant If...? 316

Section 28.3—Prenatal Care for Pregnant Teens 318

Section 28.4—Teen Parents... You're Not Alone! 320

Section 28.1

Statistics on Teen Pregnancy in the United States

This section includes text excerpted from "Reproductive
Health—Teen Pregnancy," Centers for Disease
Control and Prevention (CDC), May 4, 2017.

Teen Pregnancy in the United States

In 2015, a total of 229,715 babies were born to women aged 15–19
years, for a birth rate of 22.3 per 1,000 women in this age group. This
is another record low for U.S. teens and a drop of 8 percent from 2014.
Birth rates fell 9 percent for women aged 15–17 years and 7 percent
for women aged 18–19 years.

Although reasons for the declines are not totally clear, evidence
suggests these declines are due to more teens abstaining from sexual
activity, and more teens who are sexually active using birth control
than in previous years.

Still, the U.S. teen pregnancy rate is substantially higher than in
other western industrialized nations, and racial/ethnic and geographic
disparities in teen birth rates persist.

Disparities in Teen Birth Rates

Teen birth rates declined from 2014 to 2015 for all races and for
Hispanics. Among 15- to 19-year-olds, teen birth rates decreased:

- 10 percent for Asian/Pacific Islanders

- 9 percent for non-Hispanic blacks

- 8 percent for Hispanics

- 8 percent for non-Hispanic whites

- 6 percent for American Indian/Alaska Natives

In 2015, the birth rate of Hispanic teens were still more than two
times higher than the rate for non-Hispanic white teens. The birth rate

of non-Hispanic black teens was almost twice as high as the rate among non-Hispanic white teens, and American Indian/Alaska Native teen birth rates remained more than one and a half times higher than the non-Hispanic white teen birth rate. Geographic differences in teen birth rates persist, both within and across states. Among some states with low overall teen birth rates, some counties have high teen birth rates.

Less favorable socioeconomic conditions, such as low education and low income levels of a teen's family, may contribute to high teen birth rates. Teens in child welfare systems are at higher risk of teen pregnancy and birth than other groups. For example, young women living in foster care are more than twice as likely to become pregnant than those not in foster care.

To improve the life opportunities of adolescents facing significant health disparities and to have the greatest impact on overall U.S. teen birth rates, Centers for Disease Control and Prevention (CDC) uses data to inform and direct interventions and resources to areas with the greatest need.

The Importance of Prevention

Teen pregnancy and childbearing bring substantial social and economic costs through immediate and long-term impacts on teen parents and their children.

- In 2010, teen pregnancy and childbirth accounted for at least $9.4 billion in costs to U.S. taxpayers for increased healthcare and foster care, increased incarceration rates among children of teen parents, and lost tax revenue because of lower educational attainment and income among teen mothers.

- Pregnancy and birth are significant contributors to high school dropout rates among girls. Only about 50 percent of teen mothers receive a high school diploma by 22 years of age, whereas approximately 90 percent of women who do not give birth during adolescence graduate from high school.

- The children of teenage mothers are more likely to have lower school achievement and to drop out of high school, have more health problems, be incarcerated at some time during adolescence, give birth as a teenager, and face unemployment as a young adult.

These effects continue for the teen mother and her child even after adjusting for those factors that increased the teenager's risk for

315

pregnancy, such as growing up in poverty, having parents with low levels of education, growing up in a single-parent family, and having poor performance in school.

Section 28.2

Could I Get Pregnant If...?

This section includes text excerpted from "Could I Get Pregnant If...?" girlshealth.gov, Office on Women's Health (OWH), April 15, 2014. Reviewed November 2017.

"Can I get pregnant if I fooled around with my clothes on?" "Can I get pregnant from kissing?" "Can I get pregnant from oral sex?" We hear lots of questions like these about what causes pregnancy. (And the answers to the questions above are no, no, and no!)

What Causes Pregnancy?

Here are some basic facts of (making) life:

Pregnancy happens when a male's sperm joins with (fertilizes) a female's egg. For you to get pregnant, sperm has to get into your vagina. Sperm can get into your vagina a few different ways.

- **Sperm is in the fluid (sometimes called "ejaculate" or "cum") that spurts out when a guy ejaculates ("comes").** The main way sperm get into the vagina is when a guy ejaculates during sexual intercourse.

- **Sperm also sometimes can get into the vagina in pre-ejaculate ("pre-cum").** This is a little bit of fluid that leaks out during sex before a guy ejaculates. A guy wouldn't know that pre-ejaculate was leaking out. That means you could get pregnant even if he pulls his penis out before he ejaculates.

- **Sperm can get into your vagina even if you're not having sexual intercourse.** This can happen if sperm get on the outside of your vagina and swim inside.

For you to get pregnant, one of your eggs has to be in the right place at the right time. You can read all about how an egg is released during your menstrual cycle and how the female reproductive system works. Keep in mind that:

- It's hard to know exactly when an egg is released, which means that avoiding sex at certain times of the month is not a very reliable way to avoid pregnancy.

- You can get pregnant if you don't have regular periods.

- You can even get pregnant during your period!

What Doesn't Cause Pregnancy?

Kissing, hugging, and rubbing clothed bodies don't cause pregnancy. The only time pregnancy can happen is when sperm can get to an egg.

Of course, touching, and other kinds of fooling around are pretty personal, and they definitely can affect your feelings and relationships even if they can't cause pregnancy. Plus, it can be hard to stop before having sex if you're in the heat of the moment. It's a good idea to think in advance about what you want and don't want to do sexually.

You may have heard lots of rumors about ways to have sex to avoid pregnancy. Make sure you have reliable info. For example, you should know that:

- A plastic bag or wrap **does not** work in place of a condom.

- Jumping up and down after sex **does not** stop sperm from getting to an egg.

- Using certain positions during sex **does not** prevent pregnancy.

Section 28.3

Prenatal Care for Pregnant Teens

This section includes text excerpted from "Prenatal Care,"
Eunice Kennedy Shriver National Institute of Child Health and
Human Development (NICHD), September 2, 2017.

What Is Prenatal Care and Why Is It Important?

Having a healthy pregnancy is one of the best ways to promote a healthy birth. Getting early and regular prenatal care improves the chances of a healthy pregnancy. This care can begin even before pregnancy with a preconception care visit to a healthcare provider.

Preconception Care

A preconception care visit can help women take steps toward a healthy pregnancy before they even get pregnant.

Women can help to promote a healthy pregnancy and birth of a healthy baby by taking the following steps before they become pregnant:

- Develop a plan for their reproductive life.

- Increase their daily intake of folic acid (one of the B vitamins) to at least 400 micrograms.

- Make sure their immunizations are up to date.

- Control diabetes and other medical conditions.

- Avoid smoking, drinking alcohol, and using drugs.

- Attain a healthy weight.

- Learn about their family health history and that of their partner.

- Seek help for depression, anxiety, or other mental health issues.

Prenatal Care

Women who suspect they may be pregnant should schedule a visit to their healthcare provider to begin prenatal care. Prenatal visits to a healthcare provider usually include a physical exam, weight checks, and providing a urine sample. Depending on the stage of the pregnancy, healthcare providers may also do blood tests and imaging tests, such as ultrasound exams. These visits also include discussions about the mother's health, the fetus's health, and any questions about the pregnancy.

Preconception and prenatal care can help prevent complications and inform women about important steps they can take to protect their infant and ensure a healthy pregnancy. With regular prenatal care women can:

- Reduce the risk of pregnancy complications. Following a healthy, safe diet; getting regular exercise as advised by a healthcare provider; and avoiding exposure to potentially harmful substances such as lead and radiation can help reduce the risk for problems during pregnancy and promote fetal health and development. Controlling existing conditions, such as high blood pressure and diabetes, is important to prevent serious complications and their effects.

- Reduce the fetus's and infant's risk for complications. Tobacco smoke and alcohol use during pregnancy have been shown to increase the risk for Sudden Infant Death Syndrome (SIDS). Alcohol use also increases the risk for fetal alcohol spectrum disorders, which can cause a variety of problems such as abnormal facial features, having a small head, poor coordination, poor memory, intellectual disability, and problems with the heart, kidneys, or bones. According to one recent study supported by the National Institutes of Health (NIH), these and other long-term problems can occur even with low levels of prenatal alcohol exposure.

- In addition, taking 400 micrograms of folic acid daily reduces the risk for neural tube defects by 70 percent. Most prenatal vitamins contain the recommended 400 micrograms of folic acid as well as other vitamins that pregnant women and their developing fetus need. Folic acid has been added to foods like cereals, breads, pasta, and other grain-based foods. Although a related form (called folate) is present in orange juice and leafy, green

319

vegetables (such as kale and spinach), folate is not absorbed as well as folic acid.

- Help ensure the medications women take are safe. Women should not take certain medications, including some acne treatments and dietary and herbal supplements, during pregnancy because they can harm the fetus.

Section 28.4

Teen Parents... You're Not Alone!

This section includes text excerpted from "Tip Sheets for Parents and Caregivers," Child Welfare Information Gateway, U.S. Department of Health and Human Services (HHS), March 24, 2016.

Being a parent is a 24-hour-a-day job, and sometimes it can feel overwhelming. You may be juggling the demands of a baby, your family, school, and work. Chances are you're not able to do all of the things you enjoyed before your baby was born.

Many teen parents sometimes feel:

- **Confused and uncertain**—about their future or their skills as a parent
- **Overwhelmed**—they don't know where to begin or they feel like giving up
- **Angry**—at the baby's other parent, their friends, or even their baby
- **Lonely**—as though they are the only person dealing with so many problems
- **Depressed**—sad and unable to manage their problems

These feelings do not mean you are a bad parent!

What You Can Do

Every parent needs support sometimes. If you think stress may be affecting how you treat your baby, it's time to find some help. Try the following:

- **Join a support group.** A group for young moms or dads could give you time with new friends who have lives similar to yours. Your children can play with other children, and you can talk about your problems with people who understand. Look on the Internet (e.g., www.Meetup.com, Yahoo! groups) or call your local social services agency for information about support groups in your community.

- **Find ways to reduce stress.** Take a break while someone reliable cares for your baby. Take a walk with the baby in a stroller, or rest while your baby naps. A social worker or nurse can help you learn other ways to manage stress.

- **Become a regular at baby-friendly places in your community.** The playground and story time at the local library are great places to bond with your baby while getting to know other parents.

- **Finish school.** Even though it may be difficult, finishing high school (or getting a general educational development (GED)) is one of the most important things you can do to help your baby and yourself. A diploma will help you get a better job or take the next step in your education, such as vocational training or college.

- **Improve your parenting skills.** Don't be afraid to ask for advice from experienced parents. Classes for parents can also help you build on what you already know about raising a happy, healthy child.

- **Call a help line.** Most States have helplines for parents. Childhelp® runs a national 24-hour hotline 800-4-A-CHILD (800-422-4453) for parents who need help or parenting advice.

Chapter 29

Lesbian, Gay, Bisexual, and Transgender Youth

Historically, Youth Risk Behavior Survey (YRBS) and other studies have gathered data on lesbian, gay, and bisexual (LGB) youth but have not included questions about transgender and questioning/queer youth. As that changes and data becomes available, this content will be updated to include information regarding transgender and questioning/queer youth.

Most lesbian, gay, bisexual youth are happy and thrive during their adolescent years. Having a school that creates a safe and supportive learning environment for all students and having caring and accepting parents are especially important. Positive environments can help all youth achieve good grades and maintain good mental and physical health. However, some LGB youth are more likely than their heterosexual peers to experience negative health and life outcomes.

For youth to thrive in schools and communities, they need to feel socially, emotionally, and physically safe and supported. A positive school climate has been associated with decreased depression, suicidal feelings, substance use, and unexcused school absences among LGB students.

This chapter includes text excerpted from "Lesbian, Gay, Bisexual, and Transgender Health—LGBT Youth," Centers for Disease Control and Prevention (CDC), June 21, 2017.

Experiences with Violence

Compared with other students, negative attitudes toward LGB persons may put these youth at increased risk for experiences with violence. 'Violence' can include behaviors such as bullying, teasing, harassment, and physical assault.

According to data from the 2015 national Youth Risk Behavior Survey (YRBS), of surveyed LGB students:

- 10 percent were threatened or injured with a weapon on school property

- 34 percent were bullied on school property

- 28 percent were bullied electronically

- 23 percent of LGB students who had dated or went out with someone during the 12 months before the survey had experienced sexual dating violence in the prior year

- 18 percent of LGB students had experienced physical dating violence

- 18 percent of LGB students had been forced to have sexual intercourse at some point in their lives.

Effects on Education and Mental Health

Exposure to violence can have negative effects on the education and health of any young person and may account for some of the health-related disparities between LGB and heterosexual youth. According to the 2015 YRBS, LGB students were 140 percent (12% v. 5%) more likely to not go to school at least one day during the 30 days prior to the survey because of safety concerns, compared with heterosexual students. While not a direct measure of school performance, absenteeism has been linked to low graduation rates, which can have lifelong consequences.

A complex combination of factors can impact youth health outcomes. LGB youth are at greater risk for depression, suicide, substance use, and sexual behaviors that can place them at increased risk for human immunodeficiency virus (HIV) and other sexually transmitted diseases (STDs). Nearly one-third (29%) of LGB youth had attempted suicide at least once in the prior year compared to 6 percent of heterosexual youth. In 2014, young gay and bisexual men accounted for 8 out of 10 HIV diagnoses among youth.

What Schools Can Do

Schools can implement evidence-based policies, procedures, and activities designed to promote a healthy environment for all youth, including LGB students. For example, research has shown that in schools with LGB support groups (such as gay-straight alliances), LGB students were less likely to experience threats of violence, miss school because they felt unsafe, or attempt suicide than those students in schools without LGB support groups. A recent study found that LGB students had fewer suicidal thoughts and attempts when schools had gay-straight alliances and policies prohibiting expression of homophobia in place for 3 or more years.

To help promote health and safety among LGB youth, schools can implement the following policies and practices (with accompanying citations)

- Encourage respect for all students and prohibit bullying, harassment, and violence against all students.

- Identify "safe spaces," such as counselors' offices or designated classrooms, where LGB youth can receive support from administrators, teachers, or other school staff.

- Encourage student-led and student-organized school clubs that promote a safe, welcoming, and accepting school environment (e.g., gay-straight alliances or gender and sexuality alliances, which are school clubs open to youth of all sexual orientations and genders).

- Ensure that health curricula or educational materials include HIV, other STD, and pregnancy prevention information that is relevant to LGB youth (such as ensuring that curricula or materials use language and terminology.

- Provide trainings to school staff on how to create safe and supportive school environments for all students, regardless of sexual orientation or gender identity, and encourage staff to attend these trainings.

- Facilitate access to community-based providers who have experience providing health services, including HIV/STD testing and counseling, social, and psychological services to LGBTQ youth.

What Parents Can Do

Positive parenting practices, such as having honest and open conversations, can help reduce teen health risk behaviors. How parents engage with their LGB teen can have a tremendous impact on their adolescent's current and future mental and physical health. Supportive and accepting parents can help youth cope with the challenges of being an LGB teen. On the other hand, unsupportive parents who react negatively to learning that their daughter or son is LGB can make it harder for their teen to thrive. Parental rejection has been linked to depression, use of drugs and alcohol, and risky sexual behavior among teens.

To be supportive, parents should talk openly and supportively with their teen about any problems or concerns. It is also important for parents to watch for behaviors that might indicate their teen is a victim of bullying or violence, or that their teen may be victimizing others. If bullying, violence, or depression is suspected, parents should take immediate action, working with school personnel and other adults in the community.

Ways Parents Can Influence the Health of Their LGB Youth

More research is needed to better understand the associations between parenting and the health of LGB youth. The following are research-based steps parents can take to support the health and well-being of their LGB teen:

Talk and listen. Parents who talk with and listen to their teen in a way that invites an open discussion about sexual orientation can help their teen feel loved and supported. Parents should have honest conversations with their teens about sex and how to avoid risky behaviors and unsafe situations.

Provide support. Parents who take time to come to terms with how they feel about their teen's sexual orientation will be more able to respond calmly and use respectful language. Parents should develop common goals with their teen, including being healthy and doing well in school.

Stay involved. Parents who make an effort to know their teen's friends and know what their teen is doing can help their teen stay safe and feel cared about.

Be proactive. Parents can access many organizations and online information resources to learn more about how they can support their LGB teen, other family members, and their teen's friends.

Part Four

Common Health Concerns of Teens and Their Parents

Chapter 30

Dealing with Chronic Health Problems

Chronic medical conditions—including cardiovascular disease, cancer, diabetes, and depression—cause more than half of all deaths worldwide.

These long-term diseases affect people of all ages, both rich and poor, in every ethnic group. Many chronic diseases have genetic components, which raise disease risk in certain people or populations. The environment can also contribute to risk, and so can lifestyle choices, including your diet, physical activity, and whether or not you smoke.

Coping with Chronic Illness

Having a long-term, or chronic, illness can disrupt your life in many ways. You may often be tired and in pain. Your illness might affect your appearance or your physical abilities and independence. You may not be able to work, causing financial problems. For children, chronic

This chapter contains text excerpted from the following sources: Text in this chapter begins with excerpts from "Chronic Diseases," National Institutes of Health (NIH), December 13, 2016; Text under the heading "Coping with Chronic Illness" is excerpted from "Coping with Chronic Illness," MedlinePlus, National Institutes of Health (NIH), July 27, 2016; Text under the heading "General Supports for Youth with Chronic Conditions and Disabilities and Their Families" is excerpted from "General Supports for Youth with Chronic Conditions and Disabilities and Their Families," Office of Adolescent Health (OAH), U.S. Department of Health and Human Services (HHS), August 23, 2017.

illnesses can be frightening, because they may not understand why this is happening to them.

These changes can cause stress, anxiety, and anger. If they do, it is important to seek help. A trained counselor can help you develop strategies to regain a feeling of control. Support groups might help, too. You will find that you are not alone, and you may learn some new tips on how to cope.

You may be able to manage your illness better if learn more about it. It is important to evaluate the information that you find, to make sure that it is reliable. It is also important to find a healthcare provider that you can trust.

General Supports for Youth with Chronic Conditions and Disabilities and Their Families

First and foremost, youth with chronic conditions and/or disabilities are still youth. Sometimes, people without disabilities can focus on youth's conditions and minimize that youth with disabilities are still interested and will gain experiences in establishing their identity, building friendships and romantic relationships, and finding their place in the world. These youth benefit from the same mentorship and developmentally-appropriate information as their peers.

All youth with special healthcare needs, regardless of the severity of their condition, benefit from efforts that make it easier for them to get the care they need by helping them navigate complex health and service delivery systems.

Coordination. Coordination of care, involving healthcare providers, teachers, and community resources, can be challenging for adolescents with special healthcare needs and their families. The required time commitment alone is substantial—nearly one of every five adolescents with special healthcare needs has parents who spend at least five hours a week coordinating their care. Furthermore, three quarters of parents of adolescents with special healthcare needs report needing help with coordination of care or services, but only a little more than half of these parents had that need adequately met. Parents must learn to be effective advocates for their adolescents with disabilities, or find an advocate who can help them navigate the policies and bureaucracies related to their adolescent's needs. Some parents hire advocates to help them navigate the complex special education system, but other families don't have the financial resources to do so.

Healthcare transition. Adolescence is full of opportunities and challenges, such as graduating from high school, entering the workforce or starting college, and gaining independence. Making the transition from pediatric to adult healthcare is another task that can be especially difficult for teens with disabilities. Some youth—particularly those with complex conditions or neurological conditions—experience serious gaps in care when they transition to the adult healthcare system.

Youth, their families, and providers may have different perspectives on how transitions are best managed. Issues may include confidentiality, risky behaviors, and health insurance coverage. As noted above, adolescents with disabilities have the same interests and concerns regarding sexuality as their nondisabled peers, and they are equally likely to have had sexual experiences. Healthcare providers can support youth by ensuring that they receive age-appropriate information that is delivered in a way that matches their development.

Often, young people face an assistance "cliff" at age 21 when they lose eligibility for the Early and Periodic Screening, Diagnosis, and Treatment (EPSDT) program, which provides medically necessary services to youth with identified health problems, and for benefits under the Individuals with Disabilities Education Act (IDEA), which funds special education services and supports. These young adults also lose access to services under Title V, which is a federal program that supports families of children with special healthcare needs, especially in coordinating their care. After age 21, these young adults are still covered by the Americans with Disabilities Act (ADA).

However, in contrast with their earlier school experience where parents are the primary advocates, adolescents with disabilities who enter college must assume responsibility for identifying and advocating for their own needs. Beyond the academic setting, additional transition concerns include assuming responsibility for current care; coordinating care; planning for future healthcare; supporting autonomy, personal responsibility, and self-reliance; gaining skills in self-management and knowledge of one's condition; and getting referrals to services.

Chapter 31

Acne

Acne is a disorder that affects the skin's oil glands and hair follicles. Plugged pores and outbreaks of lesions, commonly called pimples or zits, occur on the face, neck, back, chest, and shoulders.

Acne affects the pilosebaceous units (PSUs), found over most of the body. They are most numerous on the face, upper back, and chest. PSUs consist of a sebaceous gland connected to a canal, called a follicle, which contains a fine hair. In healthy PSUs, the sebaceous glands make an oily substance called sebum that empties onto the skin surface through the opening of the follicle, called a pore. Cells called keratinocytes line the follicle.

When someone has acne, the hair, sebum and keratinocytes may plug up the pore, which keeps the sebum from reaching the surface of the skin. The mixture of oil and cells allows bacteria that normally live on the skin to grow in the plugged follicles and cause inflammation—swelling, redness, heat, and pain. When the wall of the plugged follicle breaks down, it spills the bacteria, skin cells and sebum into nearby skin, causing lesions or pimples.

For most people, acne tends to go away by the time they reach their thirties, but some people in their forties and fifties continue to have this skin problem.

This chapter includes text excerpted from "Acne," National Institute of Arthritis and Musculoskeletal and Skin Diseases (NIAMS), January 9, 2016.

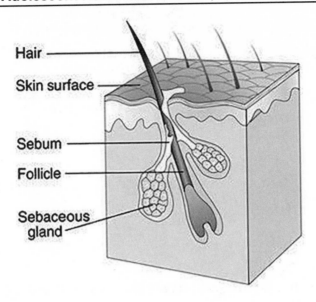

Figure 31.1. *Normal Pilosebaceous Unit*

Who Gets

People of all races and ages get acne, but it is most common in adolescents and young adults. An estimated 80 percent of all people between the ages of 11 and 30 have acne outbreaks at some point.

Types

Acne causes several types of lesions, or pimples.

- **A comedo:** enlarged and plugged hair follicle.

- **A whitehead or closed comedo:** a plugged hair follicle that stays beneath the skin and produces a white bump.

- **A blackhead or open comedo:** a plugged follicle that reaches the surface of the skin and opens up. It looks black on the skin surface because the air discolors the sebum, not because it is dirty.

- **Papules:** inflamed lesions that usually appear as small, pink bumps on the skin and can be tender to the touch.

- **Pustules or pimples:** papules topped by white or yellow pus-filled lesions that may be red at the base.

- **Nodules:** large, painful solid lesions that are lodged deep within the skin.

- **Cysts:** deep, painful, pus-filled lesions that can cause scarring.

Causes

Doctors don't know exactly what causes acne, but it probably results from several related factors. One is an increase in hormones called androgens, or male sex hormones. These increase in both boys and girls during puberty and cause the sebaceous glands to enlarge and make more sebum. Hormonal changes related to pregnancy or starting or stopping birth control pills can also cause acne.

Researchers believe that you may be more likely to get acne if your parents had acne. Certain drugs, including androgens and lithium, can also cause acne. Greasy makeup may alter the cells of the follicles and make them stick together, causing pores to get clogged.

There are many myths about what causes acne. The following do not cause acne:

- Foods you eat, such as chocolate and greasy foods.

- Dirty skin.

- Stress, but if you already have acne, stress can make it worse.

Treatment

Treatment helps heal existing lesions, stop new lesions from forming, and prevent scarring. Medicines can reduce several problems that play a part in causing acne, including abnormal clumping of cells in the follicles, increased oil production, bacteria, and inflammation. A doctor may recommend over-the-counter (OTC) or prescription medicines to take in a pill or apply to the skin.

Some over-the-counter topical medicines, which are applied to the skin, include:

- Benzoyl peroxide, which kills bacteria and may also reduce oil production.

- Resorcinol, which can help break down blackheads and whiteheads.

- Salicylic acid, which helps break down blackheads and whiteheads and also helps reduce the shedding of cells lining the hair follicles.

- Sulfur, which helps break down blackheads and whiteheads.

Topical medicines come in many forms, including gels, lotions, creams, soaps, and pads. In some people, topical medicines may cause side effects such as skin irritation, burning, or redness, which often get better or go away with continued use. If you have severe or prolonged side effects, you should report them to your doctor.

Several types of prescription medicines include:

- Antibiotics, which help slow or stop the growth of bacteria and reduce inflammation.

- Vitamin A derivatives, or retinoids, which unplug existing comedones, allowing other medicines, such as antibiotics, to enter the follicles. Some may also help decrease the formation of comedones.

- Other medicines may destroy bacteria, reduce oil production or reduce inflammation.

Who Treats

Diagnosing and treating acne may involve you and several types of health professionals, including:

- General or family physicians.

- Dermatologists, who specialize in treating skin problems.

- Internists, who specialize in the diagnosis and medical treatment of adults.

- Pediatricians, who diagnose and treat children.

Living With

If you have acne, you may want to follow some of these recommendations for taking care of your skin.

- **Clean your skin gently.** Use a mild cleanser in the morning, in the evening and after heavy exercise. Do not use strong soaps or rough scrub pads. Only use astringents if the skin is very oily, and then only on oily spots.

- **Shampoo your hair regularly.** If you have oily hair, you may want to wash it every day.

- **Avoid rubbing and touching skin lesions.** Squeezing or picking blemishes can cause scars or dark blotches to develop.

- **Shave carefully.** Make sure the blade is sharp, and soften the hair with soap and water before applying shaving cream. Shave gently and only when necessary to reduce the risk of nicking blemishes.

- **Avoid sunburn and suntan.** Many of the medicines used to treat acne can make you more prone to sunburn.

- **Choose cosmetics carefully.** All cosmetics and hair-care products should be oil free. Choose products labeled noncomedogenic, which means they don't clog pores. In some people, however, even these products may make acne worse.

Some things can make acne worse. These include:

- Changing hormone levels in teen girls and adult women two to seven days before their menstrual periods start.

- Oil from skin products (moisturizers or cosmetics) or grease in the work environment (such as a kitchen with fry vats).

- Pressure from sports helmets, tight clothes or backpacks.

- Environmental irritants, such as pollution and high humidity.

- Squeezing or picking at blemishes.

- Scrubbing your skin too hard.

- Stress.

Chapter 32

Allergies in Adolescents

What Is Allergy?

An allergy is a reaction by your immune system to something that does not bother most other people. People who have allergies often are sensitive to more than one thing. Substances that often cause reactions are:

- Pollen

- Dust mites

- Mold spores

- Pet dander

- Food

- Insect stings

- Medicines

Normally, your immune system fights germs. It is your body's defense system. In most allergic reactions, however, it is responding to a false alarm. Genes and the environment probably both play a role.

This chapter contains text excerpted from the following sources: Text under the heading "What Is Allergy?" is excerpted from "Allergy," MedlinePlus, National Institutes of Health (NIH), July 6, 2015; Text beginning with the heading "What's the Problem?" is excerpted from "Allergies," Centers for Disease Control and Prevention (CDC), September 15, 2017.

Allergies can cause a variety of symptoms such as a runny nose, sneezing, itching, rashes, swelling, or asthma. Allergies can range from minor to severe. Anaphylaxis is a severe reaction that can be life-threatening. Doctors use skin and blood tests to diagnose allergies. Treatments include medicines, allergy shots, and avoiding the substances that cause the reactions.

What's the Problem?

Allergies are the 6th leading cause of chronic illness in the United States with an annual cost in excess of $18 billion. More than 50 million Americans suffer from allergies each year. Allergies are an overreaction of the immune system to substances that generally do not affect other individuals. These substances, or allergens, can cause sneezing, coughing, and itching. Allergic reactions range from merely bothersome to life-threatening. Some allergies are seasonal, like hay fever. Allergies have also been associated with chronic conditions like sinusitis and asthma.

Who's at Risk?

Anyone may have or develop an allergy—from a baby born with an allergy to cow's milk, to a child who gets poison ivy, to a senior citizen who develops hives after taking a new medication.

Can It Be Prevented?

Allergies can generally not be prevented but allergic reactions can be. Once a person knows they are allergic to a certain substance, they can avoid contact with the allergen. Strategies for doing this include being in an air conditioned environment during peak hay fever season, avoiding certain foods, and eliminating dust mites and animal dander from the home. They can also control the allergy by reducing or eliminating the symptoms. Strategies include taking medication to counteract reactions or minimize symptoms and being immunized with allergy injection therapy.

The Bottom Line

- The most common allergic diseases include:
  - Hay fever
  - Asthma

- Conjunctivitis
- Hives
- Eczema
- Dermatitis
- Sinusitis
- Food allergies are most prevalent in young children and are frequently outgrown.
- Latex allergies are a reaction to the proteins in latex rubber, a substance used in gloves, condoms, and other products.
- Bees, hornets, wasps, yellow jackets, and fire ants can cause insect sting allergies.
- Allergies to drugs, like penicillin, can affect any tissue or organ in the body.

Anaphylaxis is the most severe allergic reaction. Symptoms include flush; tingling of the palms of the hands, soles of the feet or lips; light headedness, and chest tightness. If not treated, these can progress into seizures, cardiac arrhythmia, shock, and respiratory distress. Anaphylaxis can result in death. Food, latex, insect sting, and drug allergies can all result in anaphylaxis.

Chapter 33

Asthma and Teens

Asthma Facts[1]

Asthma is a leading chronic illness among children and adolescents in the United States. It is also one of the leading causes of school absenteeism. On average, in a classroom of 30 children, about 3 are likely to have asthma. Low-income populations, minorities, and children living in inner cities experience more emergency department visits, hospitalizations, and deaths due to asthma than the general population.

When children and adolescents are exposed to things in the environment—such as dust mites, and tobacco smoke—an asthma episode can occur. These are called asthma triggers. Asthma symptoms can be controlled by avoiding triggers and taking medications prescribed by a healthcare provider, if needed. Asthma is common but treatable; using treatment based on current scientific knowledge reduces illness and future episodes.

What Is Asthma?[2]

Asthma is a chronic (long-term) lung disease that inflames and narrows the airways. Asthma causes recurring periods of wheezing

This chapter includes text excerpted from documents published by two public domain sources. Text under heading marked 1 is excerpted from "Asthma in Schools," Centers for Disease Control and Prevention (CDC), May 9, 2017; Text under headings marked 2 are excerpted from "Asthma," National Heart, Lung, and Blood Institute (NHLBI), August 4, 2014. Reviewed November 2017.

(a whistling sound when you breathe), chest tightness, shortness of breath, and coughing. The coughing often occurs at night or early in the morning.

Asthma affects people of all ages, but it most often starts during childhood. In the United States, more than 25 million people are known to have asthma. About 7 million of these people are children.

To understand asthma, it helps to know how the airways work. The airways are tubes that carry air into and out of your lungs. People who have asthma have inflamed airways. The inflammation makes the airways swollen and very sensitive. The airways tend to react strongly to certain inhaled substances.

When the airways react, the muscles around them tighten. This narrows the airways, causing less air to flow into the lungs. The swelling also can worsen, making the airways even narrower. Cells in the airways might make more mucus than usual. Mucus is a sticky, thick liquid that can further narrow the airways.

This chain reaction can result in asthma symptoms. Symptoms can happen each time the airways are inflamed.

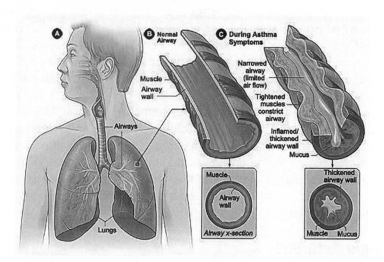

Figure 33.1. *How Asthma Affects Lungs*

Figure A shows the location of the lungs and airways in the body. Figure B shows a cross-section of a normal airway. Figure C shows a cross-section of an airway during asthma symptoms.

Sometimes asthma symptoms are mild and go away on their own or after minimal treatment with asthma medicine. Other times, symptoms continue to get worse.

When symptoms get more intense and/or more symptoms occur, you're having an asthma attack. Asthma attacks also are called flare ups or exacerbations.

Treating symptoms when you first notice them is important. This will help prevent the symptoms from worsening and causing a severe asthma attack. Severe asthma attacks may require emergency care, and they can be fatal.

Managing Asthma in Schools[1]

Asthma-friendly schools are those that make the effort to create safe and supportive learning environments for students with asthma. They have policies and procedures that allow students to successfully manage their asthma. Research and case studies that looked at ways to best manage asthma in schools found that successful school-based asthma programs:

- Establish strong links with asthma care clinicians to ensure appropriate and ongoing medical care.

- Target students who are the most affected by asthma at school to identify and intervene with those in greatest need.

- Get administrative buy-in and build a team of enthusiastic people, including a full-time school nurse, to support the program.

- Use a coordinated, multi-component and collaborative approach that includes school nursing services, asthma education for students and professional development for school staff.

- Provide appropriate school health services for students with asthma, ensuring that students take their medicines and learn to use them when appropriate.

- Provide asthma education for students with asthma and awareness programs for students, school staff, parents, and families.

- Provide a safe and healthy school environment to reduce asthma triggers.

- Offer safe and enjoyable physical education and activities for students with asthma.

- Support evaluation of school-based programs and use adequate and appropriate outcome measures.

Chapter 34

Cancer in Childhood and Adolescence

How Common Is Cancer in Children?

Although cancer in children is rare, it is the leading cause of death by disease past infancy among children in the United States. In 2017, it is estimated that 15,270 children and adolescents ages 0 to 19 years will be diagnosed with cancer and 1,790 will die of the disease in the United States. Among children ages 0 to 14 years, it is estimated that 10,270 will be diagnosed with cancer and 1,190 will die of the disease in 2017.

The most common types of cancer diagnosed in children ages 0 to 14 years in the United States are leukemias, followed by brain and other central nervous system tumors, lymphomas, soft tissue sarcomas (of which half are rhabdomyosarcoma), neuroblastoma, and kidney tumors. The most common types of cancer diagnosed in 15- to 19-year-olds are lymphomas, followed by brain and other central nervous system tumors, leukemias, gonadal (testicular and ovarian) germ cell tumors, thyroid cancer, and melanoma.

As of January 1, 2014 (the most recent date for which data exists), approximately 419,000 survivors of childhood and adolescent cancer (diagnosed at ages 0 to 19 years) were alive in the United States. The

This chapter includes text excerpted from "Cancer in Children and Adolescents," National Cancer Institute (NCI), August 24, 2017.

number of survivors will continue to increase, given that the incidence of childhood cancer has been rising slightly in recent decades and that survival rates overall are improving.

What Is the Outlook for Children with Cancer?

The overall outlook for children with cancer has improved greatly over the last half-century. In 1975, just over 50 percent of children diagnosed with cancer before age 20 years survived at least 5 years. In 2007–2013, 83 percent of children diagnosed with cancer before age 20 years survived at least 5 years.

Although survival rates for most childhood cancers have improved in recent decades, the improvement has been especially dramatic for a few cancers, particularly acute lymphoblastic leukemia, which is the most common childhood cancer. Improved treatments introduced beginning in the 1960s and 1970s raised the 5-year survival rate for children diagnosed with acute lymphoblastic leukemia before age 20 years from less than 10 percent in the 1960s to about 88 percent in 2007–2013. The 5-year survival rate for children diagnosed with non-Hodgkin lymphoma before age 20 years has also increased dramatically, from less than 50 percent in the late 1970s to about 89 percent in 2007–2013.

A notable example of how treatment advances have improved the outlook for children with leukemia is reflected in recent data showing that during 1999–2014, brain cancer replaced leukemia as the leading cause of cancer death among 1- to 19-year-olds.

By contrast, survival rates remain very low for some cancer types, for some age groups, and for some cancers within a site. For example, median survival for children with diffuse intrinsic pontine glioma (a type of brain tumor) is less than 1 year from diagnosis. Among children with Wilms tumor (a type of kidney cancer), older children (those diagnosed between ages 10 and 16 years) have worse 5-year survival rates than younger children. For soft tissue sarcomas, 5-year survival rates in 2007–2013 among children and adolescents ages 0 to 19 years ranged from 65 percent (rhabdomyosarcoma) to 95 percent (chondrosarcoma), but children with sarcomas who present with metastatic disease have much lower 5-year survival rates.

The cancer mortality rate—the number of deaths due to cancer per 100,000 people per year—among children ages 0 to 19 years declined by more than 50 percent from 1975–1977 to 2010–2014. Specifically, the mortality rate was slightly more than 5 per 100,000 children in 1975 and about 2.1 per 100,000 children in 2010–2014. However, despite the overall decrease in mortality, approximately 1,800 children die of cancer each year in the United States, indicating that new advances and continued research to identify effective treatments are required to further reduce childhood cancer mortality.

What Are the Possible Causes of Cancer in Children?

The causes of most childhood cancers are not known. About 5 percent of all cancers in children are caused by an inherited genetic mutation (a mutation that can be passed from parents to their children). For example, 25 percent to 30 percent of cases of retinoblastoma, a cancer of the eye that develops mainly in children, are caused by an inherited mutation in a gene called RB1. However, retinoblastoma accounts for only about 4 percent of all cancers in children ages 0 to 14 years. Inherited mutations associated with certain familial syndromes, such as Li-Fraumeni syndrome, Beckwith-Wiedemann syndrome, Fanconi anemia syndrome, Noonan syndrome, and von Hippel-Lindau syndrome, also increase the risk of childhood cancer.

Genetic mutations that initiate cancer development can also arise during the development of a fetus in the womb. Evidence for this comes from studies of monozygotic (identical) twins in which both twins developed leukemia with an identical leukemia-initiating gene mutation.

Children who have Down syndrome, a genetic condition caused by the presence of an extra copy of chromosome 21, are 10 to 20 times more likely to develop leukemia than children without Down syndrome. However, only a very small proportion of childhood leukemia is linked to Down syndrome.

Most cancers in children, like those in adults, are thought to develop as a result of mutations in genes that lead to uncontrolled cell growth and eventually cancer. In adults, these gene mutations are often the result of exposure to environmental factors, such as cigarette smoke, asbestos, and ultraviolet radiation from the sun. However, environmental causes of childhood cancer have been difficult to identify, partly because cancer in children is rare, and partly because it is difficult to determine what children might have been exposed to early in their development.

Many studies have shown that exposure to ionizing radiation can damage Deoxyribonucleic acid (DNA), which can lead to the development of childhood leukemia and possibly other cancers. For example, children and adolescents who were exposed to radiation from the World War II atomic bomb blasts had an elevated risk of leukemia, and children and adults who were exposed to radiation from accidents at nuclear power plants had an elevated risk for thyroid cancer. Children whose mothers had X-rays during pregnancy (that is, children who were exposed before birth) and children who were exposed after birth to diagnostic medical radiation from computed tomography scans also have an increased risk of some cancers.

Studies of other possible environmental risk factors, including parental exposure to cancer-causing chemicals, prenatal exposure to pesticides, childhood exposure to common infectious agents, and living near a nuclear power plant, have produced mixed results. Whereas some studies have found associations between these factors and risk of some cancers in children, other studies have found no such associations. Higher risks of cancer have not been seen in children who have a parent who was diagnosed with and treated for a childhood cancer that was not caused by an inherited mutation.

How Do Cancers in Adolescents and Young Adults Differ from Those in Younger Children?

Cancer occurs more frequently in adolescents and young adults ages 15 to 39 years than in younger children, although incidence in this group is still much lower than in older adults. According to National Cancer Institute's (NCI) Surveillance, Epidemiology, and End Results (SEER) program, each year in 2010–2014 there were:

- 2 cancer diagnoses per 100,000 children ages 0 to 14 years

- 71 cancer diagnoses per 100,000 adolescents and young adults ages 15 to 39 years

- 1 cancer diagnoses per 100,000 people aged 40 years or older

About 102,130 adolescents and young adults ages 15 to 39 years were diagnosed with cancer in the United States each year in 2010–2014.

Adolescents and young adults are often diagnosed with different types of cancer than either younger children or older adults. For example, adolescents and young adults are more likely than either younger children or older adults to be diagnosed with Hodgkin lymphoma and testicular cancer. However, the incidence of specific cancer types varies widely across the adolescent and young adult age continuum.

The 5-year overall survival rate among adolescents ages 15 to 19 years with cancer exceeded 80 percent in 2007–2013, similar to that among younger children [84% vs 83%]. However, for specific diagnoses, survival is lower for 15- to 19-year-olds than for younger children. For example, the 5-year survival rate for acute lymphoblastic leukemia in

2007–2013 was 91 percent for children younger than 15 years, compared with 74 percent for adolescents ages 15 to 19 years.

Some evidence suggests that adolescents and young adults with acute lymphoblastic leukemia may have better outcomes if they are treated with pediatric treatment regimens than if they receive adult treatment regimens. The improvement in 5-year survival rates for 15- to 19-year-olds with acute lymphoblastic leukemia—from approximately 50 percent in the early 1990s to 74 percent in 2007–2013—may reflect greater use of these pediatric treatment regimens.

Between 1999 and 2014, the cancer death rate dropped the most for 1- to-4-year-olds (26%), followed by that for 15- to 19-year-olds (22%), 10- to 14-year-olds (19%), and 5- to 9-year-olds (14%).

Where Do Children with Cancer Get Treated?

Children who have cancer are often treated at a children's cancer center, which is a hospital or a unit within a hospital that specializes in diagnosing and treating children and adolescents who have cancer. Most children's cancer centers treat patients up to 20 years of age. The health professionals at these centers have specific training and expertise to provide comprehensive care for children, adolescents, and their families.

Children's cancer centers also participate in clinical trials. The improvements in survival for children with cancer that have occurred over the past half century have been achieved because of treatment advances that were studied and proven to be effective in clinical trials.

More than 90 percent of children and adolescents who are diagnosed with cancer each year in the United States are cared for at a children's cancer center that is affiliated with the NCI-supported Children's Oncology Group (COG). COG is the world's largest organization that performs clinical research to improve the care and treatment of children and adolescents with cancer. Each year, approximately 4,000 children who are diagnosed with cancer enroll in a COG-sponsored clinical trial.

Every children's cancer center that participates in COG has met strict standards of excellence for childhood cancer care. A directory of COG locations is available on COG's website. Families can ask their pediatrician or family doctor for a referral to a children's cancer center. Families and health professionals can call NCI's Contact Center at 800-4-CANCER to learn more about children's cancer centers that belong to COG.

If My Child Is Treated at a Children's Cancer Center, Will He or She Automatically Be Part of a Clinical Trial?

No. Participation in a clinical trial is voluntary, and it is up to each family to decide if clinical trial participation is right for their child.

What Should Survivors of Childhood Cancer Consider after They Complete Treatment?

Survivors of childhood cancer need follow-up care and enhanced medical surveillance for the rest of their lives because of the risk of complications that can occur many years after they complete treatment for their cancer. Health problems that develop months or years after treatment has ended are known as late effects.

Long-term follow-up analysis of a cohort of survivors of childhood cancer treated between 1970 and 1986 has shown that cancer survivors remain at risk of complications and premature death as they age, with more than half of survivors having experienced a severe or disabling complication or even death by the time they reach age 50 years. Children treated in more recent decades may have lower risks of late complication or mortality due to modifications in treatment regimens to reduce exposures to radiotherapy and chemotherapy, increased efforts to detect late effects as early as possible, and improvements in medical care for late effects of therapy.

The specific late effects that a person who was treated for childhood cancer might experience depend on the type and location of his or her cancer, the type of treatment he or she received, and patient-related factors, such as age at diagnosis.

Children who were treated for bone cancer, brain tumors, and Hodgkin lymphoma, or who received radiation to their chest, abdomen, or pelvis, have the highest risk of serious late effects from their cancer treatment, including second cancers, joint replacement, hearing loss, and congestive heart failure.

It's important for childhood cancer survivors to have regular medical follow-up examinations so any health problems that occur can be identified and treated as soon as possible. The Children's Oncology Group (COG) has developed long-term follow-up guidelines for survivors of childhood, adolescent, and young adult cancers.

It is also important to keep a record of the cancer treatment that someone received as a child. This record should include:

- The type and stage of cancer

- Date of diagnosis and dates of any relapses

- Types and dates of imaging tests
- Contact information for the hospitals and doctors who provided treatment
- Names and total doses of all chemotherapy drugs used in treatment
- The parts of the body that were treated with radiation and the total doses of radiation that were given
- Types and dates of all surgeries
- Any other cancer treatments received
- Any serious complications that occurred during treatment and how those complications were treated
- The date that cancer treatment was completed

The record should be kept in a safe place, and copies of the record should be given to all doctors or other healthcare providers who are involved with the child's follow-up care, even as the child grows into adulthood.

Many children's cancer centers have follow-up clinics where survivors of childhood cancer can go for follow-up until they reach their early 20s. Some cancer centers are now creating clinics dedicated to follow-up care for long-term survivors of pediatric and adolescent cancers.

Chapter 35

Diabetes in Children and Teens

What Is Diabetes?[1]

Diabetes is a disease that occurs when your blood glucose, also called blood sugar, is too high. Blood glucose is your main source of energy and comes from the food you eat. Insulin, a hormone made by the pancreas, helps glucose from food get into your cells to be used for energy. Sometimes your body doesn't make enough—or any—insulin or doesn't use insulin well. Glucose then stays in your blood and doesn't reach your cells.

Over time, having too much glucose in your blood can cause health problems. Although diabetes has no cure, you can take steps to manage your diabetes and stay healthy.

Sometimes people call diabetes "a touch of sugar" or "borderline diabetes." These terms suggest that someone doesn't really have diabetes or has a less serious case, but every case of diabetes is serious.

This chapter includes text excerpted from documents published by two public domain sources. Text under headings marked 1 are excerpted from "What Is Diabetes?" National Institute of Diabetes and Digestive and Kidney Diseases (NIDDK), November 2016; Text under heading marked 2 is excerpted from "Diabetes in Children and Teens," MedlinePlus, National Institutes of Health (NIH), June 30, 2016.

What Are the Different Types of Diabetes?[1]

The most common types of diabetes are type 1, type 2, and gestational diabetes.

Type 1 Diabetes

If you have type 1 diabetes, your body does not make insulin. Your immune system attacks and destroys the cells in your pancreas that make insulin. Type 1 diabetes is usually diagnosed in children and young adults, although it can appear at any age. People with type 1 diabetes need to take insulin every day to stay alive.

Type 2 Diabetes

If you have type 2 diabetes, your body does not make or use insulin well. You can develop type 2 diabetes at any age, even during childhood. However, this type of diabetes occurs most often in middle-aged and older people. Type 2 is the most common type of diabetes.

Gestational Diabetes

Gestational diabetes develops in some women when they are pregnant. Most of the time, this type of diabetes goes away after the baby is born. However, if you've had gestational diabetes, you have a greater chance of developing type 2 diabetes later in life. Sometimes diabetes diagnosed during pregnancy is actually type 2 diabetes.

Other Types of Diabetes

Less common types include monogenic diabetes, which is an inherited form of diabetes, and cystic fibrosis-related diabetes.

Diabetes in Children and Teens[2]

The common type of diabetes in children and teens used to be type 1. It was called juvenile diabetes. With Type 1 diabetes, the pancreas does not make insulin. Insulin is a hormone that helps glucose, or sugar, get into your cells to give them energy. Without insulin, too much sugar stays in the blood.

But now younger people are also getting type 2 diabetes. Type 2 diabetes used to be called adult-onset diabetes. But now it is becoming more common in children and teens, due to more obesity. With type 2 diabetes, the body does not make or use insulin well.

Children have a higher risk of type 2 diabetes if they are obese, have a family history of diabetes, or are not active, and do not eat well. To lower the risk of type 2 diabetes in children:

- Have them maintain a healthy weight.

- Be sure they are physically active.

- Have them eat smaller portions of healthy foods.

- Limit time with the TV, computer, and video.

Children and teens with type 1 diabetes may need to take insulin. Type 2 diabetes may be controlled with diet and exercise. If not, patients will need to take oral diabetes medicines or insulin. A blood test called the A1C can check on how you are managing your diabetes.

How Common Is Diabetes?[1]

As of 2015, 30.3 million people in the United States, or 9.4 percent of the population, had diabetes. More than 1 in 4 of them didn't know they had the disease. Diabetes affects 1 in 4 people over the age of 65. About 90–95 percent of cases in adults are type 2 diabetes.

Who Is More Likely to Develop Type 2 Diabetes?[1]

You are more likely to develop type 2 diabetes if you are age 45 or older, have a family history of diabetes, or are overweight. Physical inactivity, race, and certain health problems such as high blood pressure also affect your chance of developing type 2 diabetes. You are also more likely to develop type 2 diabetes if you have prediabetes or had gestational diabetes when you were pregnant.

What Health Problems Can People with Diabetes Develop?[1]

Over time, high blood glucose leads to problems such as:

- heart disease

- stroke

- kidney disease

- eye problems

- dental disease

- nerve damage

- foot problems

You can take steps to lower your chances of developing these diabetes-related health problems.

Chapter 36

Growing Concerns

Chapter Contents

Section 36.1—Growing Pains 360

Section 36.2—Common Growth Disorders 363

Section 36.1

Growing Pains

"Growing Pains," © 2017 Omnigraphics.
Reviewed November 2017.

What Are Growing Pains?

"Growing pains" is the term used to describe a benign ache or throbbing in the legs commonly experienced by preschool- and school-age children. The condition generally affects kids between the ages of 3 and 4 and those from 8 to 12, and statistics show that at least 10 to 35 percent of children go through this pain at least once during childhood. Both boys and girls can suffer from growing pains, but the condition is seen slightly more often in girls.

Symptoms

The symptoms of growing pains differ for each child and can range from mild to severe, from infrequent to everyday, and can last from months to years. Some common symptoms of growing pains include:

- The pain appears in both legs.

- Pain in the muscles rather than the joints, usually in the calves, behind the thighs or knees, and in the shins.

- It often occurs late in the afternoon or at night and fades away in the morning.

- The intensity of pain may sometimes wake a child from his or her sleep.

- Stiffness can accompany the pain.

- Some children may also be susceptible to headaches or abdominal pains.

The following symptoms require the attention of a healthcare provider, since they can indicate a more serious problem:

- The pain persists for a long period.

- It does not diminish in the morning.

- The pain affects the joint and not the muscle.

- Symptoms interfere with the child's normal activities.

- Unusual rashes develop.

- The pain only affects one limb.

- The symptoms are accompanied by swelling in the legs, loss of appetite, fever, and fatigue.

Causes and Risk Factors

It was once believed that these pains were linked to the faster growth of bones in comparison with the growth of tendons. However, we now know that growing pains are not related to the process of growing at all. However, despite the new understanding, the name "growing pains" remains the common term for the condition. To date, no single specific cause for growing pains has been identified. One study suggests that children with less bone strength may experience growing pains. In some cases, it's possible that increased physical activity, such as running, jumping, and climbing, may cause the pain. In addition, some studies have linked growing pains to restless leg syndrome.

Diagnosis

To diagnose growing pains, a healthcare provider will generally ask a number of questions regarding the symptoms and medical history of the child and will conduct a physical examination. The healthcare provider will rule out other possible reasons for the symptoms before diagnosing the condition as growing pains. For example, since growing pains usually affect both legs, the problem might not be the same if the pain is only in one leg, and it does not fade by morning, and an alternative diagnosis may be necessary.

One method growing pains can be differentiated from other types of pain is by the way a child reacts to touch during the examination. Generally, a child experiencing growing pains will feel better when the area is massaged, whereas many other kinds of pain will increase when touched. In a few cases, blood tests or X-rays may help doctors with a diagnosis.

Treatment

There is no specific treatment for growing pains, and it generally subsides on its own, usually within one or two years. The healthcare provider will likely help the parents of the child understand that growing pain is not a serious condition, and ask the parents to follow certain steps to ease the child's discomfort. These steps may include:

- **Massage.** Massaging the affected area may help reduce the pain.

- **Heat treatment.** A heating pad can provide relief for aching muscles.

- **Stretching.** Stretching the legs may help ease some of the pain.

- **Medication.** The healthcare provider might prescribe ibuprofen, naproxen, or acetaminophen for pain. Aspirin should be avoided for young children, since it may increase the risk of a condition called Reye syndrome, which could be life threatening.

Growing pains are generally not serious, and most children outgrow the condition over time. However, proper management of the pain can help relieve the trauma of recurring pain, which can be upsetting to children.

References

1. "Growing Pains," Cleveland Clinic, n.d.

2. "Growing Pains," KidsHealth, June 2015.

3. "Growing Pains," WebMD, July 28, 2016.

4. "Patient Care & Health Information: Growing Pains," Mayo Clinic, August 19, 2016.

Section 36.2

Common Growth Disorders

This section contains text excerpted from the following sources:
Text in this section begins with excerpts from "Growth Disorders,"
MedlinePlus, National Institutes of Health (NIH), November 30,
2016; Text under the heading "Growth Hormone Deficiency" is
excerpted from "Growth Hormone Deficiency," Genetic and
Rate Diseases Information Center (GARD), U.S. Department of
Health and Human Services (HHS), June 3, 2016; Text
under the heading "Endocrine Diseases," is excerpted
from "Endocrine Diseases," MedlinePlus, National
Institutes of Health (NIH). September 27, 2017.

Does your child seem much shorter—or much taller—than other
kids his or her age? It could be normal. Some children may be small
for their age but still be developing normally. Some children are short
or tall because their parents are.

But some children have growth disorders. Growth disorders are
problems that prevent children from developing normal height, weight,
sexual maturity or other features.

Very slow or very fast growth can sometimes signal a gland problem
or disease.

The pituitary gland makes growth hormone, which stimulates the
growth of bone and other tissues. Children who have too little of it may
be very short. Treatment with growth hormone can stimulate growth.

People can also have too much growth hormone. Usually the cause
is a pituitary gland tumor, which is not cancer. Too much growth hormone can cause gigantism in children, where their bones and their
body grow too much. In adults, it can cause acromegaly, which makes
the hands, feet and face larger than normal. Possible treatments
include surgery to remove the tumor, medicines, and radiation therapy.

Growth Hormone Deficiency

Growth hormone deficiency (GHD) is characterized by abnormally
short height due to lack (or shortage) of growth hormone. It can be
congenital (present at birth) or acquired. Most cases are identified in

children. Although it is uncommon, growth hormone deficiency may also be diagnosed in adults. Too little growth hormone can cause short stature in children, and changes in muscle mass, cholesterol levels, and bone strength in adults. Most of the time, no single clear cause can be identified but several genetic causes of GHD have been described, such as mutations in the to POU1F1/Pit1, PROP1 GHRH, and GH1 genes. In adolescents, puberty may be delayed or absent. Treatment involves growth hormone injections.

Endocrine Diseases

Your endocrine system includes eight major glands throughout your body. These glands make hormones. Hormones are chemical messengers. They travel through your bloodstream to tissues or organs. Hormones work slowly and affect body processes from head to toe. These include:

- Growth and development
- Metabolism—digestion, elimination, breathing, blood circulation and maintaining body temperature
- Sexual function
- Reproduction
- Mood

If your hormone levels are too high or too low, you may have a hormone disorder. Hormone diseases also occur if your body does not respond to hormones the way it is supposed to. Stress, infection and changes in your blood's fluid and electrolyte balance can also influence hormone levels.

In the United States, the most common endocrine disease is diabetes. There are many others. They are usually treated by controlling how much hormone your body makes. Hormone supplements can help if the problem is too little of a hormone.

Chapter 37

Juvenile Arthritis

Juvenile arthritis is the term used to describe arthritis in children. Children can get arthritis just like adults. Arthritis is caused by inflammation of the joints. A joint is where two or more bones are joined together. Arthritis causes:

- Pain
- Swelling
- Stiffness
- Loss of motion

The most common type of arthritis in children is called juvenile idiopathic arthritis (idiopathic means "from unknown causes"). There are several other forms of arthritis affecting children.

Juvenile arthritis is a rheumatic disease, or one that causes loss of function due to an inflamed supporting structure or structures of the body. Some rheumatic diseases also can involve internal organs.

Who Gets It?

Juvenile arthritis affects children of all ages and ethnic backgrounds. About 294,000 American children under age 18 have arthritis or other rheumatic conditions.

This chapter includes text excerpted from "Juvenile Arthritis," National Institute of Arthritis and Musculoskeletal and Skin Diseases (NIAMS), June 30, 2015.

What Are the Symptoms?

The most common symptoms of juvenile arthritis are joint swelling, pain, and stiffness that don't go away. Usually it affects the knees, hands, and feet, and it's worse in the morning or after a nap. Other signs can include:

- Limping in the morning because of a stiff knee

- Excessive clumsiness

- High fever and skin rash

- Swelling in lymph nodes in the neck and other parts of the body

Most children with arthritis have times when the symptoms get better or go away (remission) and other times when they get worse (flare).

What Causes It?

Scientists are looking for the possible causes of juvenile arthritis. They are studying both genetic and environmental factors that they think are involved.

Juvenile arthritis is usually an autoimmune disorder. A healthy immune system helps a person fight off harmful bacteria and viruses. But in an autoimmune disorder, the immune system attacks some of the body's own healthy cells and tissues.

Scientists don't know why this happens or what causes the disorder in children. Some think that something in a child's genes (passed from parents to children) makes the child more likely to get arthritis, and then something else, such as a virus, sets off the arthritis.

Is There a Test?

There is no easy way a doctor can tell if a child has juvenile arthritis. Doctors usually suspect arthritis when a child has symptoms of:

- Constant joint pain or swelling

- Skin rashes that can't be explained

- Fever along with swelling of lymph nodes or inflammation in the body's organs

To be sure that it is juvenile arthritis, doctors may:

- Perform a physical exam

- Ask about family health history
- Order lab or blood tests
- Order X-rays

How Is It Treated?

Doctors who treat arthritis in children will try to make sure your child can remain physically active. They also try to make sure your child can stay involved in social activities and have an overall good quality of life.

Doctors can prescribe treatments to reduce swelling, maintain joint movement, and relieve pain. They also try to prevent, identify, and treat problems that result from the arthritis. Most children with arthritis need a blend of treatments—some treatments include medicines.

Chapter 38

Infections Often Spread in Schools

Chapter Contents

Section 38.1—Preventing Influenza in Schools.......................... 370

Section 38.2—Meningococcal Infection on Campus.................. 375

Section 38.3—Staphylococcal Infections in Teens.................... 380

Section 38.4—Mononucleosis 386

Section 38.1

Preventing Influenza in Schools

This section contains text excerpted from the following sources: Text
beginning with the heading "What Is Influenza (Flu)?" is excerpted
from "Key Facts about Influenza (Flu)," Centers for Disease Control
and Prevention (CDC), August 25, 2016; Text under the heading
"How to Clean and Disinfect Schools to Help Slow the Spread of Flu"
is excerpted from "How to Clean and Disinfect Schools to
Help Slow the Spread of Flu," Centers for Disease Control
and Prevention (CDC), October 5, 2016.

What Is Influenza (Flu)?

The flu is a contagious respiratory illness caused by influenza
viruses that infect the nose, throat, and sometimes the lungs. It can
cause mild to severe illness, and at times can lead to death. The best
way to prevent the flu is by getting a flu vaccine each year.

Signs and Symptoms of Flu

People who have the flu often feel some or all of these signs and
symptoms that usually start suddenly, not gradually:

- Fever* or feeling feverish/chills

- Cough

- Sore throat

- Runny or stuffy nose

- Muscle or body aches

- Headaches

- Fatigue (very tired)

- Some people may have vomiting and diarrhea, though this is
  more common in young children than in adults

It's important to note that not everyone with flu will have a fever.

How Flu Spreads

Most experts believe that flu viruses spread mainly by tiny droplets made when people with flu cough, sneeze or talk. These droplets can land in the mouths or noses of people who are nearby. Less often, a person might also get flu by touching a surface or object that has flu virus on it and then touching their own mouth, nose, or possibly their eyes.

Period of Contagiousness

You may be able to pass on the flu to someone else before you know you are sick, as well as while you are sick. Although people with the flu are most contagious in the first 3–4 days after their illness begins, some otherwise healthy adults may be able to infect others beginning 1 day before symptoms develop and up to 5 to 7 days after becoming sick. Some people, especially young children and people with weakened immune systems, might be able to infect others with flu viruses for an even longer time.

Onset of Symptoms

The time from when a person is exposed to flu virus and infected to when symptoms begin is about 1 to 4 days, with an average of about 2 days.

Complications of Flu

Complications of flu can include bacterial pneumonia, ear infections, sinus infections, and worsening of chronic medical conditions, such as congestive heart failure, asthma, or diabetes.

People at High Risk from Flu

Anyone can get the flu (even healthy people), and serious problems related to the flu can happen at any age, but some people are at high risk of developing serious flu-related complications if they get sick. This includes people 65 years and older, people of any age with certain chronic medical conditions (such as asthma, diabetes, or heart disease), pregnant women, and young children.

Preventing Seasonal Flu

The first and most important step in preventing flu is to get a flu vaccination each year. Centers for Disease Control and Prevention

(CDC) also recommends everyday preventive actions (like staying away from people who are sick, covering coughs and sneezes and frequent handwashing) to help slow the spread of germs that cause respiratory (nose, throat, and lungs) illnesses, like flu.

Diagnosing Flu

It is very difficult to distinguish the flu from other viral or bacterial causes of respiratory illnesses on the basis of symptoms alone. There are tests available to diagnose flu.

How to Clean and Disinfect Schools to Help Slow the Spread of Flu

Cleaning and disinfecting are part of a broad approach to preventing infectious diseases in schools. To help slow the spread of influenza (flu), the first line of defense is getting vaccinated. Other measures include staying home when sick, covering coughs and sneezes, and washing hands often. Below are tips on how to slow the spread of flu specifically through cleaning and disinfecting.

Cleaning removes germs, dirt, and impurities from surfaces or objects. Cleaning works by using soap (or detergent) and water to physically remove germs from surfaces. This process does not necessarily kill germs, but by removing them, it lowers their numbers and the risk of spreading infection.

Disinfecting kills germs on surfaces or objects. Disinfecting works by using chemicals to kill germs on surfaces or objects. This process does not necessarily clean dirty surfaces or remove germs, but by killing germs on a surface after cleaning, it can further lower the risk of spreading infection.

Sanitizing lowers the number of germs on surfaces or objects to a safe level, as judged by public health standards or requirements. This process works by either cleaning or disinfecting surfaces or objects to lower the risk of spreading infection.

Clean and Disinfect Surfaces and Objects That Are Touched Often

Follow your school's standard procedures for routine cleaning and disinfecting. Typically, this means daily sanitizing surfaces and objects that are touched often, such as desks, countertops, doorknobs, computer keyboards, hands-on learning items, faucet handles, phones, and toys. Some schools may also require daily disinfecting these items. Standard procedures often call for disinfecting specific areas of the school, like bathrooms.

Immediately clean surfaces and objects that are visibly soiled. If surfaces or objects are soiled with body fluids or blood, use gloves and other standard precautions to avoid coming into contact with the fluid. Remove the spill, and then clean and disinfect the surface.

Simply Do Routine Cleaning and Disinfecting

It is important to match your cleaning and disinfecting activities to the types of germs you want to remove or kill. Most studies have shown that the flu virus can live and potentially infect a person for up to 48 hours after being deposited on a surface. However, it is not necessary to close schools to clean or disinfect every surface in the building to slow the spread of flu. Also, if students and staff are dismissed because the school cannot function normally (e.g., high absenteeism during a flu outbreak), it is not necessary to do extra cleaning and disinfecting.

Flu viruses are relatively fragile, so standard cleaning and disinfecting practices are sufficient to remove or kill them. Special cleaning and disinfecting processes, including wiping down walls and ceilings, frequently using room air deodorizers, and fumigating, are not necessary or recommended. These processes can irritate eyes, noses, throats, and skin; aggravate asthma; and cause other serious side effects.

Clean and Disinfect Correctly

Always follow label directions on cleaning products and disinfectants. Wash surfaces with a general household cleaner to remove germs. Rinse with water, and follow with an U.S. Environmental Protection Agency (EPA)-registered disinfectant to kill germs. Read the label to make sure it states that EPA has approved the product for effectiveness against influenza A virus.

If a surface is not visibly dirty, you can clean it with an EPA-registered product that both cleans (removes germs) and disinfects (kills germs) instead. Be sure to read the label directions carefully, as there may be a separate procedure for using the product as a cleaner or as a disinfectant. Disinfection usually requires the product to remain on the surface for a certain period of time (e.g., letting it stand for 3 to 5 minutes).

Use disinfecting wipes on electronic items that are touched often, such as phones and computers. Pay close attention to the directions for using disinfecting wipes. It may be necessary to use more than one wipe to keep the surface wet for the stated length of contact time. Make sure that the electronics can withstand the use of liquids for cleaning and disinfecting.

Use Products Safely

Pay close attention to hazard warnings and directions on product labels. Cleaning products and disinfectants often call for the use of gloves or eye protection. For example, gloves should always be worn to protect your hands when working with bleach solutions.

Do not mix cleaners and disinfectants unless the labels indicate it is safe to do so. Combining certain products (such as chlorine bleach and ammonia cleaners) can result in serious injury or death.

Ensure that custodial staff, teachers, and others who use cleaners and disinfectants read and understand all instruction labels and understand safe and appropriate use. This might require that instructional materials and training be provided in other languages.

Handle Waste Properly

Follow your school's standard procedures for handling waste, which may include wearing gloves. Place no-touch waste baskets where they are easy to use. Throw disposable items used to clean surfaces and items in the trash immediately after use. Avoid touching used tissues and other waste when emptying waste baskets. Wash your hands with soap and water after emptying waste baskets and touching used tissues and similar waste.

Section 38.2

Meningococcal Infection on Campus

This section includes text excerpted from "Meningococcal," Centers
for Disease Control and Prevention (CDC), March 28, 2017.

Meningococcal disease can refer to any illness caused by the type
of bacteria called Neisseria meningitidis, also known as meningococcus. These illnesses are often severe and can be deadly. They include
infections of the lining of the brain and spinal cord (meningitis) and
bloodstream infections (bacteremia or septicemia).

These bacteria spread through the exchange of respiratory and
throat secretions like spit (e.g., by living in close quarters, kissing).
Doctors treat meningococcal disease with antibiotics, but quick medical attention is extremely important. Keeping up to date with recommended vaccines is the best defense against meningococcal disease.

Risk Factors

Certain people are at increased risk for meningococcal disease.
Some risk factors include:

- **Age**

  - Doctors more commonly diagnose meningococcal disease in
    infants, teens, and young adults.

- **Community setting**

  - Infectious diseases tend to spread wherever large groups
    of people gather together. Several college campuses have
    reported outbreaks of serogroup B meningococcal disease
    during the last several years.

- **Certain medical conditions**

  - Certain medical conditions and medications put people at
    increased risk of meningococcal disease. They include not
    having a spleen, having a complement component deficiency,
    and being infected with HIV.

- **Travel**
  - Travelers to the meningitis belt in sub-Saharan Africa may be at risk for meningococcal disease.

Causes and How It Spread to Others

Causes

Bacteria called Neisseria meningitidis cause meningococcal disease. About 1 in 10 people have these bacteria in the back of their nose and throat with no signs or symptoms of disease; this is called being 'a carrier'. But sometimes the bacteria invade the body and cause certain illnesses, which are known as meningococcal disease.

There are five serogroups (types) of Neisseria meningitidis—A, B, C, W, and Y—that cause most disease worldwide. Three of these serogroups (B, C, and Y) cause most of the illness seen in the United States.

How It Spread to Others

People spread meningococcal bacteria to other people by sharing respiratory and throat secretions (saliva or spit). Generally, it takes close (for example, coughing or kissing) or lengthy contact to spread these bacteria. Fortunately, they are not as contagious as germs that cause the common cold or the flu. People do not catch them through casual contact or by breathing air where someone with meningococcal disease has been.

Sometimes the bacteria spread to people who have had close or lengthy contact with a patient with meningococcal disease. Those at increased risk of getting sick include:

- People who live with the patient
- Anyone with direct contact with the patient's oral secretions, such as a boyfriend or girlfriend

Close contacts of someone with meningococcal disease should receive antibiotics to help prevent them from getting the disease. This is known as prophylaxis. Health departments investigate each case of meningococcal disease to identify all close contacts and make sure they receive prophylaxis. This does not mean that the contacts have the disease; it is to prevent it. People who are not a close contact of a patient with meningococcal disease do not need prophylaxis.

Signs and Symptoms

Seek medical attention immediately if you or your child develops symptoms of meningococcal disease. Symptoms of meningococcal disease can first appear as a flu-like illness and rapidly worsen. The two most common types of meningococcal infections are meningitis and septicemia. Both of these types of infections are very serious and can be deadly in a matter of hours.

Meningococcal Meningitis

Doctors call meningitis caused by the bacteria Neisseria meningitidis meningococcal meningitis. When someone has meningococcal meningitis, the bacteria infect the protective membranes covering their brain and spinal cord and cause swelling.

The most common symptoms include:

- Fever
- Headache
- Stiff neck

There are often additional symptoms, such as:

- Nausea
- Vomiting
- Photophobia (eyes being more sensitive to light)
- Altered mental status (confusion)

Newborns and babies may not have or it may be difficult to notice the classic symptoms of fever, headache, and neck stiffness. Instead, babies may be slow or inactive, irritable, vomiting, or feeding poorly. In young children, doctors may also look at the child's reflexes for signs of meningitis.

If you think you or your child has any of these symptoms, call the doctor right away.

Meningococcal Septicemia (aka Meningococcemia)

Doctors call septicemia (a bloodstream infection) caused by Neisseria meningitidis meningococcal septicemia or meningococcemia. When someone has meningococcal septicemia, the bacteria enter the bloodstream and multiply, damaging the walls of the blood vessels. This causes bleeding into the skin and organs.

377

Symptoms may include:

- Fever

- Fatigue

- Vomiting

- Cold hands and feet

- Cold chills

- Severe aches or pain in the muscles, joints, chest or abdomen (belly)

- Rapid breathing

- Diarrhea

- In the later stages, a dark purple rash

Diagnosis, Treatment, and Complications

Meningococcal disease is very serious and can be deadly in a matter of hours. Early diagnosis and treatment are very important.

Diagnosis

Meningococcal disease can be difficult to diagnose because the signs and symptoms are often similar to those of other illnesses. If a doctor suspects meningococcal disease, they will collect samples of blood or cerebrospinal fluid (fluid near the spinal cord; see image below). Doctors then test the samples to see if there is an infection and, if so, what germ is causing it. If Neisseria meningitidis bacteria are in the samples, laboratorians can grow (culture) the bacteria. Growing the bacteria in the laboratory allows doctors to know the specific type of bacteria that is causing the infection. Knowing this helps doctors decide which antibiotic will work best. Other tests can sometimes detect and identify the bacteria if the cultures do not.

Treatment

Doctors treat meningococcal disease with a number of effective antibiotics. It is important that treatment start as soon as possible. If a doctor suspects meningococcal disease, they will give the patient antibiotics right away. Antibiotics help reduce the risk of dying.

Depending on how serious the infection is, people with meningococcal disease may need other treatments, including:

- Breathing support
- Medications to treat low blood pressure
- Wound care for parts of the body with damaged skin

Complications

Even with antibiotic treatment, 10 to 15 in 100 people infected with meningococcal disease will die. About 11 to 19 in 100 survivors will have long-term disabilities, such as loss of limb(s), deafness, nervous system problems, or brain damage.

Prevention

Keeping up to date with recommended immunizations is the best defense against meningococcal disease. Maintaining healthy habits, like getting plenty of rest and not having close contact with people who are sick, also helps.

Vaccination

Vaccines help protect against all three serogroups (B, C, and Y) of Neisseria meningitidis bacteria commonly seen in the United States. Like with any vaccine, meningococcal vaccines are not 100% effective. This means there is still a chance you can develop meningococcal disease after vaccination. People should know the symptoms of meningococcal disease since early recognition and quick medical attention are extremely important.

Antibiotics

Close contacts of a person with meningococcal disease should receive antibiotics to prevent them from getting sick. This is known as prophylaxis. Examples of close contacts include:

- People in the same household or roommates
- Anyone with direct contact with a patient's oral secretions (saliva or spit), such as a boyfriend or girlfriend

Doctors or local health departments recommend who should get prophylaxis

Re-Infection

Although rare, people can get meningococcal disease more than once. A previous infection will not offer lifelong protection from future infections. Therefore, Centers for Disease Control and Prevention (CDC) recommends meningococcal vaccines for all preteens and teens. In certain situations, children and adults should also get meningococcal vaccines.

Section 38.3

Staphylococcal Infections in Teens

This section contains text excerpted from the following sources: Text in this section begins with excerpts from "Staphylococcal Infections," MedlinePlus, National Institutes of Health (NIH), August 25, 2016; Text beginning with the heading "General Information about MRSA in the Community" is excerpted from "General Information about MRSA in the Community," Centers for Disease Control and Prevention (CDC), February 9, 2016; Text beginning with the heading "Steps to Take If You Think a Student Might Have a Skin Infection" is excerpted from "Information and Advice about MRSA for School and Daycare Officials," Centers for Disease Control and Prevention (CDC), February 3, 2016; Text under the heading "What Should a Person Do If a Family Member or Close Friend Staphylococcal Infection?" is excerpted from "General Information about VISA/VRSA," Centers for Disease Control and Prevention (CDC), July 21, 2015.

Staph is short for Staphylococcus, a type of bacteria. There are over 30 types, but *Staphylococcus aureus* causes most staph infections (pronounced "staff infections"), including:

- Skin infections

- Pneumonia

- Food poisoning

- Toxic shock syndrome

- Blood poisoning (bacteremia)

Skin infections are the most common. They can look like pimples or boils. They may be red, swollen and painful, and sometimes have pus or other drainage. They can turn into impetigo, which turns into a crust on the skin, or cellulitis, a swollen, red area of skin that feels hot.

Anyone can get a staph skin infection. You are more likely to get one if you have a cut or scratch, or have contact with a person or surface that has staph bacteria. The best way to prevent staph is to keep hands and wounds clean. Most staph skin infections are easily treated with antibiotics or by draining the infection. Some staph bacteria such as MRSA (methicillin-resistant *Staphylococcus aureus*) are resistant to certain antibiotics, making infections harder to treat.

General Information about MRSA in the Community

MRSA is methicillin-resistant *Staphylococcus aureus*, a type of staph bacteria that is resistant to several antibiotics. In the general community, MRSA most often causes skin infections. In some cases, it causes pneumonia (lung infection) and other issues. If left untreated, MRSA infections can become severe and cause sepsis—a life-threatening reaction to severe infection in the body.

In a healthcare setting, such as a hospital or nursing home, MRSA can cause severe problems such as bloodstream infections, pneumonia and surgical site infections.

Who Is at Risk, and How Is MRSA Spread in the Community?

Anyone can get MRSA on their body from contact with an infected wound or by sharing personal items, such as towels or razors, that have touched infected skin. MRSA infection risk can be increased when a person is in activities or places that involve crowding, skin-to-skin contact, and shared equipment or supplies. People including athletes, daycare and school students, military personnel in barracks, and those who recently received inpatient medical care are at higher risk.

How Common Is MRSA?

Studies show that about one in three people carry staph in their nose, usually without any illness. Two in 100 people carry MRSA. There are not data showing the total number of people who get MRSA skin infections in the community.

Can I Prevent MRSA? How?

There are the steps you can take to reduce your risk of MRSA infection:

- Maintain good hand and body hygiene. Wash hands often, and clean your body regularly, especially after exercise.
- Keep cuts, scrapes and wounds clean and covered until healed.
- Avoid sharing personal items such as towels and razors.
- Get care early if you think you might have an infection.

What Are MRSA Symptoms?

Sometimes, people with MRSA skin infections first think they have a spider bite. However, unless a spider is actually seen, the irritation is likely not a spider bite. Most staph skin infections, including MRSA, appear as a bump or infected area on the skin that might be:

- Red
- Swollen
- Painful
- Warm to the touch
- Full of pus or other drainage
- Accompanied by a fever

What Should I Do If I See These Symptoms?

If you or someone in your family experiences these signs and symptoms, cover the area with a bandage, wash your hands, and contact your doctor. It is especially important to contact your doctor if signs and symptoms of an MRSA skin infection are accompanied by a fever.

What Should I do if I Think I Have a Skin Infection?

- You can't tell by looking at the skin if it is a staph infection (including MRSA).
- Contact your doctor if you think you have an infection. Finding infections early and getting care make it less likely that the infection will become severe.

- Do not try to treat the infection yourself by picking or popping the sore.

- Cover possible infections with clean, dry bandages until you can be seen by a doctor, nurse, or other healthcare provider.

How to Prevent Spreading MRSA

- Cover your wounds. Keep wounds covered with clean, dry bandages until healed. Follow your doctor's instructions about proper care of the wound. Pus from infected wounds can contain MRSA so keeping the infection covered will help prevent the spread to others. Bandages and tape can be thrown away with the regular trash. Do not try to treat the infection yourself by picking or popping the sore.

- Clean your hands often. You, your family, and others in close contact should wash their hands often with soap and water or use an alcohol-based hand rub, especially after changing the bandage or touching the infected wound.

- Do not share personal items. Personal items include towels, washcloths, razors and clothing, including uniforms.

- Wash used sheets, towels, and clothes with water and laundry detergent. Use a dryer to dry them completely.

- Wash clothes according to manufacturer's instructions on the label. Clean your hands after touching dirty clothes.

Steps to Take If You Think a Student Might Have a Skin Infection

The decision to close a school for any communicable disease should be made by school officials in consultation with local and/or state public health officials. However, in most cases, it is not necessary to close schools because of an MRSA infection in a student. It is important to note that MRSA transmission can be prevented by simple measures such as hand hygiene and covering infections.

Closing to Clean or Disinfect

In general, it is not necessary to close entire schools to "disinfect" them when MRSA infections occur. MRSA skin infections are transmitted primarily by skin-to-skin contact and by contact with surfaces that have come into contact with someone else's infection. Covering infections will greatly reduce the risks of surfaces becoming contaminated with MRSA.

Notifications

School Notifications to the School Community following an MRSA Infection. Staphylococcus (staph) bacteria, including MRSA, have been and remain a common cause of skin infections. Usually, it should not be necessary to inform the entire school community about a single MRSA infection. When an MRSA infection occurs within the school population, the school clinician should determine, based on medical judgment, whether some or all students, parents, and staff should be notified. If medical personnel are not available at the school, consultation with the local public health authorities should be used to guide this decision. Repeat cases, spread to other students, or complex cases should be reported to the health department for consultation.

Notifications to the School that a Student has an MRSA Infection. Most schools require that any communicable disease be reported to the student's teacher or administration. Consult with your school about its policy.

Excluding Students with MRSA Infections from School

- Unless directed by a physician, students with MRSA infections should not be excluded from attending school.

- Exclusion from school and sports activities should be reserved for those with wound drainage ("pus") that cannot be covered and contained with a clean, dry bandage and for those who cannot maintain good personal hygiene.

Practical Advice for Teachers

- If you observe children with open draining wounds or infections, refer the child to the school nurse. If a nurse is not available, call the child's guardian and refer them to seek medical attention.

- Enforce hand hygiene with soap and water or alcohol-based hand sanitizers (if available) before eating and after using the bathroom.

Advice for School Health Personnel

- Students with skin infections may need to be referred to a licensed healthcare provider for diagnosis and treatment. School health personnel should notify parents/guardians when possible skin infections are detected.

- Use standard precautions (e.g., hand hygiene before and after contact, wearing gloves) when caring for nonintact skin or potential infections.

- Use barriers such as gowns, masks, and eye protection if splashing of body fluids is anticipated.

What Should a Person Do If a Family Member or Close Friend Staphylococcal Infection?

VISA and VRSA are types of antibiotic-resistant staph bacteria. Therefore, as with all staph bacteria, spread occurs among people having close physical contact with infected patients or contaminated material, such as bandages. Persons having close physical contact with infected patients while they are outside of the healthcare setting should:

1. Keep their hands clean by washing thoroughly with soap and water

2. Avoid contact with other people's wounds or material contaminated from wounds

If they go to the hospital to visit a friend or family member who is infected with VISA or VRSA, they must follow the hospital's recommended precautions.

Section 38.4

Mononucleosis

This section includes text excerpted from "Epstein-Barr—
Mononucleosis," Centers for Disease Control and
Prevention (CDC), September 14, 2016.

Infectious mononucleosis, also called "mono," is a contagious disease. Epstein-Barr virus (EBV) is the most common cause of infectious mononucleosis, but other viruses can also cause this disease. It is common among teenagers and young adults, especially college students. At least one out of four teenagers and young adults who get infected with EBV will develop infectious mononucleosis.

Symptoms

Typical symptoms of infectious mononucleosis usually appear four to six weeks after you get infected with EBV. Symptoms may develop slowly and may not all occur at the same time.

These symptoms include:

- extreme fatigue
- fever
- sore throat
- head and body aches
- swollen lymph nodes in the neck and armpits
- swollen liver or spleen or both
- rash

Enlarged spleen and a swollen liver are less common symptoms. For some people, their liver or spleen or both may remain enlarged even after their fatigue ends.

Most people get better in two to four weeks; however, some people may feel fatigued for several more weeks. Occasionally, the symptoms of infectious mononucleosis can last for six months or longer.

Transmission

EBV is the most common cause of infectious mononucleosis, but other viruses can cause this disease. Typically, these viruses spread most commonly through bodily fluids, especially saliva. However, these viruses can also spread through blood and semen during sexual contact, blood transfusions, and organ transplantations.

Prevention and Treatment

There is no vaccine to protect against infectious mononucleosis. You can help protect yourself by not kissing or sharing drinks, food, or personal items, like toothbrushes, with people who have infectious mononucleosis.

You can help relieve symptoms of infectious mononucleosis by:

- drinking fluids to stay hydrated

- getting plenty of rest

- taking over-the-counter medications for pain and fever

If you have infectious mononucleosis, you should not take ampicillin or amoxicillin. Based on the severity of the symptoms, a healthcare provider may recommend treatment of specific organ systems affected by infectious mononucleosis.

Because your spleen may become enlarged as a result of infectious mononucleosis, you should avoid contact sports until you fully recover. Participating in contact sports can be strenuous and may cause the spleen to rupture.

Diagnosing Infectious Mononucleosis

Healthcare providers typically diagnose infectious mononucleosis based on symptoms.

Laboratory tests are not usually needed to diagnose infectious mononucleosis. However, specific laboratory tests may be needed to identify the cause of illness in people who do not have a typical case of infectious mononucleosis.

The blood work of patients who have infectious mononucleosis due to EBV infection may show:

- more white blood cells (lymphocytes) than normal

- unusual looking white blood cells (atypical lymphocytes)

- fewer than normal neutrophils or platelets
- abnormal liver function

Chapter 39

Malocclusion

What Is Malocclusion?

Malocclusion is the misalignment of upper and lower teeth. Normally, the teeth in the upper jaw should slightly overlap the lower teeth, and the molar points should fit into the grooves of the opposing molar. This proper alignment is known as occlusion, which enables effective chewing and distributes pressure evenly among all the teeth. When it's correct, the upper teeth protect the cheeks and lips from being bitten, and the lower teeth protect the tongue. When the upper and lower teeth do not align properly, a whole host of problems can occur, including jaw joint pain, speech issues, face disfigurement, and gum tissue problems.

Types of malocclusion include crowded teeth, crossbite, underbite, overbite, or open bite. While some minor malocclusions don't necessarily require treatment, more serious cases need to be corrected, usually by braces but sometimes with surgery. An orthodontist, a dentist who specializes in the correction of irregularities in teeth and jaws, can assess the condition and help correct the alignment or recommend other treatment.

Causes and Risk Factors of Malocclusion

According to the National Institutes of Health (NIH), only a limited number of people have perfect occlusion; therefore, a small

"Malocclusion," © 2017 Omnigraphics. Reviewed November 2017.

amount of misalignment between teeth is not unusual. There can be many causes for malocclusion; however, genetic factors seem to be the primary cause. Inherited traits can result in a difference in size between the upper and lower jaw, or disparate tooth size, which can lead to abnormal bite patterns or tooth overcrowding. The shape of the jaws or cleft lip and palate, present at birth, can also cause malocclusion.

Nongenetic causes of malocclusion can include the following:

- Dental disease.

- Thumb or finger sucking beyond the age of five.

- Tumors inside the mouth or on the jaw.

- Ill-fitting retainers, braces, crowns, or dental fillings.

- Trauma or injury to the jaw.

- An extra tooth, impacted tooth, lost tooth, or abnormally-shaped tooth.

Risk factors for malocclusion include thumb or finger sucking, tongue thrusting activity, and the use of feeding bottles or pacifiers for an unusually long time. Children who have tiny spaces between the primary teeth are also at risk of having malocclusion when their permanent teeth emerge.

Symptoms of Malocclusion

The symptoms of malocclusion can range from headaches to tooth pain and premature wear. Some common symptoms include:

- misaligned teeth

- biting and chewing difficulty

- habitual mouth breathing

- difficulty with speech

- facial disfigurement or abnormality

Malocclusion in young children often corrects itself with time, and jaw growth during the teen years can correct minor misalignment. However, malocclusion in adults generally remains the same or even worsens over time.

Diagnosing Malocclusion

Malocclusion is most commonly diagnosed during a routine dental checkup. If there is a mismatch in the bite between the upper and lower teeth, the dentist may refer the patient to an orthodontist for further diagnosis and treatment. After examining the patient, the orthodontist will likely order a set of dental X-rays—and possibly facial, head, and skull X-rays—to help identify underlying problems in the internal tissues, teeth, and bones in the mouth. An impression of the teeth may also be taken to aid in diagnosis and help the orthodontist develop a treatment plan.

Treatment for Malocclusion

An orthodontist will decide on the most beneficial kind of treatment that can be provided based on the specific type of malocclusion. Treatment is determined based on the following:

- the patient's age and medical history
- the severity of the malocclusion
- tolerance for pain, dental procedures, and therapies
- duration of treatment
- the patient's preferences

The main goal of treatment is to correct the position of the teeth. However, treating malocclusion can offer other benefits, such as:

- lower risk of tooth breakage, tooth decay, or periodontal disease
- ease of teeth cleaning
- relief of temporomandibular joint disorder (TMJ)
- reduced strain on teeth and jaws

The orthodontist may suggest that the treatment be carried out in phased manner, especially if the malocclusion is severe or the treatment plan is very complex. Some common procedures for correcting malocclusion include the following:

- **Extraction.** Certain cases require the removal of a tooth to create additional space.
- **Braces or other dental appliances.** Bands made of metal, ceramic, or plastic are placed around the teeth in the upper or

lower jaw. These bands exert pressure on the teeth and gradually help to correct their position.

- **Reshaping the tooth.** In few cases, metal bands are not required, and the tooth can be adjusted to fit into its proper groove. This is achieved by bonding, capping, or reshaping.

- **Jaw surgery.** In some cases, jaw surgery is necessary if bone issues are causing the malocclusion. This type of surgery is done by a maxillofacial surgeon.

In order for treatment to be successful, the patient may be required to avoid certain kinds of food, including sticky foods, hard nuts, ice, or gum. Following good oral hygiene (brushing and flossing) and regular dental checkups will help avoid posttreatment problems. Treatment may last from six months to two years, or in some cases, even more. Treatment outcomes are usually better for children and adolescents, as their bones are still soft, and teeth can be repositioned more easily than in adults. Possible complications may involve discomfort during treatment, difficulty in chewing or speaking, irritation inside the mouth, or tooth decay. However, these can generally be avoided by following the orthodontist's instructions carefully.

Prevention for Malocclusion

Most types of malocclusion are not preventable since the condition is largely hereditary. However, if certain habits, such as thumb or finger sucking are curbed, then the risk of other kinds of malocclusion can be reduced. In addition, good dental hygiene can help prevent tooth loss, which can also lead to malocclusion.

References

1. "Malocclusion," Stanford Children's Health, n.d.

2. "Malocclusion and Orthodontics," Emedicinehealth.com, January 2, 2013.

3. "Malocclusion of Teeth," U.S. National Library of Medicine (NLM), February 22, 2016.

4. "Malocclusion of the Teeth," Healthline.com, n.d.

Chapter 40

Scoliosis

What Is Scoliosis?

Scoliosis causes a sideways curve of your backbone, or spine. These curves are often S- or C-shaped. Scoliosis is most common in late childhood and the early teens, when children grow fast. Girls are more likely to have it than boys. It can run in families. Symptoms include leaning to one side and having uneven shoulders and hips. Sometimes it is easy to notice, but not always.

Children may get screening for scoliosis at school or during a check-up. If it looks like there is a problem, your doctor will use your medical and family history, a physical exam, and imaging tests to make a diagnosis. Treatment depends on your age, how much more you're likely to grow, how much curving there is, and whether the curve is temporary or permanent. People with mild scoliosis might only need check-ups to see if the curve is getting worse. Others might need to wear a brace or have surgery.

Who Gets It?

People of all ages can have scoliosis. The most common type has no known cause and occurs in children age 10 to 12 and in their early

This chapter contains text excerpted from the following sources: Text under the heading "What Is Scoliosis?" is excerpted from "Scoliosis," MedlinePlus, National Institutes of Health (NIH), October 18, 2016; Text beginning with the heading "Who Gets It?" is excerpted from "Scoliosis in Children and Adolescents," National Institute of Arthritis and Musculoskeletal and Skin Diseases (NIAMS), December 30, 2015.

teens. Girls are more likely than boys to have this type of scoliosis. You are more likely to have scoliosis if your parent, brother or sister have it.

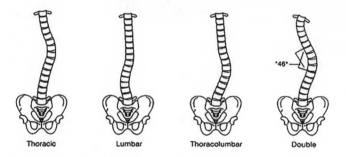

Figure 40.1. *Curve Pattern*

What Are the Symptoms?

Scoliosis is a disorder in which there is a sideways curve of the spine. Signs of scoliosis can include:

- Uneven shoulders.
- Head that is not centered.
- Sides of the body are not level with each other.
- One side of the rib cage is higher than the other when bending forward.

What Causes It?

In most people with scoliosis, the cause is not known. In some cases, there is a known cause.

Doctors classify curves as:

- **Nonstructural**, which is when the spine is structurally normal and the curve is temporary. In these cases, the doctor will try to find and correct the cause.

- **Structural**, which is when the spine has a fixed curve. The cause could be a disease, injury, infection, birth defect, or unknown.

Is There a Test?

- **Medical history** to look for medical problems that might be causing your spine to curve.

- **Physical examination** to look at your back, chest, pelvis, legs, feet, and skin.

- **X-rays** to measure the curve of the spine. This information is used to determine how to treat scoliosis.

How Is It Treated?

Your doctor may recommend the following treatments:

- **Observation**. If the curve is mild and you are still growing, your doctor will re-examine you every few months.

- **Bracing**. If the curve is moderate and you are still growing, your doctor may recommend a brace to keep the curve from getting worse. Braces are selected for the specific curve problem and fitted to each patient. Braces must be worn every day for the full number of hours prescribed by the doctor.

- **Surgery**. If you are still growing and have a severe curve that is getting worse, your doctor may suggest surgery. This often involves fusing together two or more bones in the spine. The doctor may also put in a metal rod or other device to help keep the spine straight after surgery. You should seek the advice of at least two experts, and ask about the benefits and risks of the surgery.

The following treatments have not been shown to keep curves from getting worse in scoliosis:

- Chiropractic treatment
- Electrical stimulation
- Nutritional supplements

Living with It

Exercise programs have not been shown to keep scoliosis from getting worse. But it is important for all people, including those with scoliosis, to exercise and remain physically fit. Weight-bearing exercise, such as walking, running, soccer, and gymnastics, helps keep bones strong. For both boys and girls, exercising and playing sports can improve their sense of well-being.

Part Five

Emotional, Social, and Mental Health Concerns in Adolescents

Chapter 41

Adolescent Stress

Stress is a feeling you get when faced with a challenge. Feeling stressed for a long time can take a toll on your mental and physical health. Even though it may seem hard to find ways to de-stress with all the things you have to do, it's important to find those ways. Your health depends on it.

What Is Stress?

Stress is a feeling you get when faced with a challenge. In small doses, stress can be good for you because it makes you more alert and gives you a burst of energy. For instance, if you start to cross the street and see a car about to run you over, that jolt you feel helps you to jump out of the way before you get hit. But feeling stressed for a long time can take a toll on your mental and physical health. Even though it may seem hard to find ways to de-stress with all the things you have to do, it's important to find those ways. Your health depends on it.

This chapter contains text excerpted from the following sources: Text in this chapter begins with excerpts from "Stress and Your Health," Office on Women's Health (OWH), U.S. Department of Health and Human Services (HHS), June 13, 2017; Text under the heading "How to Cope with Stress" is excerpted from "Nine Tips to Help You Cope with Stress," National Institute on Drug Abuse (NIDA) for Teens, May 16, 2016.

What Are the Most Common Causes of Stress?

Stress happens when people feel like they don't have the tools to manage all of the demands in their lives. Stress can be short- or long-term. Missing the bus or arguing with your spouse or partner can cause short-term stress. Money problems or trouble at work can cause long-term stress. Even happy events, like having a baby or getting married can cause stress. Some of the most common stressful life events include:

- Losing your job
- Major personal illness or injury
- Pregnancy
- Marriage
- Marital separation
- Divorce
- Death of a spouse
- Death of a close family member
- Spending time in jail

What Are Some Common Signs of Stress?

Everyone responds to stress a little differently. Your symptoms may be different from someone else's. Here are some of the signs to look for:

- Not eating or eating too much
- Feeling like you have no control
- Needing to have too much control
- Forgetfulness
- Headaches
- Lack of energy
- Lack of focus
- Trouble getting things done
- Poor self-esteem
- Short temper

- Trouble sleeping

- Upset stomach

- Back pain

- General aches and pains

These symptoms may also be signs of depression or anxiety, which can be caused by long-term stress.

Can Stress Affect My Health?

The body responds to stress by releasing stress hormones. These hormones make blood pressure, heart rate, and blood sugar levels go up. Long-term stress can help cause a variety of health problems, including:

- Mental health disorders, like depression and anxiety

- Obesity

- Heart disease

- High blood pressure

- Abnormal heart beats

- Menstrual problems

- Acne and other skin problems

How to Cope with Stress

We probably don't need to tell you that teens can really feel stressed out. Even when times are generally good, sometimes you may feel stress building up from pressure at school, at work, or in relationships with your family and friends.

Everybody feels stress at times. But too much stress, or feeling stress over a long period of time, can be bad for your health. It can lead you to feel depressed or make it hard to focus in class. Stress can even cause physical problems like headaches and stomachaches, or cause you to get sick more often.

Is there something you can do about it (besides downing a pint of ice cream or a bag of chips)? Yes! To fight stress in your life, you can try some of these tips, adapted from the Office of Disease Prevention and Health Promotion (ODPHP). These tips are for managing both ongoing stress and a single stressful event:

1. Plan ahead—If you have too many tasks or assignments due, make a to-do list and do the most important thing first. Make sure your plans are realistic; don't plan to accomplish more than you actually can.

2. Prepare—If you're worried about an upcoming event, try visualizing yourself there, and thinking about how you might handle different situations that could come up.

3. Breathe deeply—Sit up straight and take a few slow, deep breaths: inhale through your nose, exhale through your mouth.

4. Relax your muscles—Do some stretches or take a hot shower to help yourself relax.

5. Exercise—Exercising can help you relax, too; it even releases feel-good chemicals like endorphins and dopamine in your brain.

6. Eat healthy—Give your body energy by eating healthy foods such as vegetables, fruits, and lean sources of protein.

7. Avoid alcohol and drugs—Substance use can make it harder for you to think clearly—or, depending on the substance, can make you feel anxious.

8. Talk to someone—Tell your family and friends that you're feeling stressed. If there's something you don't want to talk about with family or friends, reach out to a teacher, school counselor, or another trusted adult.

9. Get help if you need it—If you ever feel like you're dealing with more than you can handle, talk to a trusted adult or a doctor, or contact the National Suicide Prevention Lifeline (which helps people with all sorts of issues, not just suicide) at 800-273-8255.

Chapter 42

School Pressures

Chapter Contents

Section 42.1—Test Anxiety 404

Section 42.2—Cheating 409

Section 42.3—Helping Your Child Feel Connected
            to School.. 412

Section 42.1

Test Anxiety

What Is Test Anxiety?

Test anxiety occurs when a person is excessively apprehensive about taking a test. The condition causes distress that can negatively affect performance on the exam, sometimes making the individual forget what he or she previously learned. Someone with test anxiety might lose concentration, become tense, and completely lose focus.

It is normal to be apprehensive before a test, and being nervous can actually have some benefits. For example, a small degree of stress can help you get started on a task and keep you going until you complete it. And it can help you focus better and complete the task properly. But when facing a test, some people become overly nervous to the point where performance suffers, and they experience symptoms that make it difficult to concentrate. When teens have test anxiety their mental faculties may become clouded, and studies show that all kinds of students, regardless of age or ability, can be prone to this condition. Preparation might be affected by insufficient study, lack of time, difficult material, physical exhaustion, or lack of sleep the night before the test. The feeling that you have not prepared properly and will not perform well can result in the symptoms of test anxiety.

Test anxiety is a kind of performance anxiety. This is something that people often experience when they need to go on stage or do something in front of others. In such situations, there is pressure to do well, which creates a high level of anxiety. This is commonly seen when someone has to perform in a play, give a speech, appear for a job interview, or play in front of a crowd.

Performing poorly on a test because of personal issues or crises at home should not be confused with test anxiety. Some of these issues, such as the death of a close relative, would naturally interfere with concentration in a test and would not be considered test anxiety.

What Are the Signs of Text Anxiety?

Test anxiety affects you mentally and physically. If you have the condition, you could completely forget what you learned and have difficulty concentrating. You can become overwhelmed with negative thoughts about how you are going to complete the test and what will happen if you fail. You might also dwell on how others are performing on the test, imaging them having much less trouble than you.

Physically, people with test anxiety may feel a fluttering known as "butterflies" in their stomach, and might also experience sweating and shaking. They might have a tension headache or feel like fainting or throwing up. Other symptoms associated with the condition include nausea, cramps, dry mouth, muscle tension, and increased breathing and heart rates. These symptoms can have an additional negative impact on test preparation and performance.

What Causes Test Anxiety?

Typically, anxiety occurs when you anticipate something stressful. This is the result of an evolutionary mechanism built into human beings known as the "fight-or-flight" response. The body prepares either to defend itself or flee from a potential threat by releasing a hormone known as adrenaline. Adrenaline causes the physical symptoms associated with test anxiety, such as shaking, sweating, muscle tension, heavy breathing, and a pounding heart. Negative thoughts, such as thinking that you will forget the answers or fail the test, adds to the anxiety and creates a vicious cycle that further worsens performance.

Who Can Suffer from Text Anxiety?

Anyone can be overcome with test anxiety, but perfectionists tend to be most prone to the condition. For them anything less than a perfect score is unacceptable, and they can be extremely fearful of making mistakes. They put pressure on themselves to perform better, which in turn creates a perfect environment for test anxiety. For many people, failing to prepare well enough can lead to test anxiety.

How Can You Cope with Test Anxiety?

Most students with test anxiety worry that they are not smart enough or sufficiently prepared to succeed. Such a mindset can be paralyzing when taking tests. Students must overcome these thoughts and view themselves as competent learners to overcome test anxiety.

Below are some strategies that can help teens deal with test anxiety more effectively.

1. **Mental Preparation**

    Students can do several things to prepare themselves better, some of which are listed below.

    - **Develop good study habits.** There's much more to learning than just attending classes. It is impossible to prepare for a test just by sitting in a classroom. It's equally important to develop good study habits and review schedules.

    - **Be thorough.** Rather than just memorizing, concentrate on the major ideas, main events, and most important issues covered in the material. Avoid anxiety with a solid understanding of the subject matter.

    - **Review the material.** Go over what you've learned by covering it throughout the week. This helps in committing the material to memory.

    - **Don't cram.** It is not advisable to study hard just before the exam. You cannot digest an entire chapter or term in just one night. Plan your study routine in advance, and review accordingly to avoid last-minute tension.

    - **Know the test format clearly in advance.** Doing this takes the initial shock you might experience when you see the test for the first time.

    - **Write out your own possible questions and answers before the test.** This will help you master the topics and feel more prepared.

    - **Don't think negatively.** Negative thoughts can disrupt your study schedule. Always think about positive outcomes.

    - **Don't expect perfection.** You don't have to know everything about a topic or the answer to every possible question.

    - **Arrive early.** Be at the test location well ahead of the test starting time, so you have time to relax with your friends. And don't discuss the test material. Last minute reviews can only serve to confuse you.

2. Planning

Having a strategy in place before you take the test can help reduce anxiety. Some helpful strategies include the following:

- When the test paper is handed out, it is normal to feel tense. Once you have the paper in hand, take a few seconds to calm down before you start.

- Plan your time so you can answer all the questions. Allow more time for the most difficult questions. And don't dwell on any one question. Move on to the next item, and can come back to it later.

- If you are surprised by a question, don't lose your cool. Try answering something easy, and then come back after you've calmed down and can give it more time.

- If you felt confident answering a question the first time around, don't second-guess yourself and change the answer. This fosters negativity and could just be a waste of time.

- If you don't know the answer to a question, just accept that. If you feel the questions shouldn't have been on the test, you can discuss it with your teacher later.

3. Physical Preparation

It is important to take care of your health and pay attention to how you behave prior to a test in order to avoid anxiety-related problems. For example:

- **Eat well.** Adequate nutrition is an important part of studying before tests. Feeling weak and cranky during study time can lead to frustration and anxiety.

- **Make time for physical activity.** Exercising regularly helps you maintain a positive attitude. Do not disrupt your exercise schedule during test preparation.

- **Get plenty of sleep.** Lack of sleep affects memory and concentration. Staying up late studying and then getting up early can be counterproductive at exactly the wrong time.

- **Socialize with friends and family and take regular breaks.** Social interaction minimizes anxiety and helps reenergize you for additional study. Blend with people with a positive attitude. In particular, avoid those who think negatively, especially about tests.

- **Don't procrastinate.** If you put off your study schedule, you might be setting yourself up for cramming. And it's possible that you could be waiting until the last minute so you have an excuse for not doing well.

4. **Relaxation Techniques**

   A number of relaxation techniques can help relieve anxiety, improve memory and enhance test performance. Some suggestions:

   - **When you start to feel anxious, try deep breathing exercises.** With your eyes closed, inhale slowly and deeply through your nose, and exhale very slowly through your mouth. Repeat until you feel yourself begin to feel less tense.

   - **Progressive muscle relaxation can help reduce stress.** For example, contract your shoulders for ten seconds, then slowly loosen up and let your muscles relax. Repeat with hands, arms, legs, and feet. Concentrate on how the actions feel and try to become more relaxed with each repetition.

   - **Visualization exercises may help ease anxiety.** Close your eyes and imagine yourself in a calm environment, such as a beach, a forest, or a spa. Combine this with a deep-breathing routine to increase the effect.

   - **If you regularly practice yoga, tai chi, or meditation, use these techniques to take a break from study.** They can help you return to your work in a more relaxed frame of mind.

Being Successful

It takes time and practice to learn how to reduce test anxiety. A good attitude towards studying determines how well you perform on a test, so the best way to deal with test anxiety is to study well and be prepared in all respects. Since test anxiety thrives on the unknown, it is important to use good study techniques and learn the material thoroughly. When students feel confident of their knowledge and develop effective test-taking strategies, they can overcome test anxiety.

References

1. Ehmke, Rachel. "Tips For Beating Test Anxiety," Child Mind Institute, Inc. n.d.

2. Lyness, D'Arcy, PhD. "Test Anxiety," The Nemours Foundation, July, 2013.

3. "Reducing Test Anxiety," Educational Testing Service (ETS), n.d.

4. "Reducing Test Anxiety," Pittsburg State University, n.d.

Section 42.2

Cheating

"Cheating," © 2017 Omnigraphics.
Reviewed November 2017.

What Is Cheating?

Cheating is a conscious decision to achieve desired results through dishonest means. Many children cheat as a way of gaining a favorable outcome at home, school, or while playing a game or a sport. Some examples of cheating include copying another student's answers on a test, using previously published words in a term paper, or moving too many spaces in a board game. Very young children don't really grasp concepts like lying and cheating, but by the age of five, most kids are able to understand that these behaviors are wrong.

How Prevalent Is Cheating among Teens?

Studies indicate that cheating is very common during adolescence. Middle schools place more emphasis on grades and performance than elementary schools; therefore, cheating starts to become more prevalent at this level, and by the time they enter high school, more than 80 percent of students admit to cheating at least once in the past year. It is often assumed that only struggling students cheat; however, many

409

studies show that some of the best academic performers cheat as much as other students. Another common misconception is that boys cheat more than girls, but research indicates otherwise. Modern technology has made it easier than ever for students to cheat, using cell phones during tests or plagiarizing essays or assignments from the Internet.

Why Do Students Cheat?

As children see examples of cheating among people from all walks of life, including movie stars, sport figures, politicians, and business professionals, they may come to believe that this behavior is acceptable. And since cheating is so common among their peers, students may feel completely normal about securing results in this manner. The pressure to cheat arises more often when there is pressure to excel, or when there is too much work to do and too little time to accomplish it. Other reasons for student cheating may include laziness, busyness, or feeling that cheating is the only way to pass a difficult test. Some students cheat once and never do it again, and some get caught and realize it was not worth it. Then there are those who continue cheating because it becomes habitual, and they cannot stop.

Consequences of Cheating

Cheating can have far more serious consequences than imagined by many students. If caught, cheaters can earn a bad reputation among parents, teachers, and their peers. And those who are caught cheating will likely suffer a grade reduction and be otherwise penalized for their act by teachers or parents. More serious consequences can include failing a grade level, being expelled, or having the cheating entered into the student's record, which can affect college admission. But even if students are not caught, feelings of guilt, embarrassment, or shame can overwhelm them, as can the feeling of disappointing or betraying their parents, teachers, or friends.

Steps to Avoid Indulging in Such Behavior

Students cheat for many reasons; however, unless this behavior is curbed, it can lead to more cheating and even more serious consequences. The following are a few steps that can help students, parents, and teachers ensure that cheating is avoided or stopped:

- If a student is unprepared or feeling ill before a test, he or she can talk to a teacher or parent about the situation, rather than cheating to get a passing grade.

- If a student is overwhelmed with school work, he or she needs to address this issue with teachers and parents.

- Many times, parents overreact to the fact that their child has cheated. This kind of emotional response is not likely to help. Handling the matter calmly will give the student confidence to share their feelings with parents, and encourage them to work together on a solution.

- Parents who break rules, steal or cheat on taxes, for instance, set a bad example that can give teens the impression that this behavior is acceptable.

- Teachers can discourage cheating in classrooms by creating a positive, caring environment. More accessibility and openness with teachers can help a student build trust and make him or her think twice before cheating.

- Students who cheat may tend to continue the behavior until it becomes habitual. However, it is never too late to break the habit. Through calm discussion and cooperation parents and teachers can help the student to make better choices.

References

1. Anderman, Eric M., PhD, Tripp Griesinger, and Gloria Westerfield. "Motivation and Cheating during Early Adolescence," Journal of Educational Psychology, American Psychological Association (APA), 1998.

2. Lyness, D'Arcy. "Cheating," KidsHealth, September 2013.

3. Pickhardt, Carl E., PhD. "Why Adolescents Cheat in School and What to Do," Psychology Today, June 27, 2009.

4. "Stealing, Lying, and Cheating: Why Your Child Does It and What to Do about It," One Tough Job, n.d.

5. Walker, Tim. "What Can Be Done about Student Cheating?" National Education Association (NEA), December 11, 2012.

Section 42.3

Helping Your Child Feel Connected to School

This section contains text excerpted from the following sources: Text
in this section begins with excerpts from "Adolescent and School
Health—School Connectedness," Centers for Disease Control and
Prevention (CDC), April 22, 2016; Text beginning with the heading
"Why Is It Important for Your Child to Feel Connected to School?"
is excerpted from "Helping Your Child Feel Connected to School,"
Centers for Disease Control and Prevention (CDC), July 2009.
Reviewed November 2017.

School connectedness—the belief held by students that adults and
peers in the school care about their learning as well as about them as
individuals—is an important protective factor. Research has shown
that young people who feel connected to their school are less likely to
engage in many risk behaviors, including early sexual initiation, alcohol, tobacco, and other drug use, and violence and gang involvement.

Students who feel connected to their school are also more likely to
have better academic achievement, including higher grades and test
scores, have better school attendance, and stay in school longer.

Efforts to improve child and adolescent health have typically
addressed specific health risk behaviors, such as tobacco use or violence. However, results from a growing number of studies suggest that
greater health impact might be achieved by also enhancing protective
factors that help children and adolescents avoid multiple behaviors
that place them at risk for adverse health and educational outcomes.

As a parent, you want your child to do well in school. You also want
your child to be healthy and avoid behaviors that are risky or harmful.
Through your guidance and support, you can have great influence on
your child's health and learning. But you also have important allies
in this effort—the caring adults in your child's school. Research shows
that students who feel a genuine sense of belonging at school are more
likely to do well in school, stay in school, and make healthy choices.
This sense of belonging is often described as school connectedness.
Connected students believe their parents, teachers, school staff, and
other students in their school care about them and about how well
they are learning.

Why Is It Important for Your Child to Feel Connected to School?

Scientists who study youth health and behavior have learned that strong connections at school can help young people:

- Get better grades
- Have higher test scores
- Stay in school longer
- Attend school more regularly

In addition, students who feel connected to their school are less likely to:

- Smoke cigarettes
- Drink alcohol
- Have sexual intercourse
- Carry a weapon or become involved in violence
- Be injured from drinking and driving or not wearing seat belts
- Have emotional distress or eating disorders
- Consider or attempt suicide

What Can You Do to Increase Your Child's Connection to School?

Here are some actions that you can take, at home and at school, to help your child become more connected to his or her school:

1. Encourage your child to talk openly with you, teachers, counselors, and other school staff about his or her ideas, needs, and worries.

2. Find out what the school expects your child to learn and how your child should behave in school by talking to teachers and staff, attending school meetings, and reading information the school sends home. Then, support these expectations at home.

3. Help your child with homework, and teach your child how to use his or her time well. Make sure your child has the tools—books, supplies, a quiet place to work—he or she needs to do homework at home, at the library, or at an after school program.

4. Encourage your child to help adults at home, at school, and in the community, such as helping with chores, serving as a library aide, volunteering at a hospital or clinic, or tutoring younger students after school.

5. Read school newsletters, attend parent teacher student conferences, and check out the school's website to learn what is going on at the school. Encourage your child to participate in school activities.

6. Meet regularly with your child's teachers to discuss his or her grades, behavior, and accomplishments.

7. Ask teachers if your child can participate in or lead parent teacher conferences.

8. As your schedule allows, help in your child's classroom, attend after school events, or participate in a school committee, such as a health team or parent organization. Ask whether your school offers babysitting or transportation for parents who need them.

9. Offer to share important aspects of your culture with your child's class.

10. If your first language is not English, ask for materials that are translated into the language you speak at home, and ask for interpreters to help you at school events.

11. Learn whether community organizations provide dental services, health screenings, child care, or health promotion programs at school. If not, advocate having those services offered at your school or in your school district.

12. Get involved with your child's school to help plan school policies and school wide activities.

13. Ask whether your school or school district provides—or could offer—programs or classes to help you become more involved in your child's academic and school life. For example, the school or school district might offer:

   • Training to help you talk with your child and to help manage his or her behavior.

   • Programs to help you to talk with your child's teachers and help your child learn.

- Educational programs for parents by telephone or online.

- General Education Development (GED), English as a second language, or other classes to help you work better with your child and with the adults at school.

14. Talk with teachers and school staff to suggest simple changes that can make the school a more pleasant and welcoming place. For example, the school might decorate the eating area with student made posters, allow families to use the school gym or other facilities during out of school times, or create a place in the school or on school grounds for kids and families to socialize.

Chapter 43

Adolescent Social Development and Concerns

Chapter Contents

Section 43.1—Encouraging Healthy Relationships:
Tips to Help Your Child 418
Section 43.2—Peer Pressure 421
Section 43.3—Parental Monitoring............................. 425

Section 43.1

Encouraging Healthy Relationships: Tips to Help Your Child

This section contains text excerpted from the following
sources: Text in this section begins with excerpts from "Healthy
Friendships in Developing Adolescents," U.S. Department of Health
and Human Services (HHS), September 20, 2016; Text under the
heading "Characteristics of Healthy and Unhealthy Relationships"
is excerpted from "Characteristics of Healthy and Unhealthy
Relationships," Youth.gov, February 7, 2012.
Reviewed November 2017.

Friendships play a major role in the lives of adolescents. A circle
of caring and supportive friends can help adolescents transition to
adulthood. Parents, teachers and other adult role models can help
young people learn how to make and keep good friends. Still, forming
and maintaining friendships during adolescence can be challenging.
Peer pressure—good and bad—often affects decisions young people
make. Adults can set good examples, teach interpersonal skills, and
help adolescents nurture positive friendships. One important lesson
is that friends can say "no" to each other and remain friends.

Characteristics of Healthy and Unhealthy Relationships

Respect for both oneself and others is a key characteristic of healthy
relationships. In contrast, in unhealthy relationships, one partner
tries to exert control and power over the other physically, sexually,
and/or emotionally.

Healthy Relationships

Healthy relationships share certain characteristics that teens
should be taught to expect. They include:

- **Mutual respect.** Respect means that each person values who
the other is and understands the other person's boundaries.

- **Trust.** Partners should place trust in each other and give each other the benefit of the doubt.

- **Honesty.** Honesty builds trust and strengthens the relationship.

- **Compromise.** In a dating relationship, each partner does not always get his or her way. Each should acknowledge different points of view and be willing to give and take.

- **Individuality.** Neither partner should have to compromise who he/she is, and his/her identity should not be based on a partner's. Each should continue seeing his or her friends and doing the things he/she loves. Each should be supportive of his/her partner wanting to pursue new hobbies or make new friends.

- **Good communication.** Each partner should speak honestly and openly to avoid miscommunication. If one person needs to sort out his or her feelings first, the other partner should respect those wishes and wait until he or she is ready to talk.

- **Anger control.** We all get angry, but how we express it can affect our relationships with others. Anger can be handled in healthy ways such as taking a deep breath, counting to ten, or talking it out.

- **Fighting fair.** Everyone argues at some point, but those who are fair, stick to the subject, and avoid insults are more likely to come up with a possible solution. Partners should take a short break away from each other if the discussion gets too heated.

- **Problem solving.** Dating partners can learn to solve problems and identify new solutions by breaking a problem into small parts or by talking through the situation.

- **Understanding.** Each partner should take time to understand what the other might be feeling.

- **Self-confidence.** When dating partners have confidence in themselves, it can help their relationships with others. It shows that they are calm and comfortable enough to allow others to express their opinions without forcing their own opinions on them.

- **Being a role model.** By embodying what respect means, partners can inspire each other, friends, and family to also behave in a respectful way.

- **Healthy sexual relationship.** Dating partners engage in a sexual relationship that both are comfortable with, and neither partner feels pressured or forced to engage in sexual activity that is outside his or her comfort zone or without consent.

Unhealthy Relationships

Unhealthy relationships are marked by characteristics such as disrespect and control. It is important for youth to be able to recognize signs of unhealthy relationships before they escalate. Some characteristics of unhealthy relationships include:

- **Control.** One dating partner makes all the decisions and tells the other what to do, what to wear, or who to spend time with. He or she is unreasonably jealous, and/or tries to isolate the other partner from his or her friends and family.

- **Hostility.** One dating partner picks a fight with or antagonizes the other dating partner. This may lead to one dating partner changing his or her behavior in order to avoid upsetting the other.

- **Dishonesty.** One dating partner lies to or keeps information from the other. One dating partner steals from the other.

- **Disrespect.** One dating partner makes fun of the opinions and interests of the other partner or destroys something that belongs to the partner.

- **Dependence.** One dating partner feels that he or she "cannot live without" the other. He or she may threaten to do something drastic if the relationship ends.

- **Intimidation.** One dating partner tries to control aspects of the other's life by making the other partner fearful or timid. One dating partner may attempt to keep his or her partner from friends and family or threaten violence or a break-up.

- **Physical violence.** One partner uses force to get his or her way (such as hitting, slapping, grabbing, or shoving).

- **Sexual violence.** One dating partner pressures or forces the other into sexual activity against his or her will or without consent

It is important to educate youth about the value of respect and the characteristics of healthy and unhealthy relationships before they start to date. Youth may not be equipped with the necessary skills to develop and maintain healthy relationships, and may not know how to break up in an appropriate way when necessary. Maintaining open lines of communication may help them form healthy relationships and recognize the signs of unhealthy relationships, thus preventing the violence before it starts.

Section 43.2

Peer Pressure

This section includes text excerpted from "Peer Pressure,"
The Cool Spot, National Institute on Alcohol Abuse and
Alcoholism (NIAAA), October 29, 2016.

Your classmates keep asking you to have them over because you have a pool, everyone at school is wearing silly hats so you do too, and your best friend begs you to go running with her because you both need more exercise, so you go, too. These are all examples of peer pressure. Don't get it yet?

- Pressure is the feeling that you are being pushed toward making a certain choice—good or bad.

- A peer is someone in your own age group.

- Peer pressure is—you guessed it—the feeling that someone your own age is pushing you toward making a certain choice, good or bad.

Why Peer Pressure Can Work?

Have you ever given into pressure? Like when a friend begs to borrow something you don't want to give up or to do something your parents say is off limits? Chances are you probably have given into pressure at some time in your life.

How did it feel to give into pressure? If you did something you wish you hadn't, then most likely you didn't feel too good about it. You might have felt:

- sad

- anxious

- guilty

- like a wimp or pushover

- disappointed in yourself

Everyone gives in to pressure at one time or another, but why do people sometimes do things that they really don't want to do? Here are a few reasons. They:

- are afraid of being rejected by others

- want to be liked and don't want to lose a friend

- want to appear grown up

- don't want to be made fun of

- don't want to hurt someone's feelings

- aren't sure of what they really want

- don't know how to get out of the situation

When you face pressure you can stand your ground.

How Peers Pressure?

Almost everyone faces peer pressure once in a while. Friends have a big influence on our lives, but sometimes they push us to do things that we may not want to do. Unless you want to give in every time you face this, you're going to need to learn how to handle it.

The first step to standing up to peer pressure is to understand it. In this section, you'll start by learning to recognize the different things people do when they pressure others. Soon you'll be able to spot peer pressure and deal with it!

Spoken versus Unspoken Pressure

Sometimes a friend can say something directly to you that puts a lot of pressure on you and makes it hard to say no. This is spoken pressure.

You may think you are supposed to act or dress a certain way because it seems like everyone else is doing it, or because it's the cool thing to do. When you feel this way even though nobody has said anything about it, this is unspoken pressure.

If you haven't already, you are going to face both spoken and unspoken pressure in the future. It's just part of life. The important part is to make the right choices when a peer pressure situation comes up.

Peer Pressure Bag of Tricks

Who needs you as a friend anyway? You're such a baby! It won't hurt bad!

Have your friends ever used these lines on you? Did you give in, even though you didn't want to?

These are a few of the goodies in the Peer Pressure Bag-of-Tricks. The tricks include put-downs, rejections, and reasoning, as well as pressure without words, or unspoken pressure.

The Tricks

Learn to spot the tricks. Being aware of the pressure is the first step to resisting it.

Rejection: Threatening to end a friendship or a relationship. This pressure can be hard to resist because nobody wants to lose friends. Some examples of pressure by rejection are:

- Who needs you as a friend anyway?
- If you don't drink we won't hang out anymore.
- Why don't you leave if you don't want to drink with us?

Put downs: Insulting or calling a person names to make them feel bad. Some examples of put downs are:

- You're never any fun.
- You're such a baby.
- You're such a wimp.
- You're so uncool.

Reasoning: Telling a person reasons why they should try something or why it would be OK if they did. (Nobody said these were good reasons.) Some examples of pressure by reasoning are:

- It won't hurt you.
- Your parents will never find out.
- You'll have more fun.

Unspoken pressure: This is something you feel without anyone saying anything to you. You feel unspoken pressure if you want to do the same things others doing. Some unspoken pressure tricks are:

- **The huddle:** A group of kids standing together in which everyone is talking and maybe looking at something you can't see, laughing and joking.

- **The look:** Kids who think they're cool give you a certain look that means we're cool and you're not.

- **The example:** A group of popular kids decide to get the same backpack and you want one too.

Peer Pressure Can Be Good Too

Peer pressure isn't all bad. You and your friends can pressure each other into some things that will improve your health and social life and make you feel good about your decisions.

Think of a time when a friend pushed you to do something good for yourself or to avoid something that would've been bad.

Here are some good things friends can pressure each other to do:

- Be honest
- Avoid Alcohol
- Avoid drugs
- Not smoke
- Be nice
- Respect others
- Work hard
- Exercise (together!)

You and your friends can also use good peer pressure to help each other resist bad peer pressure.

If you see a friend taking some heat, try some of these lines...

- We don't want to drink.
- We don't need to drink to have fun.
- Let's go and do something else.
- Leave her alone. She said she didn't want any.

Section 43.3

Parental Monitoring

This section contains text excerpted from the following
sources: Text in this section begins with excerpts from "Adolescent
and School Health—Positive Parenting Practices," Centers for
Disease Control and Prevention (CDC), July 7, 2017; Text beginning
with the heading "Parents: A Powerful Influence" is excerpted from
"Monitoring Your Teen's Activities—What Parents and Families
Should Know," Centers for Disease Control and Prevention (CDC)
December 2012. Reviewed November 2017; Text under the heading
"What Can Parents Do to Monitor Their Teens Effectively?" is
excerpted from "Talking with Teens about Peer Relationships: How
You Make a Difference," U.S. Department of Health and Human
Services (HHS), October 17, 2016.

Parenting a teen is not easy. Many outside influences distract our youth and add challenges to parenting efforts. Youth need adults who are there for them—people who connect with them, communicate with them, spend time with them, and show a genuine interest in them. A key parental role is helping teens understand that their health and well-being—now and in the future—are not simply a matter of chance, but a matter of choice.

By engaging in positive parenting, parents can help their adolescent make healthy choices.

Parents: A Powerful Influence

Parents are a powerful influence in the lives of their teens. When parents make a habit of knowing about their teens—what they are doing, who they are with, and where they are and setting clear expectations for behavior with regular check-ins to be sure these expectations are being met—they can reduce their teens' risks for injury, pregnancy, and drug, alcohol, and cigarette use. These parents are monitoring their teens' activities and behavior.

What Is Parental Monitoring?

Parental monitoring includes:

1. the expectations parents have for their teen's behavior;

2. the actions parents take to keep track of their teen; and

3. the ways parents respond when their teen breaks the rules.

You are using parental monitoring when you ask your teen :

- Where will you be?

- Whom will you be with?

- When will you be home?

You are also monitoring when you:

- Check in with your teen by phone.

- Get to know his or her friends and their parents.

- Talk with your teen about how he or she spends time or whether he or she is making safe choices.

- Set and enforce rules for your teen's behavior by clearly explaining the rules and consequences and following through with appropriate consequences when the rules are broken.

Monitoring should start in early childhood and continue throughout the teen years, evolving as children grow and mature. As children develop into teenagers, adults might view them as more independent and less in need of monitoring. But, consistent monitoring throughout the teen years is critical—teens' desire for independence can bring opportunities for unhealthy or unsafe behaviors.

Does Parental Monitoring Make a Difference?

Yes. Research shows that teens whose parents use effective monitoring practices are less likely to make poor decisions, such as having sex at an early age, smoking cigarettes, drinking alcohol, being physically aggressive, or skipping school. Clear communication about your expectations is especially important. Research shows that teens who believe their parents disapprove of risky behaviors are less likely to choose those behaviors.

What Can Parents Do to Monitor Their Teens Effectively?

- **Model healthy relationships with others.** The one place where teens learn about relationships is in their families. What they learn from and experience with parents and siblings has a lot of influence on how they find and get along with friends.

- **Maintain a positive relationship.** When parents have positive relationships with their teens, their teens are more likely to form more positive relationships with their peers, including healthy romantic relationships. A positive parent teen relationship is one that is warm, caring, and emotionally open while also setting boundaries and having high expectations.

- **Encourage positive friendships.** You can welcome your teen's friends to your home, support them doing things together, and encourage participation in activities with positive peer groups, such as school activities, youth programs, and religious activities.

- **Teach friendship skills.** Help your teen learn to strike up a conversation with someone new, show empathy and support to a friend, listen and ask questions, resolve conflicts, set appropriate boundaries, and other skills that lead to positive, meaningful relationships with peers.

- **Know your teen's friends.** Keep track of where teens spend time, who they're with, and what they're doing. Then you have the opportunity to ask questions or offer additional encouragement for the friendships, depending on the situation.

- **Express concerns, ask questions, and set limits, when necessary.** If you are uncomfortable with some friends and do not believe they are a positive influence, talk about your concerns with your teen, teaching him or her how to think about relationships. Be open and willing to listen to what your teen has to say about these friends, and also talk about what makes you nervous. It's best not to forbid a friendship, unless it is putting your teen in danger.

- **Create an inviting home for friends.** Make your home a place where your teen's friends like to hang out. (Snacks always help!) Get to know them while they are relaxed and open to conversation. If there are activities they want to attend together, offer to drive or supervise the outing.

- **Don't jump to conclusions based on appearances.** Don't judge your adolescent's friends based on their dress, hairstyle (or color), appearance, interests, or other external factors. Remember that teens sometimes "try on" different identities and interests as a way of expressing their independence. Over reacting with negative comments can make it less likely that friends will let you get to know them.

- **Do pay attention to warning signs.** If teens are hanging out with people who are much older, or if they are overly secretive about friends and what they are doing, monitor the situation more closely. Be less enthusiastic about these friendships, since your teen will sense your concern. If you have reason to suspect harmful activities (such as premature sexual activity, alcohol, tobacco, or other drug use), be assertive and clear about your concerns and your expectations.

- **Connect with your teen's friends' parents.** Get to know the parents or guardians of your teen's friends. You will often find that they share your values and priorities and that you can work together to ensure that the friendships are positive for everyone.

- **Practice peer pressure resistance strategies.** Role play different scenarios with teens so they have practice saying "no" in difficult situations. This strategy can help your teen be prepared and know how to respond when a sticky situation comes up. Focus on strengthening these resistance strategies:

  - **Get the person's attention.** Use the person's name. Make eye contact. Say, "Please listen to me!" Just getting the person to stop and pay attention can shift the energy and momentum, making it easier to resist the pressure.

  - **State your "no" decision.** Use "I" messages and a firm voice. Reinforce the decision with body language. You don't have to get defensive or explain everything. A firm "No, I do not want to do that" shows confidence and commitment.

  - **Use self-control.** Restate the "no" decision. Suggest an alternative subject, if appropriate. Or simply leave. Getting angry or arguing is rarely productive in the heat of the moment. Rather, your goal is to get away from the situation. If needed, discussing the issues can happen at another time when there's less pressure.

- **Recruit other help.** Chances are that you're not the only one who's uncomfortable doing things that you believe are unsafe or wrong. Your stance will often be respected, and others may follow your lead. If it's an ongoing situation, you can talk with others who share your perspective and come up with a strategy together.

- **Try other ways to say "no."** Use humor. Change the focus of the conversation. Reverse the pressure in a positive direction. Sometimes the humorous response defuses the situation, particularly if the humor follows a clear "no" statement.

- **Share your perspective with your teen.** When talking about a friend who you believe may be a negative influence, focus on the friend's behaviors, not on his personality. For example, instead of calling your teen's friend irresponsible for smoking, you could point out that the behavior has a negative effect on the friend's health and recommend ways for your teen to help the friend quit.

- **Set boundaries.** Teens can want to spend all their time with their friends or with their boyfriend or girlfriend. Insist that they also spend time at home and meet their other responsibilities. Be sure your teen participates in family gatherings and events (potentially inviting a friend to come along sometimes).

- **Investigate if your teen doesn't have friends.** Some young people are introverted and don't want or need a lot of friends. But spending a lot of time alone and not having any friends can also be a warning sign that your teen is isolated or having trouble with peer relationships. Ask about it. Check with teachers or other school personnel to see if they have concerns. (Sometimes teens interact well at school, but need alone time at home.) Losing interest in friends for several weeks may indicate depression or other issues. You may also consider seeking help from a counselor if your concerns persist.

- **Keep your relationship a top priority.** When parents have positive relationships with their teens, their teens are more likely to form more positive relationships with their peers, including healthy romantic relationships. A positive parent teen relationship is one that is warm, caring, and emotionally open while also setting boundaries and having high expectations. Even if you are concerned about friends and their influence, do not let your worries drive a wedge between you and your teen. Work hard to maintain your relationship, even while expressing your worries. When you express concerns, be sure to reinforce your love for your teen. Your influence will be greater in the long run if you do what you can to maintain a positive relationship.

Chapter 44

Facts about Mental Health Disorders in Adolescents

Important mental health habits—including coping, resilience, and good judgment—help adolescents to achieve overall well-being and set the stage for positive mental health in adulthood. Mood swings are common during adolescence. However, approximately one in five adolescents has a diagnosable mental disorder, such as depression and/or anxiety disorders. Friends and family can watch for warning signs of mental disorders and urge young people to get help. Effective treatments exist and may involve a combination of psychotherapy and medication. Unfortunately, less than half of adolescents with psychiatric disorders received any kind of treatment in the last year.

Common Mental Health Warning Signs

Mental health is not simply the presence or absence of symptoms. Mental health includes generally feeling and functioning well and resilience when faced with setbacks. Adolescents may have different symptoms than adults with the same mental health disorder and symptoms may vary from person to person. Some adolescents only experience one or two symptoms while others experience more. Furthermore,

This chapter includes text excerpted from "Adolescent Development—Mental Health in Adolescents," Office of Adolescent Health (OAH), U.S. Department of Health and Human Services (HHS), February 24, 2017.

adolescents may experience symptoms only once or infrequently, in which case they may be just experiencing emotions that are common at this age. These issues can make identification and diagnosis of mental health disorders challenging. According to the National Institute of Mental Health (NIMH), a child or teen might need help if they:

- Often feel very angry or very worried
- Have difficulty sleeping or eating
- Are unable to enjoy pleasurable activities they used to enjoy
- Isolate themselves and avoid social interactions
- Feel grief for a long time after a loss or death
- Use alcohol, tobacco, or other drugs
- Exercise, diet, and/or binge eat obsessively
- Hurt other people or destroy property
- Have low or no energy
- Feel like they can't control their emotions
- Have thoughts of suicide
- Harm themselves (e.g., burning or cutting their skin)
- Think their mind is being controlled or is out of control
- Hear voices

If you observe a teen experiencing these symptoms and need to seek help, consult your healthcare provider or mental health professional. In crisis or life-threatening situations, call 911, contact the National Suicide Prevention Lifeline, or go to your nearest hospital emergency room.

Common Mental Health Disorders in Adolescence

Common mental health disorders in adolescence include those related to anxiety, mood, attention deficit-hyperactivity, and eating disorders.

Anxiety Disorders

- Characterized by feelings of excessive uneasiness, worry, and fear

- Occur in approximately 25 percent of 13- to 18-year-olds

- Examples include generalized anxiety disorder, posttraumatic stress disorder, social anxiety disorder, obsessive-compulsive disorder, and phobias

Mood Disorders

- Characterized by extreme lows and highs in mood

- Occur in approximately 14 percent of 13- to 18-year-olds

- Examples include major depressive disorder, dysthymic disorder, and bipolar disorder

Attention Deficit-Hyperactivity Disorder (ADHD)

- Characterized by continuing inattention and/or hyperactivity-impulsivity that interferes with daily functioning or development

- Occurs in approximately 9 percent of 13- to 18-year-olds

Eating Disorders

- Characterized by extreme and abnormal eating behaviors, such as insufficient or excessive eating

- Occur in almost three percent of 13- to 18-year-olds

- Examples include anorexia nervosa, bulimia, and binge eating disorder

Co-occurring Disorders

When a person has a mental health and substance use disorder at the same time, they have co-occurring disorders. Compared to the general population, people with mental health disorders are more likely to experience a substance use disorder, repeatedly use alcohol and/or drugs to the point of impairment, and neglect major responsibilities at home, work, or school. Youth who have experienced a major depressive episode are twice as likely to start using alcohol or an illicit drug. A 2010 study found that more than 29 percent of youth who started using alcohol within the past year did so after a major depressive episode compared to only 14. percent of youth who had not experienced a major depressive episode. The same pattern also occurred with the use of illicit drugs.

Substance use shares many characteristics with mental illness. Prevention efforts and early treatment are beneficial for people who are at risk for both substance use and mental health disorders. One of the U.S. Surgeon General's report highlights the scope of substance use (including alcohol) and its negative health impacts for individuals and the nation. Because mental health and substance use disorders are complicated and involve biological, psychological, and social elements, the Substance Abuse and Mental Health Services Administration (SAMHSA) supports an integrated treatment approach to co-occurring disorders. This approach allows practitioners to comprehensively address symptoms and underlying causes, which often lowers the cost of treatment and leads to better outcomes.

Substance use is not the only disorder that occurs at the same time as mental health disorders. Different mental health disorders can occur together (like anxiety and depression) or mental health disorders can overlap with physical health disorders (like depression and diabetes). Symptoms of mental health disorders can also be similar to other conditions. For example, autism spectrum disorder (ASD) is the name for a group of developmental disorders often characterized by impairments in the ability to communicate and interact with others. ASD includes a wide range of symptoms, skills, and levels of disability. These disorders occur in about 1.5 percent of children and often co-occur with disorders such as depression, anxiety, and sensory integration disorder.

Chapter 45

Treating Mental Health Disorders in Teens

Research shows that half of all lifetime cases of mental illness begin by age 14. Scientists are discovering that changes in the body leading to mental illness may start much earlier, before any symptoms appear.

This chapter addresses common questions about treatment options for children with mental illnesses. Disorders affecting children may include anxiety disorders, attention deficit hyperactivity disorder (ADHD), autism spectrum disorders (ASD), bipolar disorder, depression, eating disorders, and schizophrenia.

Are There Treatment Options for Children?

Yes. Once a diagnosis is made, a child specialist will recommend a specific treatment. It is important to understand the various treatment choices, which often include psychotherapy or medication. Talk about the options with a healthcare professional who has experience treating the illness observed in the child. Some treatment choices have been studied experimentally, and other treatments are a part of healthcare practice. In addition, not every community has every type of service or program.

This chapter includes text excerpted from "Treatment of Children with Mental Illness," National Institute of Mental Health (NIMH), 2009. Reviewed November 2017.

What Are Psychotropic Medications?

Psychotropic medications are substances that affect brain chemicals related to mood and behavior. In recent years, research has been conducted to understand the benefits and risks of using psychotropics in children. Still, more needs to be learned about the effects of psychotropics, especially in children under six years of age. While researchers are trying to clarify how early treatment affects a growing body, families and doctors should weigh the benefits and risks of medication. Each child has individual needs, and each child needs to be monitored closely while taking medications.

Are There Treatments Other Than Medications?

Yes. Psychosocial therapies can be very effective alone and in combination with medications. Psychosocial therapies are also called "talk therapies" or "behavioral therapy," and they help people with mental illness change behavior. Therapies that teach parents and children coping strategies can also be effective.

Cognitive behavioral therapy (CBT) is a type of psychotherapy that can be used with children. It has been widely studied and is an effective treatment for a number of conditions, such as depression, obsessive-compulsive disorder, and social anxiety. A person in CBT learns to change distorted thinking patterns and unhealthy behavior. Children can receive CBT with or without their parents, as well as in a group setting. CBT can be adapted to fit the needs of each child. It is especially useful when treating anxiety disorders.

Additionally, a number of therapies exist for ADHD, oppositional defiant disorder, and conduct disorder and include behavioral parent management training (PMT) and behavioral classroom management. Some children benefit from a combination of different psychosocial approaches. An example is behavioral parent management training in combination with CBT for the child. In other cases, a combination of medication and psychosocial therapies may be most effective. Psychosocial therapies often take time, effort, and patience. However, sometimes children learn new skills that may have positive long-term benefits.

When Is It a Good Idea to Use Psychotropic Medications in Young Children?

When the benefits of treatment outweigh the risks, psychotropic medications may be prescribed. Some children need medication to manage severe and difficult problems. Without treatment, these children would suffer serious or dangerous consequences. In addition, psychosocial treatments may not always be effective by themselves. In some instances, however, they can be quite effective when combined with medication.

For some conditions, the child might be more likely to require medication (e.g., schizophrenia, bipolar disorder), but for many other conditions there are research-supported alternatives to medication (e.g., CBT for anxiety, behavioral PMT for conduct-related problems).

Ask your doctor questions about alternatives to medications and about the risks of starting and continuing on these medications. Learn everything you can about the medications prescribed for the child. Learn about possible side effects, some of which may be harmful. Know what a particular treatment is supposed to do. For example, will it change a specific behavior? If you do not see these changes while the child is taking the medication, talk to his or her doctor. Also, discuss the risks of stopping medication with your doctor.

Does Medication Affect Young Children Differently Than Older Children or Adults?

Yes. Young children handle medications differently than older children and adults. The brains of young children change and develop rapidly. Studies have found that developing brains can be very sensitive to medications. There are also developmental differences in how children metabolize—how their bodies process—medications. Therefore, doctors should carefully consider the dosage or how much medication to give each child. Much more research is needed to determine the effects and benefits of medications in children of all ages. But keep in mind that serious untreated mental disorders themselves can harm brain development.

Also, it is important to avoid drug interactions. If the child takes medicine for asthma or cold symptoms, talk to your doctor or pharmacist. Drug interactions could cause medications to not work as intended or lead to serious side effects.

How Should Medication Be Included in an Overall Treatment Plan?

Medication should be used with other treatments. It should not be the only treatment. Consider other services, such as family therapy, family support services, educational classes, and behavior management techniques. If the child's doctor prescribes medication, he or she should evaluate the child regularly to make sure the medication is working. Children need treatment plans tailored to their individual problems and needs.

What Medications Are Used for Which Kinds of Childhood Mental Disorders?

Psychotropic medications include stimulants, antidepressants, anti-anxiety medications, antipsychotics, and mood stabilizers. Dosages approved by the U.S. Food and Drug Administration (FDA) for use in children depend on body weight and age.

What Does It Mean If a Medication Is Specifically Approved for Use in Children?

When the FDA approves a medication, it means the drug manufacturer provided the agency with information showing the medication is safe and effective in a particular group of people. Based on this information, the drug's label lists proper dosage, potential side effects, and approved age. Medications approved for children follow these guidelines.

Many psychotropic medications have not been studied in children, which means they have not been approved by the FDA for use in children. But doctors may prescribe medications as they feel appropriate, even if those uses are not included on the label. This is called "off-label" use. Research shows that off-label use of some medications works well in some children. Other medications need more study in children. In particular, the use of most psychotropic medications has not been adequately studied in preschoolers.

More studies in children are needed before we can fully know the appropriate dosages, how a medication works in children, and what effects a medication might have on learning and development.

Why Haven't Many Medications Been Tested in Children?

In the past, medications were seldom studied in children because mental illness was not recognized in childhood. Also, there were ethical concerns about involving children in research. This led to a lack of knowledge about the best treatments for children. In clinical settings today, children with mental or behavioral disorders are being prescribed medications at increasingly early ages. The FDA has been urging that medications be appropriately studied in children, and Congress passed legislation in 1997 offering incentives to drug manufacturers to carry out such testing. These activities have helped increase research on the effects of medications in children. There still are ethical concerns about testing medications in children. However, strict rules protect participants in research studies. Each study must go through many types of review before, and after it begins.

What Else Can I Do to Help My Child?

Children with mental illness need guidance and understanding from their parents and teachers. This support can help the child achieve his or her full potential and succeed in school. Before the child is diagnosed, frustration, blame, and anger may have built up within a family. Parents and children may need special help to undo these unhealthy interaction patterns. Mental health professionals can counsel the child and family to help everyone develop new skills, attitudes, and ways of relating to each other.

Parents can also help by taking part in parenting skills training. This helps parents learn how to handle difficult situations and behaviors. Training encourages parents to share a pleasant or relaxing activity with their child, to notice and point out what their child does well, and to praise their child's strengths and abilities. Parents may also learn to arrange family situations in more positive ways. Also, parents may benefit from learning stress-management techniques to help them deal with frustration and respond calmly to their child's behavior.

Sometimes, the whole family may need counseling. Therapists can help family members find better ways to handle disruptive behaviors and encourage behavior changes. Finally, support groups help parents and families connect with others who have similar problems and concerns. Groups often meet regularly to share frustrations and successes, to exchange information about recommended specialists and strategies, and to talk with experts.

Where Can I Go for Help?

If you are unsure where to go for help, ask your family doctor. Others who can help are:

- Mental health specialists, such as psychiatrists, psychologists, social workers, or mental health counselors

- Health maintenance organizations

- Community mental health centers

- Hospital psychiatry departments and outpatient clinics

- Mental health programs at universities or medical schools

- State hospital outpatient clinics

- Family services, social agencies, or clergy

- Peer support groups

- Private clinics and facilities

- Employee assistance programs

- Local medical and/or psychiatric societies.

You can also check the phone book under "mental health," "health," "social services," "hotlines," or "physicians" for phone numbers and addresses. An emergency room doctor can also provide temporary help and can tell you where and how to get further help.

Chapter 46

Depression

Chapter Contents

Section 46.1—Depression in Teens 442

Section 46.2—Antidepressants and Teens 446

Section 46.1

Depression in Teens

This section includes text excerpted from "Teen Depression,"
National Institute of Mental Health (NIMH), June 11, 2015.

If you have been feeling sad, hopeless, or irritable for what seems like a long time, you might have depression.

• Depression is a real, treatable brain illness, or health problem.

• Depression can be caused by big transitions in life, stress, or changes in your body's chemicals that affect your thoughts and moods.

• Even if you feel hopeless, depression gets better with treatment.

• There are lots of people who understand and want to help you.

• Ask for help as early as you can so you can get back to being yourself.

You are not alone. There are ways you can feel better.

Regular Sadness and Depression Are Not the Same

Regular Sadness

Feeling moody, sad, or grouchy? Who doesn't once in awhile? It's easy to have a couple of bad days. Your schoolwork, activities, and family, and friend drama, all mixed with not enough sleep, can leave you feeling overwhelmed. On top of that, teen hormones can be all over the place and also make you moody or cry about the smallest thing. Regular moodiness and sadness usually go away quickly though, within a couple of days.

Depression

Untreated depression is a more intense feeling of sadness, hopelessness, and anger or frustration that lasts much longer, such as for weeks, months, or longer. These feelings make it hard for you to function as you normally would or participate in your usual activities. You may also have trouble focusing and feel like you have little to no motivation or energy. You may not even feel like seeing your best friends. Depression can make you feel like it is hard to enjoy life or even get through the day.

Know the Signs and Symptoms of Depression

Most of the day or nearly every day you may feel one or all of the following:

- Sad
- Empty
- Hopeless
- Angry, cranky, or frustrated, even at minor things

You also may:

- Not care about things or activities you used to enjoy.
- Have weight loss when you are not dieting or weight gain from eating too much.
- Have trouble falling asleep or staying asleep, or sleep much more than usual.
- Move or talk more slowly.
- Feel restless or have trouble sitting still.
- Feel very tired or like you have no energy.
- Feel worthless or very guilty.
- Have trouble concentrating, remembering information, or making decisions.
- Think about dying or suicide or try suicide.

Not everyone experiences depression the same way. And depression can occur at the same time as other mental health problems, such as anxiety, an eating disorder, or substance abuse.

If You Think You Are Depressed, Ask for Help as Early as You Can

1. Talk to:
   - Your parents or guardian

- Your teacher or counselor

- Your doctor

- A helpline, such as 800-273-TALK (800-273-8255), free 24-hour help

- Or call 911 if you are in a crisis or want to hurt yourself.

2. Ask your parent or guardian to make an appointment with your doctor for a checkup. Your doctor can make sure that you do not have another health problem that is causing your depression. If your doctor finds that you do not have another health problem, he or she can treat your depression or refer you to a mental health professional. A mental health professional can give you a thorough evaluation and also treat your depression.

3. Talk to a mental health professional, such as a psychiatrist, counselor, psychologist, or other therapist. These mental health professionals can diagnose and treat depression and other mental health problems.

There Are Ways You Can Feel Better

Effective treatments for depression include talk therapy or a combination of talk therapy and medicine.

Talk Therapy

A therapist, such as a psychiatrist, a psychologist, a social worker, or counselor can help you understand and manage your moods and feelings. You can talk out your emotions to someone who understands and supports you. You can also learn how to stop thinking negatively and start to look at the positives in life. This will help you build confidence and feel better about yourself. Research has shown that certain types of talk therapy or psychotherapy can help teens deal with depression. These include cognitive behavioral therapy, which focuses on thoughts, behaviors, and feelings related to depression, and interpersonal psychotherapy, which focuses on working on relationships.

Medicines

If your doctor thinks you need medicine to help your depression, he or she can prescribe an antidepressant. There are a few antidepressants that have been widely studied and proven to help teens. If your doctor recommends medicine, it is important to see your doctor regularly and tell your parents or guardian about your feelings, especially if you start feeling worse or have thoughts of hurting yourself.

Be Good to Yourself

Besides seeing a doctor and a counselor, you can also help your depression by being patient with yourself and good to yourself. Don't expect to get better immediately, but you will feel yourself improving gradually over time.

- Daily exercise, getting enough sleep, spending time outside in nature and in the sun, or eating healthy foods can also help you feel better.

- Your counselor may teach you how to be aware of your feelings and teach you relaxation techniques. Use these when you start feeling down or upset.

- Try to spend time with supportive family members. Talking with your parents, guardian, or other family members who listen and care about you gives you support and they can make you laugh.

- Try to get out with friends and try fun things that help you express yourself.

Depression Can Affect Relationships

It's understandable that you don't want to tell other people that you have been struggling with depression. But know that depression can affect your relationships with family and friends, and how you perform at school. Maybe your grades have dropped because you find it hard to concentrate and stay on top of school. Teachers may think that you aren't trying in class. Maybe because you're feeling hopeless, peers think you are too negative and start giving you a hard time.

Know that their misunderstanding won't last forever because you are getting better with treatment. Think about talking with people you trust to help them understand what you are going through.

Depression Is Not Your Fault or Caused by Something You Did Wrong

Depression is a real, treatable brain illness, or health problem. Depression can be caused by big transitions in life, stress, or changes in your body's chemicals that affect your thoughts and moods. Depression can run in families. Maybe you haven't realized that you have depression and have been blaming yourself for being negative. Remember that depression is not your fault!

Section 46.2

Antidepressants and Teens

This section includes text excerpted from "Antidepressant Medications for Children and Adolescents: Information for Parents and Caregivers," National Institute of Mental Health (NIMH), June 21, 2017.

Depression

Depression is a serious disorder that can cause significant problems in mood, thinking, and behavior at home, in school, and with peers. It is estimated that major depressive disorder (MDD) affects about 5 percent of adolescents.

Treatment for Depression

Research has shown that, as in adults, depression in children and adolescents is treatable. Certain antidepressant medications, called selective serotonin reuptake inhibitors (SSRIs), can be beneficial to children and adolescents with MDD. Certain types of psychological therapies also have been shown to be effective. However, the knowledge of antidepressant treatments in youth, though growing substantially, is limited compared to what is known about treating depression in adults.

There has been some concern that the use of antidepressant medications themselves may induce suicidal behavior in youths. Following a thorough and comprehensive review of all the available published and unpublished controlled clinical trials of antidepressants in children and adolescents, the U.S. Food and Drug Administration (FDA) issued a public warning in October 2004 about an increased risk of suicidal thoughts or behavior (suicidality) in children and adolescents treated with SSRI antidepressant medications. In 2006, an advisory committee to the FDA recommended that the agency extend the warning to include young adults up to age 25.

Results of a comprehensive review of pediatric trials conducted between 1988 and 2006 suggested that the benefits of antidepressant medications likely outweigh their risks to children and adolescents with major depression and anxiety disorders. The study, partially funded by National Institute of Mental Health (NIMH), was published in the April 18, 2007, issue of the *Journal of the American Medical Association* (JAMA).

What Did the U.S. Food and Drug Administration (FDA) Review Find?

In the FDA review, no completed suicides occurred among nearly 2,200 children treated with SSRI medications. However, about 4 percent of those taking SSRI medications experienced suicidal thinking or behavior, including actual suicide attempts—twice the rate of those taking placebo, or sugar pills.

In response, the FDA adopted a "black box" label warning indicating that antidepressants may increase the risk of suicidal thinking and behavior in some children and adolescents with MDD. A blackbox warning is the most serious type of warning in prescription drug labeling.

The warning also notes that children and adolescents taking SSRI medications should be closely monitored for any worsening in depression, emergence of suicidal thinking or behavior, or unusual changes in behavior, such as sleeplessness, agitation, or withdrawal from normal social situations. Close monitoring is especially important during the first four weeks of treatment. SSRI medications usually have few side effects in children and adolescents, but for unknown reasons, they may trigger agitation and abnormal behavior in certain individuals.

What Do We Know about Antidepressant Medications?

The SSRIs include:

- fluoxetine (Prozac)
- sertraline (Zoloft)
- paroxetine (Paxil)

- citalopram (Celexa)

- escitalopram (Lexapro)

- fluvoxamine (Luvox)

Another antidepressant medication, venlafaxine (Effexor), is not an SSRI but is closely related. SSRI medications are considered an improvement over older antidepressant medications because they have fewer side effects and are less likely to be harmful if taken in an overdose, which is an issue for patients with depression already at risk for suicide. They have been shown to be safe and effective for adults.

However, use of SSRI medications among children and adolescents ages 10 to 19 has risen dramatically in the past several years. Fluoxetine (Prozac) is the only medication approved by the FDA for use in treating depression in children ages 8 and older. The other SSRI medications and the SSRI-related antidepressant venlafaxine have not been approved for treatment of depression in children or adolescents, but doctors still sometimes prescribe them to children on an "off-label" basis. In June 2003, however, the FDA recommended that paroxetine not be used in children and adolescents for treating MDD.

Fluoxetine can be helpful in treating childhood depression, and can lead to significant improvement of depression overall. However, it may increase the risk for suicidal behaviors *in a small subset of adolescents*. As with all medical decisions, doctors and families should weigh the risks and benefits of treatment for each individual patient.

What Should You Do for a Child with Depression?

A child or adolescent with MDD should be carefully and thoroughly evaluated by a doctor to determine if medication is appropriate. Psychotherapy often is tried as an initial treatment for mild depression. Psychotherapy may help to determine the severity and persistence of the depression and whether antidepressant medications may be warranted. Types of psychotherapies include "cognitive behavioral therapy," which helps people learn new ways of thinking and behaving, and "interpersonal therapy," which helps people understand and work through troubled personal relationships.

Those who are prescribed an SSRI medication should receive ongoing medical monitoring. Children already taking an SSRI medication should remain on the medication if it has been helpful, but should be carefully monitored by a doctor for side effects. Parents should promptly seek medical advice and evaluation if their child or adolescent experiences suicidal thinking or behavior, nervousness, agitation, irritability, mood instability, or sleeplessness that either emerges or worsens during treatment with SSRI medications.

Once started, treatment with these medications should not be abruptly stopped. Although they are not habit-forming or addictive, abruptly ending an antidepressant can cause withdrawal symptoms or lead to a relapse. Families should not discontinue treatment without consulting their doctor.

All treatments can be associated with side effects. Families and doctors should carefully weigh the risks and benefits, and maintain appropriate follow-up and monitoring to help control for the risks.

Chapter 47

Other Common Mental Health Disorders Affecting Adolescents

Chapter Contents

Section 47.1—Anxiety Disorders.. 452

Section 47.2—Attention Deficit Hyperactivity
Disorder (ADHD).. 457

Section 47.3—Behavior or Conduct Problems........................ 464

Section 47.4—Bipolar Disorder in Children and
Teens... 467

Section 47.5—Borderline Personality Disorder 472

Section 47.6—Eating Disorders 478

Section 47.7—Obsessive-Compulsive Disorder (OCD) 482

Section 47.8—Schizophrenia 486

Section 47.9—Tics and Tourette Syndrome in Youth.............. 490

Section 47.1

Anxiety Disorders

This section includes text excerpted from "Anxiety Disorders,"
National Institute of Mental Health (NIMH), March 2016.

Occasional anxiety is a normal part of life. You might feel anxious
when faced with a problem at work, before taking a test, or making an
important decision. But anxiety disorders involve more than temporary worry or fear. For a person with an anxiety disorder, the anxiety
does not go away and can get worse over time. The feelings can interfere with daily activities such as job performance, school work, and
relationships. There are several different types of anxiety disorders.
Examples include generalized anxiety disorder, panic disorder, and
social anxiety disorder.

Signs and Symptoms

Generalized Anxiety Disorder (GAD)

People with generalized anxiety disorder display excessive anxiety
or worry for months and face several anxiety-related symptoms.
Generalized anxiety disorder symptoms include:

- Restlessness or feeling wound-up or on edge

- Being easily fatigued

- Difficulty concentrating or having their minds go blank

- Irritability

- Muscle tension

- Difficulty controlling the worry

- Sleep problems (difficulty falling or staying asleep or restless,
  unsatisfying sleep)

Panic Disorder

People with panic disorder have recurrent unexpected panic attacks,
which are sudden periods of intense fear that may include palpitations,

pounding heart, or accelerated heart rate; sweating; trembling or shaking; sensations of shortness of breath, smothering, or choking; and feeling of impending doom.

Panic disorder symptoms include:

- Sudden and repeated attacks of intense fear

- Feelings of being out of control during a panic attack

- Intense worries about when the next attack will happen

- Fear or avoidance of places where panic attacks have occurred in the past

Social Anxiety Disorder (SAD)

People with social anxiety disorder (sometimes called "social phobia") have a marked fear of social or performance situations in which they expect to feel embarrassed, judged, rejected, or fearful of offending others.

Social anxiety disorder symptoms include:

- Feeling highly anxious about being with other people and having a hard time talking to them

- Feeling very self-conscious in front of other people and worried about feeling humiliated, embarrassed, or rejected, or fearful of offending others

- Being very afraid that other people will judge them

- Worrying for days or weeks before an event where other people will be

- Staying away from places where there are other people

- Having a hard time making friends and keeping friends

- Blushing, sweating, or trembling around other people

- Feeling nauseous or sick to your stomach when other people are around

Evaluation for an anxiety disorder often begins with a visit to a primary care provider. Some physical health conditions, such as an overactive thyroid or low blood sugar, as well as taking certain medications, can imitate or worsen an anxiety disorder. A thorough mental health evaluation is also helpful, because anxiety disorders often coexist with other related conditions, such as depression or obsessive-compulsive disorder (OCD).

Risk Factors

Researchers are finding that genetic and environmental factors, frequently in interaction with one another, are risk factors for anxiety disorders. Specific factors include:

- Shyness, or behavioral inhibition, in childhood
- Being female
- Having few economic resources
- Being divorced or widowed
- Exposure to stressful life events in childhood and adulthood
- Anxiety disorders in close biological relatives
- Parental history of mental disorders
- Elevated afternoon cortisol levels in the saliva (specifically for social anxiety disorder)

Treatments and Therapies

Anxiety disorders are generally treated with psychotherapy, medication, or both.

Psychotherapy

Psychotherapy or "talk therapy" can help people with anxiety disorders. To be effective, psychotherapy must be directed at the person's specific anxieties and tailored to his or her needs. A typical "side effect" of psychotherapy is temporary discomfort involved with thinking about confronting feared situations.

Cognitive Behavioral Therapy (CBT)

CBT is a type of psychotherapy that can help people with anxiety disorders. It teaches a person different ways of thinking, behaving, and reacting to anxiety-producing and fearful situations. CBT can also help people learn and practice social skills, which is vital for treating social anxiety disorder.

Two specific stand-alone components of CBT used to treat social anxiety disorder are **cognitive therapy** and **exposure therapy**. Cognitive therapy focuses on identifying, challenging, and then neutralizing unhelpful thoughts underlying anxiety disorders.

Exposure therapy focuses on confronting the fears underlying an anxiety disorder in order to help people engage in activities they have been avoiding. Exposure therapy is used along with relaxation exercises and/or imagery. One study, called a meta-analysis because it pulls together all of the previous studies and calculates the statistical magnitude of the combined effects, found that cognitive therapy was superior to exposure therapy for treating social anxiety disorder.

CBT may be conducted individually or with a group of people who have similar problems. Group therapy is particularly effective for social anxiety disorder. Often "homework" is assigned for participants to complete between sessions.

Self-Help or Support Groups

Some people with anxiety disorders might benefit from joining a self-help or support group and sharing their problems and achievements with others. Internet chat rooms might also be useful, but any advice received over the Internet should be used with caution, as Internet acquaintances have usually never seen each other and false identities are common. Talking with a trusted friend or member of the clergy can also provide support, but it is not necessarily a sufficient alternative to care from an expert clinician.

Stress Management Techniques

Stress management techniques and meditation can help people with anxiety disorders calm themselves and may enhance the effects of therapy. While there is evidence that aerobic exercise has a calming effect, the quality of the studies is not strong enough to support its use as treatment. Since caffeine, certain illicit drugs, and even some over-the-counter cold medications can aggravate the symptoms of anxiety disorders, avoiding them should be considered. Check with your physician or pharmacist before taking any additional medications.

The family can be important in the recovery of a person with an anxiety disorder. Ideally, the family should be supportive but not help perpetuate their loved one's symptoms.

Medication

Medication does not cure anxiety disorders but often relieves symptoms. Medication can only be prescribed by a medical doctor (such as a psychiatrist or a primary care provider), but a few states allow psychologists to prescribe psychiatric medications.

Medications are sometimes used as the initial treatment of an anxiety disorder, or are used only if there is insufficient response to a course of psychotherapy. In research studies, it is common for patients treated with a combination of psychotherapy and medication to have better outcomes than those treated with only one or the other.

The most common classes of medications used to combat anxiety disorders are antidepressants, antianxiety drugs, and beta blockers. Be aware that some medications are effective only if they are taken regularly and that symptoms may recur if the medication is stopped.

Antidepressants

Antidepressants are used to treat depression, but they also are helpful for treating anxiety disorders. They take several weeks to start working and may cause side effects such as headache, nausea, or difficulty sleeping. The side effects are usually not a problem for most people, especially if the dose starts off low and is increased slowly over time.

Antianxiety Medications

Antianxiety medications help reduce the symptoms of anxiety, panic attacks, or extreme fear and worry. The most common antianxiety medications are called benzodiazepines. Benzodiazepines are first-line treatments for generalized anxiety disorder. With panic disorder or social phobia (social anxiety disorder), benzodiazepines are usually second-line treatments, behind antidepressants.

Beta Blockers

Beta blockers, such as propranolol and atenolol, are also helpful in the treatment of the physical symptoms of anxiety, especially social anxiety. Physicians prescribe them to control rapid heartbeat, shaking, trembling, and blushing in anxious situations.

Choosing the right medication, medication dose, and treatment plan should be based on a person's needs and medical situation, and done under an expert's care. Only an expert clinician can help you decide whether the medication's ability to help is worth the risk of a side effect. Your doctor may try several medicines before finding the right one.

You and your doctor should discuss:

• How well medications are working or might work to improve your symptoms

- Benefits and side effects of each medication

- Risk for serious side effects based on your medical history

- The likelihood of the medications requiring lifestyle changes

- Costs of each medication

- Other alternative therapies, medications, vitamins, and supplements you are taking and how these may affect your treatment

- How the medication should be stopped. Some drugs can't be stopped abruptly but must be tapered off slowly under a doctor's supervision.

Section 47.2

Attention Deficit Hyperactivity Disorder (ADHD)

This section includes text excerpted from "Attention Deficit Hyperactivity Disorder," National Institute of Mental Health (NIMH), March 2016.

Attention deficit hyperactivity disorder (ADHD) is a brain disorder marked by an ongoing pattern of inattention and/or hyperactivity-impulsivity that interferes with functioning or development.

- **Inattention** means a person wanders off task, lacks persistence, has difficulty sustaining focus, and is disorganized; and these problems are not due to defiance or lack of comprehension.

- **Hyperactivity** means a person seems to move about constantly, including in situations in which it is not appropriate; or excessively fidgets, taps, or talks. In adults, it may be extreme restlessness or wearing others out with constant activity.

- **Impulsivity** means a person makes hasty actions that occur in the moment without first thinking about them and that may have high potential for harm; or a desire for immediate rewards or inability to delay gratification. An impulsive person may be socially intrusive and excessively interrupt others or make important decisions without considering the long-term consequences.

Signs and Symptoms

Inattention and hyperactivity/impulsivity are the key behaviors of ADHD. Some people with ADHD only have problems with one of the behaviors, while others have both inattention and hyperactivity-impulsivity. Most children have the combined type of ADHD.

In preschool, the most common ADHD symptom is hyperactivity.

It is normal to have some inattention, unfocused motor activity and impulsivity, but for people with ADHD, these behaviors:

- are more severe

- occur more often

- interfere with or reduce the quality of how they functions socially, at school, or in a job

Inattention

People with symptoms of inattention may often:

- Overlook or miss details, make careless mistakes in schoolwork, at work, or during other activities

- Have problems sustaining attention in tasks or play, including conversations, lectures, or lengthy reading

- Not seem to listen when spoken to directly

- Not follow through on instructions and fail to finish schoolwork, chores, or duties in the workplace or start tasks but quickly lose focus and get easily sidetracked

- Have problems organizing tasks and activities, such as what to do in sequence, keeping materials and belongings in order, having messy work and poor time management, and failing to meet deadlines

- Avoid or dislike tasks that require sustained mental effort, such as schoolwork or homework, or for teens and older adults, preparing reports, completing forms or reviewing lengthy papers

- Lose things necessary for tasks or activities, such as school supplies, pencils, books, tools, wallets, keys, paperwork, eyeglasses, and cell phones

- Be easily distracted by unrelated thoughts or stimuli

- Be forgetful in daily activities, such as chores, errands, returning calls, and keeping appointments

Hyperactivity-Impulsivity

People with symptoms of hyperactivity-impulsivity may often:

- Fidget and squirm in their seats

- Leave their seats in situations when staying seated is expected, such as in the classroom or in the office

- Run or dash around or climb in situations where it is inappropriate or, in teens and adults, often feel restless

- Be unable to play or engage in hobbies quietly

- Be constantly in motion or "on the go," or act as if "driven by a motor"

- Talk nonstop

- Blurt out an answer before a question has been completed, finish other people's sentences, or speak without waiting for a turn in conversation

- Have trouble waiting his or her turn

- Interrupt or intrude on others, for example in conversations, games, or activities

Diagnosis of ADHD requires a comprehensive evaluation by a licensed clinician, such as a pediatrician, psychologist, or psychiatrist with expertise in ADHD. For a person to receive a diagnosis of ADHD, the symptoms of inattention and/or hyperactivity-impulsivity must be chronic or long-lasting, impair the person's functioning, and cause the person to fall behind normal development for his or her age. The doctor will also ensure that any ADHD symptoms are not due to another medical or psychiatric condition. Most children with ADHD receive a diagnosis during the elementary school years. For an adolescent or adult to receive a diagnosis of ADHD, the symptoms need to have been present prior to age 12.

ADHD symptoms can appear as early as between the ages of 3 and 6 and can continue through adolescence and adulthood. Symptoms of ADHD can be mistaken for emotional or disciplinary problems or missed entirely in quiet, well-behaved children, leading to a delay in diagnosis. Adults with undiagnosed ADHD may have a history of poor academic performance, problems at work, or difficult or failed relationships.

ADHD symptoms can change over time as a person ages. In young children with ADHD, hyperactivity-impulsivity is the most predominant symptom. As a child reaches elementary school, the symptom of inattention may become more prominent and cause the child to struggle academically. In adolescence, hyperactivity seems to lessen and may show more often as feelings of restlessness or fidgeting, but inattention and impulsivity may remain. Many adolescents with ADHD also struggle with relationships and antisocial behaviors. Inattention, restlessness, and impulsivity tend to persist into adulthood.

Risk Factors

Scientists are not sure what causes ADHD. Like many other illnesses, a number of factors can contribute to ADHD, such as:

- Genes

- Cigarette smoking, alcohol use, or drug use during pregnancy

- Exposure to environmental toxins during pregnancy

- Exposure to environmental toxins, such as high levels of lead, at a young age

- Low birth weight

- Brain injuries

ADHD is more common in males than females, and females with ADHD are more likely to have problems primarily with inattention. Other conditions, such as learning disabilities, anxiety disorder, conduct disorder, depression, and substance abuse, are common in people with ADHD.

Treatment and Therapies

While there is no cure for ADHD, currently available treatments can help reduce symptoms and improve functioning. Treatments include medication, psychotherapy, education or training, or a combination of treatments.

Medication

For many people, ADHD medications reduce hyperactivity and impulsivity and improve their ability to focus, work, and learn. Medication also may improve physical coordination. Sometimes several different medications or dosages must be tried before finding the right one that works for a particular person. Anyone taking medications must be monitored closely and carefully by their prescribing doctor.

Stimulants

The most common type of medication used for treating ADHD is called a "stimulant." Although it may seem unusual to treat ADHD with a medication that is considered a stimulant, it works because it increases the brain chemicals dopamine and norepinephrine, which play essential roles in thinking and attention.

Under medical supervision, stimulant medications are considered safe. However, there are risks and side effects, especially when misused or taken in excess of the prescribed dose. For example, stimulants can raise blood pressure and heart rate and increase anxiety. Therefore, a person with other health problems, including high blood pressure, seizures, heart disease, glaucoma, liver or kidney disease, or an anxiety disorder should tell their doctor before taking a stimulant.

Talk with a doctor if you see any of these side effects while taking stimulants:

- decreased appetite
- sleep problems
- tics (sudden, repetitive movements or sounds)
- personality changes
- increased anxiety and irritability
- stomachaches
- headaches

Nonstimulants

A few other ADHD medications are nonstimulants. These medications take longer to start working than stimulants, but can also improve focus, attention, and impulsivity in a person with ADHD. Doctors may prescribe a nonstimulant: when a person has bothersome side effects from stimulants; when a stimulant was not effective; or in combination with a stimulant to increase effectiveness.

Although not approved by the U.S. Food and Drug Administration (FDA) specifically for the treatment of ADHD, some antidepressants are sometimes used alone or in combination with a stimulant to treat ADHD. Antidepressants may help all of the symptoms of ADHD and can be prescribed if a patient has bothersome side effects from stimulants. Antidepressants can be helpful in combination with stimulants if a patient also has another condition, such as an anxiety disorder, depression, or another mood disorder.

Doctors and patients can work together to find the best medication, dose, or medication combination.

Psychotherapy

Adding psychotherapy to treat ADHD can help patients and their families to better cope with everyday problems.

Behavioral therapy is a type of psychotherapy that aims to help a person change his or her behavior. It might involve practical assistance, such as help organizing tasks or completing schoolwork, or working through emotionally difficult events. Behavioral therapy also teaches a person how to:

- monitor his or her own behavior

- give oneself praise or rewards for acting in a desired way, such as controlling anger or thinking before acting

Parents, teachers, and family members also can give positive or negative feedback for certain behaviors and help establish clear rules, chore lists, and other structured routines to help a person control his or her behavior. Therapists may also teach children social skills, such as how to wait their turn, share toys, ask for help, or respond to teasing. Learning to read facial expressions and the tone of voice in others, and how to respond appropriately can also be part of social skills training.

Cognitive behavioral therapy can also teach a person mindfulness techniques, or meditation. A person learns how to be aware and accepting of one's own thoughts and feelings to improve focus and concentration. The therapist also encourages the person with ADHD to adjust to the life changes that come with treatment, such as thinking before acting, or resisting the urge to take unnecessary risks.

Family and marital therapy can help family members and spouses find better ways to handle disruptive behaviors, to encourage behavior changes, and improve interactions with the patient.

Education and Training

Children and adults with ADHD need guidance and understanding from their parents, families, and teachers to reach their full potential and to succeed. For school-age children, frustration, blame, and anger may have built up within a family before a child is diagnosed. Parents and children may need special help to overcome negative feelings. Mental health professionals can educate parents about ADHD and how it affects a family. They also will help the child and his or her parents develop new skills, attitudes, and ways of relating to each other.

Parenting skills training (behavioral parent management training) teaches parents the skills they need to encourage and reward positive behaviors in their children. It helps parents learn how to use a system of rewards and consequences to change a child's behavior. Parents are taught to give immediate and positive feedback for behaviors they want to encourage, and ignore or redirect behaviors that they want to discourage. They may also learn to structure situations in ways that support desired behavior.

Stress management techniques can benefit parents of children with ADHD by increasing their ability to deal with frustration so that they can respond calmly to their child's behavior.

Support groups can help parents and families connect with others who have similar problems and concerns. Groups often meet regularly to share frustrations and successes, to exchange information about recommended specialists and strategies, and to talk with experts.

Tips to Help Kids with ADHD Stay Organized

Parents and teachers can help kids with ADHD stay organized and follow directions with tools such as:

- **Keeping a routine and a schedule.** Keep the same routine every day, from wake-up time to bedtime. Include times for homework, outdoor play, and indoor activities. Keep the schedule on the refrigerator or on a bulletin board in the kitchen. Write changes on the schedule as far in advance as possible.

- **Organizing everyday items.** Have a place for everything, and keep everything in its place. This includes clothing, backpacks, and toys.

- **Using homework and notebook organizers.** Use organizers for school material and supplies. Stress to your child the importance of writing down assignments and bringing home the necessary books.

- **Being clear and consistent.** Children with ADHD need consistent rules they can understand and follow.

- **Giving praise or rewards when rules are followed.** Children with ADHD often receive and expect criticism. Look for good behavior, and praise it.

Section 47.3

Behavior or Conduct Problems

This section includes text excerpted from "Children's Mental Health—Behavior or Conduct Problems," Centers for Disease Control and Prevention (CDC), March 23, 2017.

Children sometimes argue, are aggressive, or act angry, or defiant around adults. A behavior disorder may be diagnosed when these disruptive behaviors are uncommon for the child's age at the time, persist over time, or are severe. Because behavior disorders involve acting out and showing unwanted behavior towards others they are often called externalizing disorders.

Oppositional Defiant Disorder

When children act out persistently so that it causes serious problems at home, in school, or with peers, they may be diagnosed with Oppositional Defiant Disorder (ODD). ODD usually starts before 8 years of age, but no later than by about 12 years of age. Children with ODD are more likely to act oppositional or defiant around people they know well, such as family members, a regular care provider, or a teacher. Children with ODD show these behaviors more often than other children their age.

Examples of ODD behaviors include:

- Often being angry or losing one's temper

- Often arguing with adults or refusing to comply with adults' rules or requests

- Often resentful or spiteful

- Deliberately annoying others or becoming annoyed with others

- Often blaming other people for one's own mistakes or misbehavior

Conduct Disorder

Conduct disorder (CD) is diagnosed when children show an ongoing pattern of aggression toward others, and serious violations of rules and social norms at home, in school, and with peers. These rule violations may involve breaking the law and result in arrest. Children with CD are more likely to get injured and may have difficulties getting along with peers.

Examples of CD behaviors include:

- Breaking serious rules, such as running away, staying out at night when told not to, or skipping school

- Being aggressive in a way that causes harm, such as bullying, fighting, or being cruel to animals

- Lying, stealing, or damaging other people's property on purpose

Treatment for Disruptive Behavior Disorders

Starting treatment early is important. Treatment is most effective if it fits the needs of the specific child and family. The first step to treatment is to talk with a healthcare provider. A comprehensive evaluation by a mental health professional may be needed to get the right diagnosis. Some of the signs of behavior problems, such as not following rules in school, could be related to learning problems which may need additional intervention.

For younger children, the treatment with the strongest evidence is behavior therapy training for parents, where a therapist helps the parent learn effective ways to strengthen the parent child relationship and respond to the child's behavior. For school age children and teens, an often used effective treatment is a combination of training and therapy that includes the child, the family, and the school.

Managing Symptoms: Staying Healthy

Being healthy is important for all children and can be especially important for children with behavior or conduct problems. In addition to behavioral therapy and medication, practicing certain healthy lifestyle behaviors may reduce challenging and disruptive behaviors your child might experience. Here are some healthy behaviors that may help:

- Engaging in regular physical activity, including aerobic and vigorous exercise

- Eating a healthful diet centered on fruits, vegetables, whole grains, legumes (for example, beans, peas, and lentils), lean protein sources, and nuts and seeds

- Getting the recommended amount of sleep each night based on age

- Strengthening relationships with family members

Prevention of Disruptive Behavior Disorders

It is not known exactly why some children develop disruptive behavior disorders. Many factors may play a role, including biological and social factors. It is known that children are at greater risk when they are exposed to other types of violence and criminal behavior, when they experience maltreatment or harsh or inconsistent parenting, or when their parents have mental health conditions like substance use disorders, depression, or attention deficit hyperactivity disorder (ADHD). The quality of early childhood care also can impact whether a child develops behavior problems.

Although these factors appear to increase the risk for disruptive behavior disorders, there are ways to decrease the chance that children experience them.

Section 47.4

Bipolar Disorder in Children and Teens

This section includes text excerpted from "Bipolar Disorder in Children and Teens," National Institute of Mental Health (NIMH), 2015.

Does your child go through intense mood changes? Does your child have extreme behavior changes? Does your child get much more excited and active than other kids his or her age? Do other people say your child is too excited or too moody? Do you notice he or she has highs and lows much more often than other children? Do these mood changes affect how your child acts at school or at home?

Some children and teens with these symptoms may have **bipolar disorder**, a serious mental illness.

What Is Bipolar Disorder?

Bipolar disorder is a serious brain illness. It is also called manic-depressive illness or manic depression. Children with bipolar disorder go through unusual mood changes. Sometimes they feel very happy or "up," and are much more energetic and active than usual, or than other kids their age. This is called a **manic episode**. Sometimes children with bipolar disorder feel very sad and "down," and are much less active than usual. This is called depression or a **depressive episode**.

Bipolar disorder is not the same as the normal ups and downs every kid goes through. Bipolar symptoms are more powerful than that. The mood swings are more extreme and are accompanied by changes in sleep, energy level, and the ability to think clearly. Bipolar symptoms are so strong, they can make it hard for a child to do well in school or get along with friends and family members. The illness can also be dangerous. Some young people with bipolar disorder try to hurt themselves or attempt suicide.

Children and teens with bipolar disorder should get treatment. With help, they can manage their symptoms and lead successful lives.

Who Develops Bipolar Disorder?

Anyone can develop bipolar disorder, including children and teens. However, most people with bipolar disorder develop it in their late teen or early adult years. The illness usually lasts a lifetime.

Why Does Someone Develop Bipolar Disorder?

Doctors do not know what causes bipolar disorder, but several things may contribute to the illness. Family genes may be one factor because bipolar disorder sometimes runs in families. However, it is important to know that just because someone in your family has bipolar disorder, it does not mean other members of the family will have it as well.

Another factor that may lead to bipolar disorder is the brain structure or the brain function of the person with the disorder. Scientists are finding out more about the disorder by studying it. Their research may help doctors do a better job of treating people. Also, this research may help doctors to predict whether a person will get bipolar disorder. One day, doctors may be able to prevent the illness in some people.

What Are the Symptoms of Bipolar Disorder?

Bipolar "mood episodes" include unusual mood changes along with unusual sleep habits, activity levels, thoughts, or behavior. In a child, these mood and activity changes must be very different from their usual behavior and from the behavior of other children. A person with bipolar disorder may have manic episodes, depressive episodes, or "mixed" episodes. A mixed episode has both manic and depressive symptoms. These mood episodes cause symptoms that last a week or two or sometimes longer. During an episode, the symptoms last every day for most of the day.

Children and teens having a manic episode may:

- Feel very happy or act silly in a way that's unusual for them and for other people their age

- Have a very short temper

- Talk really fast about a lot of different things

- Have trouble sleeping but not feel tired

- Have trouble staying focused

- Talk and think about sex more often
- Do risky things

Children and teens having a depressive episode may:

- Feel very sad
- Complain about pain a lot, such as stomachaches and headaches
- Sleep too little or too much
- Feel guilty and worthless
- Eat too little or too much
- Have little energy and no interest in fun activities
- Think about death or suicide

Can Children and Teens with Bipolar Disorder Have Other Problems?

Young people with bipolar disorder can have several problems at the same time. These include:

- **Substance abuse.** Both adults and kids with bipolar disorder are at risk of drinking or taking drugs.
- **Attention deficit hyperactivity disorder (ADHD).** Children who have both bipolar disorder and ADHD may have trouble staying focused.
- **Anxiety disorders, like separation anxiety.**

Sometimes behavior problems go along with mood episodes. Young people may take a lot of risks, such as driving too fast or spending too much money. Some young people with bipolar disorder think about suicide. **Watch for any signs of suicidal thinking. Take these signs seriously and call your child's doctor.**

How Is Bipolar Disorder Diagnosed?

An experienced doctor will carefully examine your child. There are no blood tests or brain scans that can diagnose bipolar disorder. Instead, the doctor will ask questions about your child's mood and sleeping patterns. The doctor will also ask about your child's energy and behavior. Sometimes doctors need to know about medical problems in your family, such as depression or alcoholism. The doctor may use tests to see if something other than bipolar disorder is causing your child's symptoms.

How Is Bipolar Disorder Treated?

Right now, there is no cure for bipolar disorder. Doctors often treat children who have the illness in much the same way they treat adults. Treatment can help control symptoms. Steady, dependable treatment works better than treatment that starts and stops. Treatment options include:

- **Medication.** There are several types of medication that can help. Children respond to medications in different ways, so the right type of medication depends on the child. Some children may need more than one type of medication because their symptoms are so complex. Sometimes they need to try different types of medicine to see which are best for them. Children should take the fewest number of medications and the smallest doses possible to help their symptoms. A good way to remember this is "start low, go slow." Medications can cause side effects. **Always tell your child's doctor about any problems with side effects.** Do not stop giving your child medication without a doctor's help. Stopping medication suddenly can be dangerous, and it can make bipolar symptoms worse.

- **Therapy.** Different kinds of psychotherapy, or "talk" therapy, can help children with bipolar disorder. Therapy can help children change their behavior and manage their routines. It can also help young people get along better with family and friends. Sometimes therapy includes family members.

What Can Children and Teens Expect from Treatment?

With treatment, children and teens with bipolar disorder can get better over time. It helps when doctors, parents, and young people work together.

Sometimes a child's bipolar disorder changes. When this happens, treatment needs to change too. For example, your child may need to try a different medication. The doctor may also recommend other treatment changes. Symptoms may come back after a while, and more adjustments may be needed. Treatment can take time, but sticking with it helps many children and teens have fewer bipolar symptoms.

You can help treatment be more effective. Try keeping a chart of your child's moods, behaviors, and sleep patterns. This is called a "daily life chart" or "mood chart." It can help you and your child understand and track the illness. A chart can also help the doctor see whether treatment is working.

How Can I Help My Child or Teen?

Help begins with the right diagnosis and treatment. If you think your child may have bipolar disorder, make an appointment with your family doctor to talk about the symptoms you notice.

If your child has bipolar disorder, here are some basic things you can do:

- Be patient.

- Encourage your child to talk, and listen to your child carefully.

- Be understanding about mood episodes.

- Help your child have fun.

- Help your child understand that treatment can make life better.

How Does Bipolar Disorder Affect Parents and Family?

Taking care of a child or teenager with bipolar disorder can be stressful for you, too. You have to cope with the mood swings and other problems, such as short tempers and risky activities. This can challenge any parent. Sometimes the stress can strain your relationships with other people, and you may miss work or lose free time.

If you are taking care of a child with bipolar disorder, take care of yourself too. Find someone you can talk to about your feelings. Talk with the doctor about support groups for caregivers. If you keep your stress level down, you will do a better job. It might help your child get better too.

Where Do I Go for Help?

If you're not sure where to get help, call your family doctor. You can also check the phone book for mental health professionals. Hospital doctors can help in an emergency.

I Know Someone Who Is in Crisis. What Do I Do?

If you know someone who might be thinking about hurting himself or herself or someone else, get help quickly.

- Do not leave the person alone.
- Call your doctor.
- Call 911 or go to the emergency room.
- Call National Suicide Prevention Lifeline, toll-free: 800-273-TALK (800-273-8255). The TTY number is 800-799-4TTY (800-799-4889).

Section 47.5

Borderline Personality Disorder

This section includes text excerpted from "Borderline Personality Disorder," National Institute of Mental Health (NIMH), August 2016.

Borderline personality disorder (BPD) is a serious mental disorder marked by a pattern of ongoing instability in moods, behavior, self-image, and functioning. These experiences often result in impulsive actions and unstable relationships. A person with BPD may experience intense episodes of anger, depression, and anxiety that may last from only a few hours to days.

Some people with BPD also have high rates of co-occurring mental disorders, such as mood disorders, anxiety disorders, and eating disorders, along with substance abuse, self-harm, suicidal thinking and behaviors, and suicide. While mental health experts now generally agree that the label "borderline personality disorder" is very misleading, a more accurate term does not exist yet.

Signs and Symptoms of Borderline Personality Disorder (BPD)

People with BPD may experience extreme mood swings and can display uncertainty about who they are. As a result, their interests and values can change rapidly.

Other symptoms include:

- Frantic efforts to avoid real or imagined abandonment
- A pattern of intense and unstable relationships with family, friends, and loved ones, often swinging from extreme closeness and love (idealization) to extreme dislike or anger (devaluation)
- Distorted and unstable self-image or sense of self
- Impulsive and often dangerous behaviors, such as spending sprees, unsafe sex, substance abuse, reckless driving, and binge eating
- Recurring suicidal behaviors or threats or self-harming behavior, such as cutting
- Intense and highly changeable moods, with each episode lasting from a few hours to a few days
- Chronic feelings of emptiness
- Inappropriate, intense anger, or problems controlling anger
- Having stress-related paranoid thoughts
- Having severe dissociative symptoms, such as feeling cut off from oneself, observing oneself from outside the body, or losing touch with reality

Seemingly ordinary events may trigger symptoms. For example, people with BPD may feel angry and distressed over minor separations—such as vacations, business trips, or sudden changes of plans—from people to whom they feel close. Studies show that people with this disorder may see anger in an emotionally neutral face and have a stronger reaction to words with negative meanings than people who do not have the disorder.

Some of these signs and symptoms may be experienced by people with other mental health problems—and even by people without mental illness—and do not necessarily mean that they have BPD. It is important that a qualified and licensed mental health professional conduct a thorough assessment to determine whether or not a diagnosis of BPD or other mental disorder is warranted, and to help guide treatment options when appropriate.

Tests and Diagnosis of BPD

Unfortunately, BPD is often underdiagnosed or misdiagnosed. A licensed mental health professional experienced in diagnosing and treating mental disorders—such as a psychiatrist, psychologist, or clinical social worker—can diagnose BPD based on a thorough interview and a comprehensive medical exam, which can help rule out other possible causes of symptoms.

The licensed mental health professional may ask about symptoms and personal and family medical histories, including any history of mental illnesses. This information can help the mental health professional decide on the best treatment. In some cases, co-occurring mental illnesses may have symptoms that overlap with BPD, making it difficult to distinguish BPD from other mental illnesses. For example, a person may describe feelings of depression but may not bring other symptoms to the mental health professional's attention.

Research funded by National Institute of Mental Health (NIMH) is underway to look for ways to improve diagnosis of and treatments for BPD, and to understand the various components of BPD and other personality disorders such as impulsivity, relationship problems, and emotional instability.

Risk Factors of BPD

The causes of BPD are not yet clear, but research suggests that genetic, brain, environmental and social factors are likely to be involved.

- **Genetics.** BPD is about five times more likely to occur if a person has a close family member (first-degree biological relatives) with the disorder.

- **Environmental and Social Factors.** Many people with BPD report experiencing traumatic life events, such as abuse or abandonment during childhood. Others may have been exposed to unstable relationships and hostile conflicts. However, some people with BPD do not have a history of trauma. And, many people with a history of traumatic life events do not have BPD.

- **Brain Factors.** Studies show that people with BPD have structural and functional changes in the brain, especially in the areas that control impulses and emotional regulation. However, some people with similar changes in the brain do not have BPD. More research is needed to understand the relationship between brain structure and function and BPD.

Treatments and Therapies of BPD

BPD has historically been viewed as difficult to treat. However, with newer and proper treatment, many people with BPD experience fewer or less severe symptoms and an improved quality of life. Many factors affect the length of time it takes for symptoms to improve once treatment begins, so it is important for people with BPD and their loved ones to be patient and to receive appropriate support during treatment. People with BPD can recover.

Psychotherapy

Psychotherapy (or "talk therapy") is the main treatment for people with BPD. Psychotherapy can be provided one-on-one between the therapist and the patient or in a group setting. Therapist-led group sessions may help teach people with BPD how to interact with others and how to express themselves effectively. It is important that people in therapy get along with and trust their therapist. The very nature of BPD can make it difficult for people with this disorder to maintain a comfortable and trusting bond with their therapist.

Types of psychotherapy used to treat BPD include:

- **Cognitive Behavioral Therapy (CBT):** Cognitive behavioral therapy (CBT) can help people with BPD identify and change core beliefs and/or behaviors that underlie inaccurate perceptions of themselves and others and problems interacting with others. CBT may help reduce a range of mood and anxiety symptoms and reduce the number of suicidal or self-harming behaviors.

- **Dialectical Behavior Therapy (DBT):** This type of therapy utilizes the concept of mindfulness, or being aware of and attentive to the current situation and moods. DBT also teaches skills to control intense emotions, reduce self-destructive behaviors, and improve relationships. DBT differs from CBT in that it integrates traditional CBT elements with mindfulness, acceptance, and techniques to improve a person's ability to tolerate stress and control his or her emotions. DBT recognizes the dialectical tension between the need for acceptance and the need for change.

- **Schema-Focused Therapy:** This type of therapy combines elements of CBT with other forms of psychotherapy that focus on reframing schemas, or the ways people view themselves.

This approach is based on the idea that BPD stems from a dysfunctional self-image—possibly brought on by negative childhood experiences—that affects how people react to their environment, interact with others, and cope with problems or stress.

- **Systems Training for Emotional Predictability and Problem Solving (STEPPS):** This is a type of group therapy that aims to educate family members, significant others, and healthcare professionals about BPD and gives them guidance on how to interact consistently with the person with the disorder using the STEPPS approach and terminology. STEPPS is designed to supplement other treatments the patient may be receiving, such as medication or individual psychotherapy.

Families of people with BPD may also benefit from therapy. The challenges of dealing with a loved one with BPD on a daily basis can be very stressful, and family members may unknowingly act in ways that worsen their relative's symptoms. Some therapies include family members in treatment sessions. These types of programs help families develop skills to better understand and support a relative with BPD. Other therapies focus on the needs of family members and help them understand the obstacles and strategies for caring for a loved one with BPD.

Other types of psychotherapy may be helpful for some people with BPD. Therapists often adapt psychotherapy to better meet a person's needs. Therapists may also switch from one type of psychotherapy to another, mix techniques from different therapies, or use a combination of psychotherapies.

Medications

Medications should not be used as the primary treatment for BPD as the benefits are unclear. However, in some cases, a mental health professional may recommend medications to treat specific symptoms, such as mood swings, depression, or other disorders that may occur with BPD.

Treatment with medications may require care from more than one medical professional. Because of the high risk of suicide among people with BPD, healthcare providers should exercise caution when prescribing medications that may be lethal in the event of an overdose. Certain medications can cause different side effects in different people. Talk to your doctor about what to expect from a particular medication.

Other Treatments

Some people with BPD experience severe symptoms and require intensive, often inpatient, care. Others may use some outpatient treatments but never need hospitalization or emergency care. Although in rare cases, some people who develop this disorder may improve without any treatment, most people benefit from and improve their quality of life by seeking treatment.

How Can I Help a Friend or Relative Who Has BPD?

If you know someone who has BPD, it affects you too. The first and most important thing you can do is help your friend or relative get the right diagnosis and treatment. You may need to make an appointment and go with your friend or relative to see the doctor. Encourage him or her to stay in treatment or to seek different treatment if symptoms do not appear to improve with the current treatment.

To help a friend or relative you can:

- Offer emotional support, understanding, patience, and encouragement—change can be difficult and frightening to people with BPD, but it is possible for them to get better over time.

- Learn about mental disorders, including BPD, so you can understand what your friend or relative is experiencing.

- With written permission from your friend or loved one, talk with his or her therapist to learn about therapies that may involve family members. Alternatively, you can encourage your loved one who is in treatment for BPD to ask about family therapy.

- Seek counseling from your own therapist about helping a loved one with BPD. It should not be the same therapist that your loved one with BPD is seeing.

Never ignore comments about someone's intent or plan to harm himself or herself or someone else. Report such comments to the person's therapist or doctor. In urgent or potentially life-threatening situations, you may need to call the police or dial 911.

How Can I Help Myself If I Have BPD?

Although it may take some time, you can get better with treatment. To help yourself:

- Talk to your doctor about treatment options and stick with treatment.

- Try to maintain a stable schedule of meals and sleep times.

- Engage in mild activity or exercise to help reduce stress.

- Set realistic goals for yourself.

- Break up large tasks into small ones, set some priorities, and do what you can, as you can.

- Try to spend time with other people and confide in a trusted friend or family member.

- Tell others about events or situations that may trigger symptoms.

- Expect your symptoms to improve gradually over time, not immediately. Be patient.

- Identify and seek out comforting situations, places, and people.

- Continue to educate yourself about this disorder.

- Don't drink alcohol or use illicit drugs—they will likely make things worse

Section 47.6

Eating Disorders

This section includes text excerpted from "Eating Disorders,"
National Institute of Mental Health (NIMH), February 2016.

There is a commonly held view that eating disorders are a lifestyle choice. Eating disorders are actually serious and often fatal illnesses that cause severe disturbances to a person's eating behaviors. Obsessions with food, body weight, and shape may also signal an eating disorder. Common eating disorders include anorexia nervosa, bulimia nervosa, and binge eating disorder.

Common Eating Disorders and Their Symptoms

Anorexia Nervosa

People with anorexia nervosa may see themselves as overweight, even when they are dangerously underweight. People with anorexia nervosa typically weigh themselves repeatedly, severely restrict the amount of food they eat, and eat very small quantities of only certain foods. Anorexia nervosa has the highest mortality rate of any mental disorder. While many young women and men with this disorder die from complications associated with starvation, others die of suicide. In women, suicide is much more common in those with anorexia than with most other mental disorders.

Symptoms include:

- Extremely restricted eating

- Extreme thinness (emaciation)

- A relentless pursuit of thinness and unwillingness to maintain a normal or healthy weight

- Intense fear of gaining weight

- Distorted body image, a self-esteem that is heavily influenced by perceptions of body weight and shape, or a denial of the seriousness of low body weight

Other symptoms may develop over time, including:

- Thinning of the bones (osteopenia or osteoporosis)

- Mild anemia and muscle wasting and weakness

- Brittle hair and nails

- Dry and yellowish skin

- Growth of fine hair all over the body (lanugo)

- Severe constipation

- Low blood pressure, slowed breathing and pulse

- Damage to the structure and function of the heart

- Brain damage

- Multiorgan failure

- Drop in internal body temperature, causing a person to feel cold all the time

- Lethargy, sluggishness, or feeling tired all the time
- Infertility

Bulimia Nervosa

People with bulimia nervosa have recurrent and frequent episodes of eating unusually large amounts of food and feeling a lack of control over these episodes. This binge eating is followed by behavior that compensates for the overeating such as forced vomiting, excessive use of laxatives or diuretics, fasting, excessive exercise, or a combination of these behaviors. Unlike anorexia nervosa, people with bulimia nervosa usually maintain what is considered a healthy or relatively normal weight.

Symptoms include:

- Chronically inflamed and sore throat
- Swollen salivary glands in the neck and jaw area
- Worn tooth enamel and increasingly sensitive and decaying teeth as a result of exposure to stomach acid
- Acid reflux disorder and other gastrointestinal problems
- Intestinal distress and irritation from laxative abuse
- Severe dehydration from purging of fluids
- Electrolyte imbalance (too low or too high levels of sodium, calcium, potassium, and other minerals) which can lead to stroke or heart attack

Binge Eating Disorder

People with binge eating disorder lose control over his or her eating. Unlike bulimia nervosa, periods of binge eating are not followed by purging, excessive exercise, or fasting. As a result, people with binge eating disorder often are overweight or obese. Binge eating disorder is the most common eating disorder in the United States.

Symptoms include:

- Eating unusually large amounts of food in a specific amount of time
- Eating even when you're full or not hungry
- Eating fast during binge episodes

- Eating until you're uncomfortably full
- Eating alone or in secret to avoid embarrassment
- Feeling distressed, ashamed, or guilty about your eating
- Frequently dieting, possibly without weight loss

Risk Factors

Eating disorders frequently appear during the teen years or young adulthood but may also develop during childhood or later in life. These disorders affect both genders, although rates among women are higher than among men. Like women who have eating disorders, men also have a distorted sense of body image. For example, men may have muscle dysmorphia, a type of disorder marked by an extreme concern with becoming more muscular.

Researchers are finding that eating disorders are caused by a complex interaction of genetic, biological, behavioral, psychological, and social factors. Researchers are using the latest technology and science to better understand eating disorders.

One approach involves the study of human genes. Eating disorders run in families. Researchers are working to identify deoxyribonucleic acid (DNA) variations that are linked to the increased risk of developing eating disorders.

Brain imaging studies are also providing a better understanding of eating disorders. For example, researchers have found differences in patterns of brain activity in women with eating disorders in comparison with healthy women. This kind of research can help guide the development of new means of diagnosis and treatment of eating disorders.

Treatments and Therapies

Adequate nutrition, reducing excessive exercise, and stopping purging behaviors are the foundations of treatment. Treatment plans are tailored to individual needs and may include one or more of the following:

- Individual, group, and/or family psychotherapy
- Medical care and monitoring
- Nutritional counseling
- Medications

Psychotherapies

Psychotherapies such as a family based therapy called the Maudsley approach, where parents of adolescents with anorexia nervosa assume responsibility for feeding their child, appear to be very effective in helping people gain weight and improve eating habits and moods.

To reduce or eliminate binge eating and purging behaviors, people may undergo cognitive behavioral therapy (CBT), which is another type of psychotherapy that helps a person learn how to identify distorted or unhelpful thinking patterns and recognize and change inaccurate beliefs.

Medications

Evidence also suggests that medications such as antidepressants, antipsychotics, or mood stabilizers approved by the U.S. Food and Drug Administration (FDA) may also be helpful for treating eating disorders and other co-occurring illnesses such as anxiety or depression.

Section 47.7

Obsessive-Compulsive Disorder (OCD)

This section includes text excerpted from "Obsessive-Compulsive Disorder," National Institute of Mental Health (NIMH), January 2016.

Obsessive-compulsive disorder (OCD) is a common, chronic and long-lasting disorder in which a person has uncontrollable, reoccurring thoughts (obsessions) and behaviors (compulsions) that he or she feels the urge to repeat over and over.

Signs and Symptoms of Obsessive-Compulsive Disorder (OCD)

People with OCD may have symptoms of obsessions, compulsions, or both. These symptoms can interfere with all aspects of life, such as work, school, and personal relationships.

Obsessions are repeated thoughts, urges, or mental images that cause anxiety. Common symptoms include:

- Fear of germs or contamination
- Unwanted forbidden or taboo thoughts involving sex, religion, and harm
- Aggressive thoughts towards others or self
- Having things symmetrical or in a perfect order

Compulsions are repetitive behaviors that a person with OCD feels the urge to do in response to an obsessive thought. Common compulsions include:

- Excessive cleaning and/or handwashing
- Ordering and arranging things in a particular, precise way
- Repeatedly checking on things, such as repeatedly checking to see if the door is locked or that the oven is off
- Compulsive counting

Not all rituals or habits are compulsions. Everyone double checks things sometimes. But a person with OCD generally:

- Can't control his or her thoughts or behaviors, even when those thoughts or behaviors are recognized as excessive
- Spends at least 1 hour a day on these thoughts or behaviors
- Doesn't get pleasure when performing the behaviors or rituals, but may feel brief relief from the anxiety the thoughts cause
- Experiences significant problems in their daily life due to these thoughts or behaviors

Some individuals with OCD also have a tic disorder. Motor tics are sudden, brief, repetitive movements, such as eye blinking and other eye movements, facial grimacing, shoulder shrugging, and head or shoulder jerking. Common vocal tics include:

- repetitive throat-clearing
- sniffing
- grunting sounds

Symptoms may come and go, ease over time, or worsen. People with OCD may try to help themselves by avoiding situations that trigger their obsessions, or they may use alcohol or drugs to calm themselves. Although most adults with OCD recognize that what they are doing doesn't make sense, some adults and most children may not realize that their behavior is out of the ordinary. Parents or teachers typically recognize OCD symptoms in children.

If you think you have OCD, talk to your doctor about your symptoms. If left untreated, OCD can interfere in all aspects of life.

Risk Factors

OCD is a common disorder that affects adults, adolescents, and children all over the world. Most people are diagnosed by about age 19, typically with an earlier age of onset in boys than in girls, but onset after age 35 does happen.

The causes of OCD are unknown, but risk factors include:

Genetics

Twin and family studies have shown that people with first degree relatives (such as a parent, sibling, or child) who have OCD are at a higher risk for developing OCD themselves. The risk is higher if the first degree relative developed OCD as a child or teen. Ongoing research continues to explore the connection between genetics and OCD and may help improve OCD diagnosis and treatment.

Brain Structure and Functioning

Imaging studies have shown differences in the frontal cortex and subcortical structures of the brain in patients with OCD. There appears to be a connection between the OCD symptoms and abnormalities in certain areas of the brain, but that connection is not clear. Research is still underway. Understanding the causes will help determine specific, personalized treatments to treat OCD.

Environment

People who have experienced abuse (physical or sexual) in childhood or other trauma are at an increased risk for developing OCD.

In some cases, children may develop OCD or OCD symptoms following a streptococcal infection—this is called Pediatric Autoimmune Neuropsychiatric Disorders Associated with Streptococcal Infections (PANDAS).

Treatments and Therapies

OCD is typically treated with medication, psychotherapy or a combination of the two. Although most patients with OCD respond to treatment, some patients continue to experience symptoms.

Sometimes people with OCD also have other mental disorders, such as anxiety, depression, and body dysmorphic disorder, a disorder in which someone mistakenly believes that a part of their body is abnormal. It is important to consider these other disorders when making decisions about treatment.

Medication

Serotonin reuptake inhibitors (SRIs) and selective serotonin reuptake inhibitors (SSRIs) are used to help reduce OCD symptoms. Examples of medications that have been proven effective in both adults and children with OCD include clomipramine, which is a member of an older class of "tricyclic" antidepressants, and several newer "selective serotonin reuptake inhibitors (SSRIs)," including:

- fluoxetine
- fluvoxamine
- sertraline

SRIs often require higher daily doses in the treatment of OCD than of depression, and may take 8 to 12 weeks to start working, but some patients experience more rapid improvement.

If symptoms do not improve with these types of medications, research shows that some patients may respond well to an antipsychotic medication (such as risperidone). Although research shows that an antipsychotic medication may be helpful in managing symptoms for people who have both OCD and a tic disorder, research on the effectiveness of antipsychotics to treat OCD is mixed.

If you are prescribed a medication, be sure you:

- Talk with your doctor or a pharmacist to make sure you understand the risks and benefits of the medications you're taking.

- Do not stop taking a medication without talking to your doctor first. Suddenly stopping a medication may lead to "rebound" or worsening of OCD symptoms. Other uncomfortable or potentially dangerous withdrawal effects are also possible.

- Report any concerns about side effects to your doctor right away. You may need a change in the dose or a different medication.

- Report serious side effects to the U.S. Food and Drug Administration (FDA) MedWatch Adverse Event Reporting program online at (www.fda.gov/Safety/MedWatch) or by phone at 800-332-1088. You or your doctor may send a report.

Psychotherapy

Psychotherapy can be an effective treatment for adults and children with OCD. Research shows that certain types of psychotherapy, including cognitive behavior therapy (CBT) and other related therapies (e.g., habit reversal training) can be as effective as medication for many individuals. Research also shows that a type of CBT called Exposure and Response Prevention (EX/RP) is effective in reducing compulsive behaviors in OCD, even in people who did not respond well to SRI medication. For many patients EX/RP is the add on treatment of choice when SRIs or SSRIs medication does not effectively treat OCD symptoms.

Other Treatment Options

National Institute of Mental Health (NIMH) is supporting research into new treatment approaches for people whose OCD does not respond well to the usual therapies. These new approaches include combination and add on (augmentation) treatments, as well as novel techniques such as deep brain stimulation (DBS).

Section 47.8

Schizophrenia

This section includes text excerpted from "Schizophrenia,"
National Institute of Mental Health (NIMH), February 2016.

Schizophrenia is a chronic and severe mental disorder that affects how a person thinks, feels, and behaves. People with schizophrenia may seem like they have lost touch with reality. Although schizophrenia is not as common as other mental disorders, the symptoms can be very disabling.

Signs and Symptoms

Symptoms of schizophrenia usually start between ages 16 and 30. In rare cases, children have schizophrenia too.

The symptoms of schizophrenia fall into three categories: positive, negative, and cognitive.

Positive symptoms: "Positive" symptoms are psychotic behaviors not generally seen in healthy people. People with positive symptoms may "lose touch" with some aspects of reality. Symptoms include:

- Hallucinations

- Delusions

- Thought disorders (unusual or dysfunctional ways of thinking)

- Movement disorders (agitated body movements)

Negative symptoms: "Negative" symptoms are associated with disruptions to normal emotions and behaviors. Symptoms include:

- "Flat affect" (reduced expression of emotions via facial expression or voice tone)

- Reduced feelings of pleasure in everyday life

- Difficulty beginning and sustaining activities

- Reduced speaking

Cognitive symptoms: For some patients, the cognitive symptoms of schizophrenia are subtle, but for others, they are more severe and patients may notice changes in their memory or other aspects of thinking. Symptoms include:

- Poor "executive functioning" (the ability to understand information and use it to make decisions)

- Trouble focusing or paying attention

- Problems with "working memory" (the ability to use information immediately after learning it)

Risk Factors

There are several factors that contribute to the risk of developing schizophrenia.

Genes and environment: Scientists have long known that schizophrenia sometimes runs in families. However, there are many people who have schizophrenia who don't have a family member with the disorder and conversely, many people with one or more family members with the disorder who do not develop it themselves.

Scientists believe that many different genes may increase the risk of schizophrenia, but that no single gene causes the disorder by itself. It is not yet possible to use genetic information to predict who will develop schizophrenia.

Scientists also think that interactions between genes and aspects of the individual's environment are necessary for schizophrenia to develop. Environmental factors may involve:

- Exposure to viruses

- Malnutrition before birth

- Problems during birth

- Psychosocial factors

Different brain chemistry and structure: Scientists think that an imbalance in the complex, interrelated chemical reactions of the brain involving the neurotransmitters (substances that brain cells use to communicate with each other) dopamine and glutamate, and possibly others, plays a role in schizophrenia.

Some experts also think problems during brain development before birth may lead to faulty connections. The brain also undergoes major changes during puberty, and these changes could trigger psychotic symptoms in people who are vulnerable due to genetics or brain differences.

Treatments and Therapies

Because the causes of schizophrenia are still unknown, treatments focus on eliminating the symptoms of the disease. Treatments include:

Antipsychotics

Antipsychotic medications are usually taken daily in pill or liquid form. Some antipsychotics are injections that are given once or twice a month. Some people have side effects when they start taking medications, but most side effects go away after a few days. Doctors and patients can work together to find the best medication or medication combination, and the right dose.

Psychosocial Treatments

These treatments are helpful after patients and their doctor find a medication that works. Learning and using coping skills to address the everyday challenges of schizophrenia helps people to pursue their life goals, such as attending school or work. Individuals who participate in regular psychosocial treatment are less likely to have relapses or be hospitalized.

Coordinated Specialty Care (CSC)

This treatment model integrates medication, psychosocial therapies, case management, family involvement, and supported education and employment services, all aimed at reducing symptoms and improving quality of life. The National Institute of Mental Health (NIMH) Recovery after an Initial Schizophrenia Episode (RAISE) research project seeks to fundamentally change the trajectory and prognosis of schizophrenia through coordinated specialty care treatment in the earliest stages of the disorder. RAISE is designed to reduce the likelihood of long-term disability that people with schizophrenia often experience and help them lead productive, independent lives.

How Can I Help Someone I Know with Schizophrenia?

Caring for and supporting a loved one with schizophrenia can be hard. It can be difficult to know how to respond to someone who makes strange or clearly false statements. It is important to understand that schizophrenia is a biological illness.

Here are some things you can do to help your loved one:

- Get them treatment and encourage them to stay in treatment

- Remember that their beliefs or hallucinations seem very real to them

- Tell them that you acknowledge that everyone has the right to see things their own way

- Be respectful, supportive, and kind without tolerating dangerous or inappropriate behavior

- Check to see if there are any support groups in your area

Section 47.9

Tics and Tourette Syndrome in Youth

This section includes text excerpted from "Facts about Tourette Syndrome," Centers for Disease Control and Prevention (CDC), May 11, 2017.

Tourette Syndrome (TS) is a condition of the nervous system. TS causes people to have "tics."

Tics are sudden twitches, movements, or sounds that people do repeatedly. People who have tics cannot stop their body from doing these things. For example, a person might keep blinking over and over again. Or, a person might make a grunting sound unwillingly.

Having tics is a little bit like having hiccups. Even though you might not want to hiccup, your body does it anyway. Sometimes people can stop themselves from doing a certain tic for awhile, but it's hard. Eventually the person has to do the tic.

Types of Tics

There are two types of tics—motor and vocal:

1. Motor Tics

Motor tics are movements of the body. Examples of motor tics include blinking, shrugging the shoulders, or jerking an arm.

2. Vocal Tics

Vocal tics are sounds that a person makes with his or her voice. Examples of vocal tics include humming, clearing the throat, or yelling out a word or phrase.

Tics can be either simple or complex:

Simple Tics

Simple tics involve just a few parts of the body. Examples of simple tics include squinting the eyes or sniffing.

Complex Tics

Complex tics usually involve several different parts of the body and can have a pattern. An example of a complex tic is bobbing the head while jerking an arm, and then jumping up.

Symptoms

The main symptoms of TS are tics. Symptoms usually begin when a child is 5 to 10 years of age. The first symptoms often are motor tics that occur in the head and neck area. Tics usually are worse during times that are stressful or exciting. They tend to improve when a person is calm or focused on an activity.

The types of tics and how often a person has tics changes a lot over time. Even though the symptoms might appear, disappear, and reappear, these conditions are considered chronic.

In most cases, tics decrease during adolescence and early adulthood, and sometimes disappear entirely. However, many people with TS experience tics into adulthood and, in some cases, tics can become worse during adulthood.

Although the media often portray people with TS as involuntarily shouting out swear words (called coprolalia) or constantly repeating the words of other people (called echolalia), these symptoms are rare, and are not required for a diagnosis of TS.

Diagnosis

There is no single test, like a blood test, to diagnose TS. Health professionals look at the person's symptoms to diagnose TS and other tic disorders. The tic disorders differ from each other in terms of the type of tic present (motor or vocal, or combination of the both), and how long the symptoms have lasted. TS can be diagnosed if a person has both motor and vocal tics, and has had tic symptoms for at least a year.

Treatments

Although there is no cure for TS, there are treatments available to help manage the tics. Many people with TS have tics that do not get in the way of their daily life and, therefore, do not need any treatment. However, medication and behavioral treatments are available if tics cause pain or injury; interfere with school, work, or social life; or cause stress.

Other Concerns and Conditions

TS often occurs with other conditions (called co-occurring conditions). Among children diagnosed with TS, 86 percent also have been diagnosed with at least one additional mental, behavioral, or developmental condition. The two most common conditions are attention deficit hyperactivity disorder (ADHD) and obsessive-compulsive disorder (OCD). It is important to find out if a person with TS has any other conditions, and treat those conditions properly.

Risk Factors and Causes

Doctors and scientists do not know the exact cause of TS. Research suggests that it is an inherited genetic condition. That means it is passed on from parent to child through *genes*.

Who Is Affected?

In the United States, 1 of every 360 children 6 through 17 years of age have been diagnosed with TS. TS can affect people of all racial and ethnic groups. Boys are affected three to five times more often than girls.

Chapter 48

Understanding Self-Harm

Self-harm, sometimes called self-injury, is when a person purposely hurts his or her own body. There are many types of self-injury, and cutting is one type that you may have heard about. If you are hurting yourself, you can learn to stop. Make sure you talk to an adult you trust, and keep reading to learn more.

What Are Ways People Hurt Themselves?

Some types of injury leave permanent scars or cause serious health problems, sometimes even death. These are some forms of self-injury:

- Cutting yourself (such as using a razorblade, knife, or other sharp object)
- Punching yourself or punching things (like a wall)
- Burning yourself with cigarettes, matches, or candles
- Pulling out your hair
- Poking objects into body openings
- Breaking your bones or bruising yourself
- Poisoning yourself

This chapter includes text excerpted from "Cutting and Self-Harm," girlshealth. gov, Office on Women's Health (OWH), February 12, 2015.

The Dangers of Self-Injury

Some teens think self-injury is not a big deal, but it is. Self-injury comes with many risks. For example, cutting can lead to infections, scars, and even death. Sharing tools for cutting puts a person at risk of diseases like human immunodeficiency virus (HIV) and hepatitis. Also, once you start self-injuring, it may be hard to stop. And teens who keep hurting themselves are less likely to learn how to deal with their feelings in healthy ways.

Who Hurts Themselves?

People from all different kinds of backgrounds hurt themselves. Among teens, girls may be more likely to do it than boys.

People of all ages hurt themselves, too, but self-injury most often starts in the teen years.

People who hurt themselves sometimes have other problems like depression, eating disorders, or drug or alcohol abuse.

Why Do Some Teens Hurt Themselves?

Some teens who hurt themselves keep their feelings bottled up inside. The physical pain then offers a sense of relief, like the feelings are getting out. Some people who hold back strong emotions begin to feel like they have no emotions, and the injury helps them at least feel something.

Some teens say that when they hurt themselves, they are trying to stop feeling painful emotions, like rage, loneliness, or hopelessness. They may injure to distract themselves from the emotional pain. Or they may be trying to feel some sense of control over what they feel.

If you are depressed, angry, or having a hard time coping, talk with an adult you trust. You also can contact a helpline. Remember, you have a right to be safe and happy!

If you are hurting yourself, please get help. It is possible to get past the urge to hurt yourself. There are other ways to deal with your feelings. You can talk to your parents, your doctor, or another trusted adult, like a teacher or religious leader. Therapy can help you find healthy ways to handle problems. You can read more about ways to stop cutting.

What Are Signs of Self-Injury in Others?

- Having cuts, bruises, or scars
- Wearing long sleeves or pants even in hot weather
- Making excuses about injuries
- Having sharp objects around for no clear reason

How Can I Help a Friend Who Is Self-Injuring?

If you think a friend may be hurting herself, try to get your friend to talk to a trusted adult. Your friend may need professional help. A therapist can suggest ways to cope with problems without turning to self-injury. If your friend won't get help, you should talk to an adult. This is too much for you to handle alone.

What If Someone Pressures Me to Hurt Myself?

If someone pressures you to hurt yourself, think about whether you really want a friend who tries to cause you pain. Try to hang out with other people who don't treat you this way. Try to hang out with people who make you feel good about yourself.

Chapter 49

Teen Suicide

Suicide is a serious public health problem that affects many young people. Suicide is the third leading cause of death for youth between the ages of 10 and 24, and results in approximately 4,600 lives lost each year.

Deaths from youth suicide are only part of the problem. More young people survive suicide attempts than actually die. A nationwide survey of high school students in the United States found that 16 percent of students reported seriously considering suicide, 13 percent reported creating a plan, and 8 percent reporting trying to take their own life in the 12 months preceding the survey. Each year, approximately 157,000 youth between the ages of 10 and 24 are treated Emergency Departments across the United States for self-inflicted injuries.

Suicide Risk among Teens

Suicide among teens and young adults has nearly tripled since the 1940's. Several factors can put a young person at risk for suicide; however, having risk factors does not always mean that a young person will attempt suicide. Risk factors include: family history of suicide; history of depression, other mental health problems, or incarceration;

This chapter contains text excerpted from the following sources: Text in this chapter begins with excerpts from "Suicide among Youth," Centers for Disease Control and Prevention (CDC), September 15, 2017; Text beginning with the heading "Warning Signs" is excerpted from "Suicide Prevention," Youth.gov, September 10, 2014. Reviewed November 2017.

easy access to lethal means; alcohol and drug use; exposure to previous suicidal behavior by others; and residential mobility that might lessen opportunities for developing healthy social connections and supports.

Suicide affects all youth, but some groups are at higher risk than others. Boys are more likely than girls to die from suicide. Of the reported suicides in the 10 to 24 age group, 81 percent of the deaths were males and 19 percent were females. Girls, however, are more likely to report attempting suicide than boys. Native American/Alaskan Native youth have the highest rates of suicide-related fatalities. A nationwide survey high school students in the United States found Hispanic youth were more likely to report attempting suicide than their black and white, non-Hispanic peers.

Warning Signs

Knowing the warning signs is also critical. Warning signs for those at risk of suicide include: talking about wanting to die, feeling hopeless, having no reason to live, feeling trapped or in unbearable pain, seeking revenge, and being a burden on others; looking for methods and making plans such as searching online or buying a gun; increasing use of alcohol or drugs; acting anxious or agitated; behaving recklessly; sleeping too little or too much; withdrawal or isolation; and displaying rage and extreme mood swings. The risk of suicide is greater if a behavior is new or has increased and if it seems related to a painful event, loss, or change. Paying attention to warning signs for mental health challenges that can be associated with increased risk for suicide is also important.

No one person (parent, teacher, counselor, administrator, mentor, etc.) can implement suicide prevention efforts on their own. The participation, support, and active involvement of families, schools, and communities are essential. Youth focused suicide prevention strategies are available. Promotion and prevention services are also available to address mental health issues. Schools, where youth spend the majority of their time, are a natural setting to support mental health.

Teen Suicide Prevention

Developmentally, the years between childhood and adulthood represent a critical period of transition and significant cognitive, mental, emotional, and social change. While adolescence is a time of tremendous growth and potential, navigating new milestones in preparation for adult roles involving education, employment, relationships, and living circumstances can be difficult. These transitions can lead to various mental health challenges that can be associated with increased risk for suicide.

Despite how common suicidal thoughts and attempts (as well as mental health disorders which can be associated with increased risk for suicide) are among youth, there is a great deal known about prevention as well as caring for youth and communities after an attempt or death. Parents, guardians, family members, friends, teachers, school administrators, coaches, extracurricular activity leaders, mentors, service providers, and many others can play a role in preventing suicide and supporting youth.

Part Six

Substance Abuse and Adolescents

Chapter 50

Addiction and the Adolescent Brain

The Human Brain

The human brain is the most complex organ in the body. This three-pound mass of gray and white matter sits at the center of all human activity—you need it to drive a car, to enjoy a meal, to breathe, to create an artistic masterpiece, and to enjoy everyday activities. In brief, the brain regulates your body's basic functions; enables you to interpret and respond to everything you experience; and shapes your thoughts, emotions, and behavior.

The brain is made up of many parts that all work together as a team. Different parts of the brain are responsible for coordinating and performing specific functions. Drugs can alter important brain areas that are necessary for life-sustaining functions and can drive the compulsive drug abuse that marks addiction. Brain areas affected by drug abuse include:

- The brain stem, which controls basic functions critical to life, such as heart rate, breathing, and sleeping.

- The cerebral cortex, which is divided into areas that control specific functions. Different areas process information from our

This chapter includes text excerpted from "Drugs, Brains, and Behavior: The Science of Addiction," National Institute on Drug Abuse (NIDA), July 2014. Reviewed November 2017.

senses, enabling us to see, feel, hear, and taste. The front part of the cortex, the frontal cortex or forebrain, is the thinking center of the brain; it powers our ability to think, plan, solve problems, and make decisions.

- The limbic system, which contains the brain's reward circuit. It links together a number of brain structures that control and regulate our ability to feel pleasure. Feeling pleasure motivates us to repeat behaviors that are critical to our existence. The limbic system is activated by healthy, life-sustaining activities such as eating and socializing—but it is also activated by drugs of abuse. In addition, the limbic system is responsible for our perception of other emotions, both positive and negative, which explains the mood-altering properties of many drugs.

How Do the Parts of the Brain Communicate?

The brain is a communications center consisting of billions of neurons, or nerve cells. Networks of neurons pass messages back and forth among different structures within the brain, the spinal cord, and nerves in the rest of the body (the peripheral nervous system). These nerve networks coordinate and regulate everything we feel, think, and do.

- **Neuron to neuron.** Each nerve cell in the brain sends and receives messages in the form of electrical and chemical signals. Once a cell receives and processes a message, it sends it on to other neurons.

- **Neurotransmitters—The brain's chemical messengers.** The messages are typically carried between neurons by chemicals called neurotransmitters.

- **Receptors—The brain's chemical receivers.** The neurotransmitter attaches to a specialized site on the receiving neuron called a receptor. A neurotransmitter and its receptor operate like a "key and lock," an exquisitely specific mechanism that ensures that each receptor will forward the appropriate message only after interacting with the right kind of neurotransmitter.

- **Transporters—The brain's chemical recyclers.** Located on the neuron that releases the neurotransmitter, transporters recycle these neurotransmitters (that is, bring them back into the neuron that released them), thereby shutting off the signal between neurons.

How Do Drugs Work in the Brain?

Drugs are chemicals that affect the brain by tapping into its communication system and interfering with the way neurons normally send, receive, and process information. Some drugs, such as marijuana and heroin, can activate neurons because their chemical structure mimics that of a natural neurotransmitter. This similarity in structure "fools" receptors and allows the drugs to attach onto and activate the neurons. Although these drugs mimic the brain's own chemicals, they don't activate neurons in the same way as a natural neurotransmitter, and they lead to abnormal messages being transmitted through the network.

Other drugs, such as amphetamine or cocaine, can cause the neurons to release abnormally large amounts of natural neurotransmitters or prevent the normal recycling of these brain chemicals. This disruption produces a greatly amplified message, ultimately disrupting communication channels.

How Do Drugs Work in the Brain to Produce Pleasure?

Most drugs of abuse directly or indirectly target the brain's reward system by flooding the circuit with dopamine. Dopamine is a neurotransmitter present in regions of the brain that regulate movement, emotion, motivation, and feelings of pleasure. When activated at normal levels, this system rewards our natural behaviors. Overstimulating the system with drugs, however, produces euphoric effects, which strongly reinforce the behavior of drug use—teaching the user to repeat it.

How Does Stimulation of the Brain's Pleasure Circuit Teach Us to Keep Taking Drugs?

Our brains are wired to ensure that we will repeat life-sustaining activities by associating those activities with pleasure or reward. Whenever this reward circuit is activated, the brain notes that something important is happening that needs to be remembered, and teaches us to do it again and again without thinking about it. Because drugs of abuse stimulate the same circuit, we learn to abuse drugs in the same way.

Why Are Drugs More Addictive Than Natural Rewards?

When some drugs of abuse are taken, they can release 2 to 10 times the amount of dopamine that natural rewards such as eating and sex do. In some cases, this occurs almost immediately (as when drugs are smoked or injected), and the effects can last much longer than those produced by natural rewards. The resulting effects on the brain's pleasure circuit dwarf those produced by naturally rewarding behaviors. The effect of such a powerful reward strongly motivates people to take drugs again and again. This is why scientists sometimes say that drug abuse is something we learn to do very, very well.

What Happens to Your Brain If You Keep Taking Drugs?

For the brain, the difference between normal rewards and drug rewards can be described as the difference between someone whispering into your ear and someone shouting into a microphone. Just as we turn down the volume on a radio that is too loud, the brain adjusts to the overwhelming surges in dopamine (and other neurotransmitters) by producing less dopamine or by reducing the number of receptors that can receive signals. As a result, dopamine's impact on the reward circuit of the brain of someone who abuses drugs can become abnormally low, and that person's ability to experience any pleasure is reduced.

This is why a person who abuses drugs eventually feels flat, lifeless, and depressed, and is unable to enjoy things that were previously pleasurable. Now, the person needs to keep taking drugs again and again just to try and bring his or her dopamine function back up to normal—which only makes the problem worse, like a vicious cycle. Also, the person will often need to take larger amounts of the drug to produce the familiar dopamine high—an effect known as tolerance.

How Does Long-Term Drug Taking Affect Brain Circuits?

The same sort of mechanisms involved in the development of tolerance can eventually lead to profound changes in neurons and brain circuits, with the potential to severely compromise the long-term health of the brain. For example, glutamate is another neurotransmitter that influences the reward circuit and the ability to learn. When the optimal concentration of glutamate is altered by drug abuse, the brain attempts to compensate for this change, which can cause impairment in cognitive function. Similarly, long-term drug abuse can trigger adaptations in habit or nonconscious memory systems. Conditioning is one example of this type of learning, in which cues in a person's daily routine or environment become associated with the drug experience and can trigger uncontrollable cravings whenever the person is exposed to these cues, even if the drug itself is not available. This learned "reflex" is extremely durable and can affect a person who once used drugs even after many years of abstinence.

What Other Brain Changes Occur with Abuse?

Chronic exposure to drugs of abuse disrupts the way critical brain structures interact to control and inhibit behaviors related to drug use. Just as continued abuse may lead to tolerance or the need for higher drug dosages to produce an effect, it may also lead to addiction, which can drive a user to seek out and take drugs compulsively. Drug addiction erodes a person's self-control and ability to make sound decisions, while producing intense impulses to take drugs.

Chapter 51

Preventing and Treating Substance Abuse

Drug Abuse: A Painful Experience

Drug abuse can be a painful experience—for the person who has the problem, and for family and friends who may feel helpless in the face of the disease. But there are things you can do if you know or suspect that someone close to you has a drug problem.

Certain drugs can change the structure and inner workings of the brain. With repeated use, they affect a person's self-control and interfere with the ability to resist the urge to take the drug. Not being able to stop taking a drug even though you know it's harmful is the hallmark of addiction.

A drug doesn't have to be illegal to cause this effect. People can become addicted to alcohol, nicotine, or even prescription drugs when they use them in ways other than prescribed or use someone else's prescription.

People are particularly vulnerable to using drugs when going through major life transitions. For adults, this might mean during a divorce or after losing a job. For children and teens, this can mean changing schools or other major upheavals in their lives.

This chapter includes text excerpted from "Dealing with Drug Problems," *NIH News in Health*, National Institutes of Health (NIH), June 2017.

Drug Abuse among Teenagers

But kids may experiment with drug use for many different reasons. "It could be a greater availability of drugs in a school with older students, or it could be that social activities are changing, or that they are trying to deal with stress," says Dr. Bethany Deeds, a National Institutes of Health (NIH) expert on drug abuse prevention. Parents may need to pay more attention to their children during these periods.

The teenage years are a critical time to prevent drug use. Trying drugs as a teenager increases your chance of developing substance use disorders. The earlier the age of first use, the higher the risk of later addiction. But addiction also happens to adults. Adults are at increased risk of addiction when they encounter prescription pain-relieving drugs after a surgery or because of a chronic pain problem. People with a history of addiction should be particularly careful with opioid pain relievers and make sure to tell their doctors about past drug use.

There are many signs that may indicate a loved one is having a problem with drugs. They might lose interest in things that they used to enjoy or start to isolate themselves. Teens' grades may drop. They may start skipping classes.

"They may violate curfew or appear irritable, sedated, or disheveled," says child psychiatrist Dr. Geetha Subramaniam, an NIH expert on substance use. Parents may also come across drug paraphernalia, such as water pipes or needles, or notice a strange smell.

"Once drug use progresses, it becomes less of a social thing and more of a compulsive thing—which means the person spends a lot of time using drugs," Subramaniam says.

If a loved one is using drugs, encourage them to talk to their primary care doctor. It can be easier to have this conversation with a doctor than a family member. Not all drug treatment requires long stays in residential treatment centers. For someone in the early stages of a substance use problem, a conversation with a doctor or another professional may be enough to get them the help they need. Doctors can help the person think about their drug use, understand the risk for addiction, and come up with a plan for change.

Treatment Options

Substance use disorder can often be treated on an outpatient basis. But that doesn't mean it's easy to treat. Substance use disorder is a complicated disease. Drugs can cause changes in the brain that make it extremely difficult to quit without medical help.

For certain substances, it can be dangerous to stop the drug without medical intervention. Some people may need to be in a hospital for a short time for detoxification, when the drug leaves their body. This can help keep them as safe and comfortable as possible. Patients should talk with their doctors about medications that treat addiction to alcohol or opioids, such as heroin and prescription pain relievers.

Recovering from a substance use disorder requires retraining the brain. A person who's been addicted to drugs will have to relearn all sorts of things, from what to do when they're bored to who to hang out with. NIH has developed a customizable wallet card to help people identify and learn to avoid their triggers, the things that make them feel like using drugs.

"You have to learn ways to deal with triggers, learn about negative peers, learn about relapse, [and] learn coping skills," Subramaniam says.

NIH-funded scientists are studying ways to stop addiction long before it starts—in childhood. Dr. Daniel Shaw at the University of Pittsburgh is looking at whether teaching healthy caregiving strategies to parents can help promote self-regulation skills in children and prevent substance abuse later on.

Starting when children are two years old, Shaw's study enrolls families at risk of substance use problems in a program called the Family Checkup. It's one of several parenting programs that have been studied by NIH-funded researchers.

During the program, a parenting consultant visits the home to observe the parents' relationship with their child. Parents complete several questionnaires about their own and their family's well-being. This includes any behavior problems they are experiencing with their child. Parents learn which of their children's problem behaviors might lead to more serious issues, such as substance abuse, down the road. The consultant also talks with the parents about possible ways to change how they interact with their child. Many parents then meet with the consultants for follow-up sessions about how to improve their parenting skills.

Children whose parents are in the program have fewer behavioral problems and do better when they get to school. Shaw and his colleagues are now following these children through their teenage years to see how the program affects their chances of developing a substance abuse problem.

Even if their teen has already started using drugs, parents can still step in. They can keep closer tabs on who their children's friends are and what they're doing. Parents can also help by finding new activities that will introduce their children to new friends and fill up the after-school hours—prime time for getting into trouble. "They don't like it at first," Shaw says. But finding other teens with similar interests can help teens form new habits and put them on a healthier path.

A substance use problem is a chronic disease that requires lifestyle adjustments and long-term treatment, like diabetes or high blood pressure. Even relapse can be a normal part of the process—not a sign of failure, but a sign that the treatment needs to be adjusted. With good care, people who have substance use disorders can live healthy, productive lives.

Ask Your Doctor

Questions to ask when choosing a treatment program:

- Does the program use treatments backed by scientific evidence? Effective programs usually combine medical and behavioral treatments.

- Does the program tailor treatment to the needs of each patient? No single treatment is right for everyone.

- Does the program adapt treatment as the patient's needs change? A person in treatment may need different services at different times.

- Is the length of treatment sufficient? Most addicted people need at least three months in treatment.

Wise Choices

People with drug problems may act differently than they used to. They might:

- spend a lot of time alone
- lose interest in their favorite things
- get messy—for instance, not bathe, change clothes, or brush their teeth
- be really tired and sad
- be very energetic, talk fast, or say things that don't make sense
- be nervous or cranky (in a bad mood)

- quickly change between feeling bad and feeling good
- sleep at strange hours
- miss important appointments
- have problems at work
- eat a lot more or a lot less than usual

Chapter 52

Smoking and Nicotine Use among Adolescents

Chapter Contents

Section 52.1—Nicotine Addiction.. 516

Section 52.2—Smokeless Tobacco 520

Section 52.3—Hookah (Water Pipe) Smoking........................... 523

Section 52.4—Smoking and How to Quit 526

Section 52.1

Nicotine Addiction

This section contains text excerpted from the following sources:
Text beginning with the heading "What Is Nicotine?" is excerpted
from "Nicotine and Addiction," Smokefree.gov, U.S. Department
of Health and Human Services (HHS), September 16, 2017; Text
under the heading "Nicotine Addiction and Youth" is excerpted
from "Preventing Tobacco Use among Youth and Young Adults Fact
Sheet," Surgeongeneral.gov, U.S. Department of Health and Human
Services (HHS), March 8, 2012. Reviewed November 2017; Text
beginning with the heading "Why Is Nicotine Addictive?" is
excerpted from "Nicotine Addiction and Your Health,"
BeTobaccoFree.gov, U.S. Department of Health and
Human Services (HHS), November 15, 2012.
Reviewed November 2017.

What Is Nicotine?

Nicotine is the chemical found in tobacco products that is
responsible for addiction. When you use tobacco, nicotine is quickly
absorbed into your body and goes directly to your brain. Nicotine
activates areas of the brain that make you feel satisfied and happy.
Whether you smoke, vape, or dip, the nicotine you are putting in
your body is dangerously addictive and can be harmful to your
developing brain.

What Does Nicotine Addiction Look Like?

Nicotine addiction can look different from person to person. Even
if you only use tobacco once in awhile, you can be addicted and can
have a hard time quitting.

Some signs of nicotine addiction include:

- Cravings, or feeling like you really need to use tobacco.

- Going out of your way to get tobacco.

- Feeling anxious or irritable if you want to use tobacco but can't.

- Continuing to use tobacco because you find it hard to stop.

If you're addicted to nicotine, you may experience symptoms of nicotine withdrawal after you stop using tobacco. Craving cigarettes, feeling sad or irritable, or having trouble sleeping are some common symptoms of withdrawal. These symptoms are usually strongest in the first week after quitting, but they are only temporary.

Why Is Nicotine Dangerous?

Nicotine can lead to addiction, which puts you at risk of becoming a lifelong smoker and exposing you to the many harmful chemicals in tobacco. These chemicals cause cancer and harm almost every organ in your body. Teens are especially sensitive to nicotine's addictive effects because their brains are still developing. This makes it easier to get hooked. Using nicotine during your teen years can also rewire your brain to become more easily addicted to other drugs.

Nicotine can have other long-lasting effects on your brain development, making it harder for you to concentrate, learn, and control your impulses.

Nicotine Addiction and Youth

Tobacco use by youth and young adults causes both immediate and long-term damage. One of the most serious health effects is nicotine addiction, which prolongs tobacco use and can lead to severe health consequences. The younger youth are when they start using tobacco, the more likely they'll be addicted.

- Early cardiovascular damage is seen in most young smokers; those most sensitive die very young.

- Smoking reduces lung function and retards lung growth. Teens who smoke are not only short of breath today, they may end up as adults with lungs that will never grow to full capacity. Such damage is permanent and increases the risk of chronic obstructive pulmonary disease.

- Youth are sensitive to nicotine and can feel dependent earlier than adults. Because of nicotine addiction, about three out of four teen smokers end up smoking into adulthood, even if they intend to quit after a few years.

- Among youth who persist in smoking, a third will die prematurely from smoking.

Youth are vulnerable to social and environmental influences to use tobacco; messages and images that make tobacco use appealing to them are everywhere.

- Young people want to fit in with their peers. Images in tobacco marketing make tobacco use look appealing to this age group.

- Youth and young adults see smoking in their social circles, movies they watch, video games they play, websites they visit, and many communities where they live. Smoking is often portrayed as a social norm, and young people exposed to these images are more likely to smoke.

- Youth identify with peers they see as social leaders and may imitate their behavior; those whose friends or siblings smoke are more likely to smoke.

- Youth who are exposed to images of smoking in movies are more likely to smoke. Those who get the most exposure to onscreen smoking are about twice as likely to begin smoking as those who get the least exposure. Images of smoking in movies have declined over the past decade; however, in 2010 nearly a third of top-grossing movies produced for children—those with ratings of G, PG, or PG-13—contained images of smoking.

Why Is Nicotine Addictive?

When you use tobacco products, nicotine is quickly absorbed into your bloodstream. Within 10 seconds of entering your body, the nicotine reaches your brain. It causes the brain to release adrenaline, creating a buzz of pleasure and energy.

The buzz fades quickly though, and leaves you feeling tired, a little down, and wanting the buzz again. This feeling is what makes you light up the next cigarette. Since your body is able to build up a high tolerance to nicotine, you'll need to smoke more and more cigarettes in order to get the nicotine's pleasurable effects and prevent withdrawal symptoms.

This up and down cycle repeats over and over, leading to addiction. Addiction keeps people smoking even when they want to quit. Breaking addiction is harder for some people than others. Many people need more than one try in order to quit.

Research suggests that children and teens may be especially sensitive to nicotine, making it easier for them to become addicted. The younger smokers are when they start, the more likely they are to become addicted. In fact, about three out of four high school smokers will become adult smokers.

Why Are Cigarettes Addictive?

Cigarette makers know that nicotine addiction helps sell their products. Cigarettes today deliver more nicotine more quickly than ever before. Tobacco companies also use additives and chemicals to make them more addictive.

Why Are Smokeless Tobacco Products Addictive?

Nicotine, found in all tobacco products, is a highly addictive drug that acts in the brain and throughout the body. Dip and chew contain more nicotine than cigarettes.

- Holding an average-sized dip in your mouth for 30 minutes can give you as much nicotine as smoking three cigarettes.

- Using two cans of snuff a week gives you as much nicotine as someone who smokes one and a half packs of cigarettes a day.

When Happens When I Quit?

Tobacco and nicotine are addictive like alcohol, cocaine, and heroin. When you stop smoking or cutback your tobacco use, you experience withdrawal. When going through withdrawal you may experience:

- Anxiety
- Irritability
- Headache
- Hunger
- Cravings for cigarettes and other sources of nicotine

Nicotine withdrawal is short-lived and symptoms pass in time, usually less than a week. Withdrawal is the most uncomfortable part of quitting, but the real challenge is beating long-term cravings and staying away from tobacco.

Section 52.2

Smokeless Tobacco

This section contains text excerpted from the following sources: Text beginning with the heading "What Is Smokeless Tobacco?" is excerpted from "Smokeless Tobacco: Get the Facts," Smokefree.gov, U.S. Department of Health and Human Services (HHS), January 22, 2017; Text beginning with the heading "What's the Problem?" is excerpted from "Smokeless Tobacco (Dip, Chew, Snuff)," Centers for Disease Control and Prevention (CDC), September 15, 2017.

What Is Smokeless Tobacco?

Smokeless tobacco is tobacco that's not burned. It's also known as chewing tobacco, oral tobacco, spit or spitting tobacco, dip, chew, and snuff.

Most people chew or suck (dip) the tobacco in their mouth and spit out the tobacco juices that build up. There's also "spitless" smokeless tobacco.

There are two main types:

- **Chewing tobacco.** This is available as loose leaves, plugs (bricks), or twists of rope. A piece of tobacco is placed between the cheek and lower lip, typically near the back of the mouth. It's either chewed or held in place. Saliva is spit out or swallowed.

- **Snuff.** This can be finely cut or powdered tobacco. It may be sold in different scents and flavors. It's packaged moist or dry—most American snuff is moist. It's available loose or in small pouches similar to tea bags. People take a pinch or pouch of moist snuff and put it between the cheek and gums—or behind the lips. In the United States, dip or dipping tobacco and snus are common forms of moist snuff.

Is It Addictive?

Yes. Smokeless tobacco contains nicotine, which is addictive. People who use smokeless tobacco and people who smoke have similar levels of nicotine in their blood.

With smokeless tobacco, nicotine is absorbed through the mouth and gets into the blood. Then it goes to the brain.

Even after people take tobacco out of their mouths, nicotine is still being absorbed into their blood. Research shows that nicotine stays in the blood longer for people who use smokeless tobacco than for smokers.

Is It Harmful?

Yes. Smokeless tobacco has high levels of chemicals and other substances that can cause cancer. People who use smokeless tobacco have a high risk of mouth and throat cancer.

People who use smokeless tobacco have more dental problems than people who smoke or people who don't use tobacco products. The sugar in smokeless tobacco can cause decay and painful mouth sores. Dip and chew can cause people's gums to pull away from their teeth. This leads to loose teeth. Smokeless tobacco can also cause leathery white patches that can turn into cancer.

What's the Problem?

Smokeless tobacco is a significant health risk and is not a safe substitute for smoking cigarettes. Smokeless tobacco contains 28 cancer-causing agents (carcinogens). Smokeless tobacco use can lead to nicotine addiction and dependence. Adolescents who use smokeless tobacco are more likely to become cigarette smokers.

The two main types of smokeless tobacco in the United States are chewing tobacco and snuff. Chewing tobacco comes in the form of loose leaf, plug, or twist. Snuff is finely ground tobacco that can be dry, moist, or in sachets (tea bag-like pouches). Although some forms of snuff can be used by sniffing or inhaling into the nose, most smokeless tobacco users place the product in their cheek or between their gum and cheek. Users then suck on the tobacco and spit out the tobacco juices, which is why smokeless tobacco is often referred to as spit or spitting tobacco.

It is a known cause of human cancer, as it increases the risk of developing cancer of the oral cavity.

Who's at Risk?

- Smokeless tobacco use in the United States is higher among young white males; American Indians/Alaska Natives; people living in southern and north central states; and people who are employed in blue collar occupations, service/laborer jobs, or who are unemployed.

- Nationally, an estimated 3 percent of adults are current smokeless tobacco users. Smokeless tobacco use is much higher among men (6%) than women (<1%).

- In the United States, 9 percent of American Indian/Alaska Natives, 4 percent of whites, 2 percent of African Americans, 1 percent of Hispanics, and <1% of Asian-American adults are current smokeless tobacco users.

- An estimated 8 percent of high school students are current smokeless tobacco users. Smokeless tobacco is more common among males (13.6%) than female high school students (2.2%). Estimates by race/ethnicity are 10.2 percent for white, 5.1 percent for Hispanic, and 1.7 percent for African-American high school students.

- An estimated 3 percent of middle school students are current smokeless tobacco users. Smokeless tobacco is more common among male (4%) than female (2%)middle school students. Estimates by race/ethnicity are 3 percent for white, 1 percent for Asian, 2 percent for African-American, and 4 percent for Hispanic middle school students.

Can It Be Prevented?

Yes. Hopefully by clarifying that smokeless tobacco is not safe, we can help people make an informed decision about its use. School-based programs are an opportunity to discourage youth on the use of smokeless tobacco. The film industry can also influence the public by not glamorizing any form of tobacco use. More community-wide efforts aimed at prevention and cessation of smokeless tobacco use among young people are needed. In addition, opportunities for intervention occur in all clinical settings and require knowledgeable and committed healthcare professionals. Training programs for healthcare providers should include components to help make smokeless tobacco counseling a higher priority.

Section 52.3

Hookah (Water Pipe) Smoking

This section includes text excerpted from "Smoking and
Tobacco Use—Hookahs," Centers for Disease Control and
Prevention (CDC), December 1, 2016.

Hookahs are water pipes that are used to smoke specially made
tobacco that comes in different flavors, such as apple, mint, cherry,
chocolate, coconut, licorice, cappuccino, and watermelon. Although
many users think it is less harmful, hookah smoking has many of the
same health risks as cigarette smoking. Hookah is also called *narghile,
argileh, shisha, hubble-bubble,* and *goza.*

Hookahs vary in size, shape, and style. A typical modern hookah
has a head (with holes in the bottom), a metal body, a water bowl, and
a flexible hose with a mouthpiece. Hookah smoking is typically done
in groups, with the same mouthpiece passed from person to person.
Tobacco users should quit all tobacco products to reduce health risks.
Hookah smoking is NOT a safe alternative to smoking cigarettes.

Hookah Use

* Hookah use began centuries ago in ancient Persia and India.

* Hookah cafés are gaining in popularity around the world, including Britain, France, Russia, the Middle East, and the United
  States.

* Hookah use by youth and college students is increasing.

* In 2010, the Monitoring the Future survey found that among
  high school seniors in the United States, about 1 in 5 boys (17%)
  and 1 in 6 girls (15%) had used a hookah in the past year.

* Other small studies of young adults have found high prevalence
  of hookah use among college students in the United States. These
  studies show past-year use ranging from 22 percent to 40 percent.

* New forms of electronic hookah smoking, including steam stones
  and hookah pens, have been introduced.

- These products are battery powered and turn liquid containing nicotine, flavorings, and other chemicals into a vapor, which is inhaled.

- Very little information is currently available on the health risks of electronic tobacco products.

Health Effects

Using a hookah to smoke tobacco poses serious health risks to smokers and others exposed to the smoke from the hookah.

Hookah Smoke and Cancer

- The charcoal used to heat the tobacco can raise health risks by producing high levels of carbon monoxide, metals, and cancer-causing chemicals.

- Even after it has passed through water, the smoke from a hookah has high levels of these toxic agents.

- Hookah tobacco and smoke contain several toxic agents known to cause lung, bladder, and oral cancers.

- Tobacco juices from hookahs irritate the mouth and increase the risk of developing oral cancers.

Other Health Effects of Hookah Smoke

- Hookah tobacco and smoke contain many toxic agents that can cause clogged arteries and heart disease.

- Infections may be passed to other smokers by sharing a hookah.

- Babies born to women who smoked water pipes every day while pregnant weigh less at birth (at least 3½ ounces less) than babies born to nonsmokers.

- Babies born to hookah smokers are also at increased risk for respiratory diseases.

Hookah Smoking Compared with Cigarette Smoking

- While many hookah smokers may think this practice is less harmful than smoking cigarettes, hookah smoking has many of the same health risks as cigarette smoking.

- Water pipe smoking delivers nicotine—the same highly addictive drug found in other tobacco products.

- The tobacco in hookahs is exposed to high heat from burning charcoal, and the smoke is at least as toxic as cigarette smoke.

- Because of the way a hookah is used, smokers may absorb more of the toxic substances also found in cigarette smoke than cigarette smokers do.

  - An hour-long hookah smoking session involves 200 puffs, while smoking an average cigarette involves 20 puffs.

  - The amount of smoke inhaled during a typical hookah session is about 90,000 milliliters (ml), compared with 500–600 ml inhaled when smoking a cigarette.

- Hookah smokers may be at risk for some of the same diseases as cigarette smokers. These include:

  - Oral cancer

  - Lung cancer

  - Stomach cancer

  - Cancer of the esophagus

  - Reduced lung function

  - Decreased fertility

Hookahs and Secondhand Smoke

Secondhand smoke from hookahs can be a health risk for nonsmokers. It contains smoke from the tobacco as well as smoke from the heat source (e.g., charcoal) used in the hookah.

Nontobacco Hookah Products

- Some sweetened and flavored nontobacco products are sold for use in hookahs.

- Labels and ads for these products often claim that users can enjoy the same taste without the harmful effects of tobacco.

- Studies of tobacco-based shisha and "herbal" shisha show that smoke from both preparations contain carbon monoxide and other toxic agents known to increase the risks for smoking-related cancers, heart disease, and lung disease.

Section 52.4

Smoking and How to Quit

This section contains text excerpted from the following sources: Text under the heading "Health Risks of Smoking and Ways to Quit" is excerpted from "Cigarette Smoking: Health Risks and How to Quit (PDQ®)—Patient Version," National Cancer Institute (NCI), September 15, 2017; Text under the heading "Smokefree Mobile Apps" is excerpted from "Smokefree Apps," Smokefree.gov, U.S. Department of Health and Human Services (HHS), June 29, 2016.

Health Risks of Smoking and Ways to Quit

Quitting Smoking Improves Health

The risk of most health problems from smoking, including cancer and heart and lung disease, can be lowered by stopping smoking. People of all ages can improve their health if they quit smoking. Quitting at a younger age will improve a person's health even more. People who quit smoking cut their risk of lung cancer by 30 percent to 50 percent after 10 years compared to people who keep smoking, and they cut their risk of cancer of the mouth or esophagus in half within 5 years after quitting.

The damage caused by smoking is even worse for people who have had cancer. They have an increased risk of cancer recurrence, new cancers, and long-term side effects from cancer treatment. Quitting smoking and stopping other unhealthy behaviors can improve long-term health and quality of life.

The Public Health Service has a set of guidelines called Treating Tobacco Use and Dependence. It asks healthcare professionals to talk to their patients about the health problems caused by smoking and the importance of quitting smoking.

Different Ways to Quit Smoking

The following are the most common methods used to help smokers quit:

Counseling

People who have even a short counseling session with a healthcare professional are more likely to quit smoking. Your doctor or other healthcare professional may take the following steps to help you quit:

- Ask about your smoking habits at every visit
- Advise you to stop smoking
- Ask you how willing you are to quit
- Help you plan to quit smoking by:
  - setting a date to quit smoking
  - giving you self-help materials
  - recommending drug treatment
- Plan follow-up visits with you

The Lung Health Study found that heavy smokers who received counseling from a doctor, took part in group sessions with other smokers to change their behavior, and used nicotine gum were more likely to quit smoking compared with smokers who did not receive counseling from a doctor, take part in group sessions, and use nicotine gum. They also had a lower risk of lung cancer, other cancers, heart disease, and respiratory disease.

Childhood cancer survivors who smoke may be more likely to quit when they take part in programs that use peer-counseling. In these programs, childhood cancer survivors are trained in ways to give support to other childhood cancer survivors who smoke and want to quit. More people quit smoking with peer-counseling than with self-help programs. If you are a childhood cancer survivor and you smoke, talk to your doctor about peer-counseling programs.

Drug Treatment

Treatment with drugs is also used to help people quit smoking. These include nicotine replacement products and non-nicotine medicines. People who use any type of drug treatment are more likely to quit smoking after 6 months than those who use a placebo or no drug treatment at all.

Nicotine replacement products have nicotine in them. You slowly reduce the use of the nicotine product in order to reduce the amount of nicotine you take in. Using a nicotine replacement product can help break the addiction to nicotine. It lessens the side effects of nicotine withdrawal, such as feeling depressed or nervous, having trouble thinking clearly, or having trouble sleeping. Nicotine replacement products, used alone or in combination, have been shown to help people quit smoking. These include:

- Nicotine gum
- Nicotine patches
- Nicotine nasal spray
- Nicotine inhalers
- Nicotine lozenges

Nicotine replacement products can cause problems in some people, especially:

- Women who are pregnant or breast-feeding
- Teenagers
- People with any of the following medical problems:
  - Heart rhythm problems
  - High blood pressure that is not controlled
  - Esophagitis
  - Ulcers
  - Insulin-dependent diabetes
  - Asthma

Other medicines that do not have nicotine in them are used to help people quit smoking. These include:

- Bupropion (also called Zyban).
- Varenicline (also called Chantix).

These medicines lessen nicotine craving and nicotine withdrawal symptoms. It is important to know that bupropion and varenicline may cause serious psychiatric problems. Symptoms include:

- Aggressive behavior
- Anxiety

- Changes in behavior

- Depression

- Nervousness

- Suicidal thoughts and attempted suicide

Varenicline may also cause serious heart problems. Before starting to take bupropion or varenicline, talk to your doctor about the important health benefits of quitting smoking and the small but serious risk of problems with the use of these drugs.

Smoking Reduction

When smokers do not quit smoking completely but smoke fewer cigarettes (smoking reduction) they may still benefit. The more you smoke, the higher your risk of lung cancer and other cancers related to smoking. Studies show that smokers who cut back are more likely to stop smoking in the future.

Smoking less is not as helpful as quitting smoking altogether, and is harmful if you inhale more deeply or smoke more of each cigarette to try to control nicotine cravings. In smokers who do not plan to quit smoking completely, nicotine replacement products have been shown to help them cut down the number of cigarettes they smoke, but this effect does not appear to last over time.

Different Types of Tobacco and Nicotine Products

The use of new or different types of tobacco products and devices that deliver nicotine is increasing rapidly in the United States, especially the use of electronic-cigarettes (e-cigarettes).

Examples of new and different tobacco and nicotine products and devices include the following:

- E-cigarettes

- Small cigars

- Water pipes (hookahs) for smoking tobacco

- Flavored smokeless tobacco products

Smokefree Mobile Apps

Get 24/7 help with a Smokefree app for your smartphone. These free apps give you the support and skills you need to get ready to quit and stay smokefree. Explore the apps to discover the features that will be most helpful for your smokefree journey.

QuitGuide

QuitGuide is a free app that helps you understand your smoking patterns and build the skills needed to become and stay smokefree. New to QuitGuide in 2016 is the ability to track cravings by time of day and location. Get inspirational messages for each craving you track, which keep you focused and motivated on your smokefree journey.

QuitGuide helps you:

- Track craving and slips by times of day and location
- Track your mood and smoking triggers
- Stay motivated with inspirational messages
- Identify your reasons for quitting
- Get tips and distractions for dealing with cravings and bad moods
- Monitor your progress toward achieving smokefree milestones
- Create journal entries

quitSTART

quitSTART is a free app made for teens who want to quit smoking, but adults can use it too. This app takes the information you provide about your smoking history and gives you tailored tips, inspiration, and challenges to help you become smokefree and live a healthier life.

quitStart App helps you:

- Get ready to quit with tips and information to prepare you for becoming smokefree
- Monitor your progress and earn badges for smokefree milestones and other achievements
- Get back on track if you slip and smoke
- Manage cravings and bad moods in healthy ways
- Distract yourself from cravings with games and challenges
- Store helpful tips, inspirations, and challenges in your Quit Kit
- Share your progress and favorite tips through social media

Chapter 53

Alcohol Use among Adolescents

Chapter Contents

Section 53.1—Underage Drinking 532

Section 53.2—Talk to Your Child about Alcohol 534

Section 53.1

Underage Drinking

This section includes text excerpted from "Fact Sheets—
Underage Drinking," Centers for Disease Control and
Prevention (CDC), October 20, 2016.

Alcohol is the most commonly used and abused drug among youth
in the United States.

- Excessive drinking is responsible for more than 4,300 deaths
  among underage youth each year, and cost the U.S. $24 billion
  in economic costs in 2010.

- Although drinking by persons under the age of 21 is illegal, people aged 12 to 20 years drink 11 percent of all alcohol consumed
  in the United States. More than 90 percent of this alcohol is consumed in the form of binge drinks.

- On average, underage drinkers consume more drinks per drinking occasion than adult drinkers.

- In 2010, there were approximately 189,000 emergency rooms
  visits by persons under age 21 for injuries and other conditions
  linked to alcohol.

Drinking Levels among Youth

The *2015 Youth Risk Behavior Survey* found that among high school
students, during the past 30 days:

- 33 percent drank some amount of alcohol.
- 18 percent binge drank.
- 8 percent drove after drinking alcohol.
- 20 percent rode with a driver who had been drinking alcohol.

Other national surveys:

- In 2015, the *National Survey on Drug Use and Health* reported
  that 20 percent of youth aged 12 to 20 years drink alcohol and
  13 percent reported binge drinking in the past 30 days.

- In 2015, the *Monitoring the Future Survey* reported that 10 percent of 8th graders and 35 percent of 12th graders drank during the past 30 days, and 5 percent of 8th graders and 17 percent of 12th graders binge drank during the past 2 weeks.

Consequences of Underage Drinking

Youth who drink alcohol are more likely to experience:

- School problems, such as higher absence and poor or failing grades.
- Social problems, such as fighting and lack of participation in youth activities.
- Legal problems, such as arrest for driving or physically hurting someone while drunk.
- Physical problems, such as hangovers or illnesses.
- Unwanted, unplanned, and unprotected sexual activity.
- Disruption of normal growth and sexual development.
- Physical and sexual assault.
- Higher risk for suicide and homicide.
- Alcohol-related car crashes and other unintentional injuries, such as burns, falls, and drowning.
- Memory problems.
- Abuse of other drugs.
- Changes in brain development that may have lifelong effects.
- Death from alcohol poisoning.

In general, the risk of youth experiencing these problems is greater for those who binge drink than for those who do not binge drink.

Youth who start drinking before age 15 years are six times more likely to develop alcohol dependence or abuse later in life than those who begin drinking at or after age 21 years.

Prevention of Underage Drinking

Reducing underage drinking will require community-based efforts to monitor the activities of youth and decrease youth access to alcohol. The publications by the Surgeon General and the Institute of Medicine has outlined many prevention strategies for the prevention of underage drinking, such as enforcement of minimum legal drinking age laws, national media campaigns targeting youth and adults, increasing alcohol excise taxes, reducing youth exposure to alcohol advertising, and development of comprehensive community-based programs.

Section 53.2

Talk to Your Child about Alcohol

This section includes text excerpted from "Parenting to Prevent
Childhood Alcohol Use," National Institute on Alcohol Abuse and
Alcoholism (NIAAA), February 2017.

Drinking alcohol undoubtedly is a part of American culture, as are conversations between parents and children about its risks and potential benefits. However, information about alcohol can seem contradictory. Alcohol affects people differently at different stages of life—small amounts may have health benefits for certain adults, but for children and adolescents, alcohol can interfere with normal brain development. Alcohol's differing effects and parents' changing role in their children's lives as they mature and seek greater independence can make talking about alcohol a challenge. Parents may have trouble setting concrete family policies for alcohol use. And they may find it difficult to communicate with children and adolescents about alcohol-related issues.

Research shows, however, that teens and young adults do believe their parents should have a say in whether they drink alcohol. Parenting styles are important—teens raised with a combination of encouragement, warmth, and appropriate discipline are more likely to respect their parents' boundaries. Understanding parental influence on children through conscious and unconscious efforts, as well as when and how to talk with children about alcohol, can help parents have more influence than they might think on a child's alcohol use. Parents can play an important role in helping their children develop healthy attitudes toward drinking while minimizing its risk.

Alcohol Use by Young People

Adolescent alcohol use remains a pervasive problem. The percentage of teenagers who drink alcohol is slowly declining; however, numbers are still quite high. About 22.8 percent of adolescents report drinking by 8th grade, and about 46.3 percent report being drunk at least once by 12th grade.

Parenting Style

Accumulating evidence suggests that alcohol use—and in particular binge drinking—may have negative effects on adolescent development and increase the risk for alcohol dependence later in life. This underscores the need for parents to help delay or prevent the onset of drinking as long as possible. Parenting styles may influence whether their children follow their advice regarding alcohol use. Every parent is unique, but the ways in which each parent interacts with his or her children can be broadly categorized into four styles:

- Authoritarian parents typically exert high control and discipline with low warmth and responsiveness. For example, they respond to bad grades with punishment but let good grades go unnoticed.

- Permissive parents typically exert low control and discipline with high warmth and responsiveness. For example, they deem any grades at all acceptable and fail to correct behavior that may lead to bad grades.

- Neglectful parents exert low control and discipline as well as low warmth and responsiveness. For example, they show no interest at all in a child's school performance.

- Authoritative parents exert high control and discipline along with high warmth and responsiveness. For example, they offer praise for good grades and use thoughtful discipline and guidance to help improve low grades.

Regardless of the developmental outcome examined—body image, academic success, or substance abuse—children raised by authoritative parents tend to fare better than their peers. This is certainly true when it comes to the issue of underage drinking, in part because children raised by such parents learn approaches to problem solving and emotional expression that help protect against the psychological dysfunction that often precedes alcohol misuse. The combination of discipline and support by authoritative parents promotes healthy decision making about alcohol and other potential threats to healthy development.

Modeling

Some parents wonder whether allowing their children to drink in the home will help them develop an appropriate relationship with alcohol. According to most studies this does not appear to be the case. In a study of 6th, 7th, and 8th graders, researchers observed that students whose parents allowed them to drink at home and/or provided them with alcohol experienced the steepest escalation in drinking. Other studies suggest that adolescents who are allowed to drink at home drink more heavily outside of the home. In contrast, adolescents are less likely to drink heavily if they live in homes where parents have specific rules against drinking at a young age and also drink responsibly themselves. However, not all studies suggest that parental provision of alcohol to teens leads to trouble. For instance, one study showed that drinking with a parent in the proper context (such as a sip of alcohol at an important family function) can be a protective factor against excessive drinking. In other contexts, parental provision of alcohol serves as a direct risk factor for excessive drinking, as is the case when parents provide alcohol for parties attended or hosted by their adolescents. Collectively, the literature suggests that permissive attitudes toward adolescent drinking, particularly when combined with poor communication and unhealthy modeling, can lead teens into unhealthy relationships with alcohol.

Genetics

Regardless of what parents may teach their children about alcohol, some genetic factors are present from birth and cannot be changed. Genes appear to influence the development of drinking behaviors in several ways. Some people, particularly those of Asian ancestry, have a natural and unpleasant response to alcohol that helps prevent them from drinking too much. Other people have a naturally high tolerance to alcohol, meaning that to feel alcohol's effects, they must drink more than others. Some personality traits are genetic, and those, like impulsivity, can put a person at risk for problem drinking. Psychiatric problems may be caused by genetic traits, and such problems can increase risk for alcohol abuse and dependence. Finally, having a parent with a drinking problem increases a child's risk for developing an alcohol problem of his or her own.

Do Teens Listen?

Adolescents do listen to their parents when it comes to issues such as drinking and smoking, particularly if the messages are conveyed consistently and with authority. Research suggests that only 19 percent of teens feel that parents should have a say in the music they listen to, and 26 percent believe their parents should influence what clothing they wear. However, the majority—around 80 percent—feel that parents should have a say in whether they drink alcohol. Those who do not think that parents have authority over these issues are four times more likely than other teens to drink alcohol and three times more likely to have plans to drink if they have not already started.

Whether teens defer to parents on the issue of drinking is statistically linked to how parents parent. Specifically, authoritative parents—those who provide a healthy and consistent balance of discipline and support—are the most likely to have teenagers who respect the boundaries they have established around drinking and other behaviors; whereas adolescents exposed to permissive, authoritarian, or neglectful parenting are less influenced by what their parents say about drinking.

Research suggests that, regardless of parenting styles, adolescents who are aware that their parents would be upset with them if they drank are less likely to do so, highlighting the importance of communication between parents and teens as a protective measure against underage alcohol use.

What Can Parents Do?

Parents influence whether and when adolescents begin drinking as well as how their children drink. Family policies about adolescent drinking in the home and the way parents themselves drink are important. For instance, if you choose to drink, always model responsible alcohol consumption. But what else can parents do to help minimize the likelihood that their adolescent will choose to drink and that such drinking, if it does occur, will become problematic? Studies have shown that it is important to:

- Talk early and often, in developmentally appropriate ways, with children and teens about your concerns—and theirs—regarding alcohol. Adolescents who know their parents' opinions about youth drinking are more likely to fall in line with their expectations.

- Establish policies early on, and be consistent in setting expectations and enforcing rules. Adolescents do feel that parents should have a say in decisions about drinking, and they maintain this deference to parental authority as long as they perceive the message to be legitimate. Consistency is central to legitimacy.

- Work with other parents to monitor where kids are gathering and what they are doing. Being involved in the lives of adolescents is key to keeping them safe.

- Work in and with the community to promote dialogue about underage drinking and the creation and implementation of action steps to address it.

- Be aware of your State's laws about providing alcohol to your own children.

- Never provide alcohol to someone else's child.

Children and adolescents often feel competing urges to comply with and resist parental influences. During childhood, the balance usually tilts toward compliance, but during adolescence, the balance often shifts toward resistance as teens prepare for the autonomy of adulthood. With open, respectful communication and explanations of boundaries and expectations, parents can continue to influence their children's decisions well into adolescence and beyond. This is especially important in young people's decisions regarding whether and how to drink—decisions that can have lifelong consequences.

Chapter 54

Marijuana Use among Adolescents

Marijuana is a green, brown, or gray mixture of dried, shredded leaves, stems, seeds, and flowers of the hemp plant (*Cannabis sativa*). Cannabis is a term that refers to marijuana and other drugs made from the same plant. Strong forms of cannabis include sinsemilla, hashish ("hash" for short), and hash oil. There are many different slang terms for marijuana and, as with other drugs, they change quickly and vary from region to region. But no matter its form or label, all cannabis products contain the psychoactive (mind-altering) chemical *delta-9-tetrahydrocannabinol* (THC). They also contain more than 400 other chemicals.

How Do People Use Marijuana?

People who use marijuana may roll loose marijuana leaves into a cigarette (called a joint) or smoke it in a pipe or a water pipe, often referred to as a bong. Some people mix marijuana into foods (often called "edibles") or use it to brew a tea. Another method is to slice open a cigar and replace some or all of the tobacco with marijuana, creating what is known as a blunt. To avoid inhaling smoke, more people are vaping—using vaporizers that allow the person to inhale vapor and not smoke. Another popular method on the rise is smoking or vaping

This chapter includes text excerpted from "Marijuana: Facts Parents Need to Know," National Institute on Drug Abuse (NIDA), June 2016.

THC-rich resins extracted from the marijuana plant, a practice called dabbing. Some popular e-cigarette devices can be used to vape marijuana or extracts.

How Many Teens Use Marijuana?

National Institute on Drug Abuse (NIDA)'s annual Monitoring the Future survey reports that among students from 8th, 10th, and 12th grades, marijuana use has remained stable over the past few years. For the three grades combined, about 24 percent of students reported past-year use in 2015. About 7 percent of 8th graders reported current (past-month) use. Among 10th graders, 15 percent reported current use, and current use for 12th graders was 21 percent.

Researchers have found that the use of marijuana and other drugs usually peaks in the late teens and early twenties, then declines in later years. Therefore, marijuana use among young people remains a natural concern for parents and is the focus of continuing research, particularly regarding its impact on brain development, which continues into a person's early twenties. Some studies suggest that the effects of heavy use that begins as a teen can be long lasting, even many years after use discontinues.

How Does Marijuana Work?

When people smoke marijuana, they feel its effects almost immediately. THC (marijuana's psychoactive ingredient) rapidly reaches every organ in the body, including the brain, and attaches to specific receptors on nerve cells. Activation of these receptors in the brain affects pleasure, memory, thinking, concentration, movement, coordination, appetite, pain, and sensory and time perception. THC is chemically similar to chemicals that the body produces naturally, called *endocannabinoids*, and marijuana disrupts the normal function of these chemicals. Because of this system's wide-ranging influence over many critical functions, it's not surprising that marijuana can have multiple effects—not just on the brain, but on a person's general health. Some of these effects last only as long as marijuana is in the body while others may build up over time to cause longer-lasting problems, including addiction. The effects of smoked marijuana can last from 1 to 3 hours. If consumed in foods, the effects come on slower and may not last as long. However, because edibles containing marijuana are often unlabeled or poorly labeled, teens can use too much waiting for the "high" and end up in the emergency room with side effects.

What Are Marijuana's Short-Term Effects?

The short-term effects of marijuana can include:

- **Euphoria (high).** THC activates the reward system in a similar way to other drugs of abuse, resulting in the release of the chemical dopamine.

- **Memory impairment.** THC alters how information is processed in the hippocampus and frontal cortex, brain areas involved in memory and concentration.

- **Negative mental reactions in some.** These include anxiety, fear, distrust, or panic, particularly in people new to the drug or those taking it in a strange setting; some may even experience psychosis.

- **Physical changes.** People who use marijuana may have red or bloodshot eyes, increased appetite ("the munchies"), increased heart rate, and sleep issues.

What Determines How Marijuana Affects an Individual?

Like any other drug, marijuana's effects on a person depends on a number of factors, including the person's previous experience with the drug or other drugs, biology (e.g., genes), gender, how the drug is taken, and the drug's potency (its strength).

How Important Is Marijuana Potency?

Potency—determined by the amount of THC contained in the marijuana—has received much attention lately because it's been increasing steadily in the past few decades. These findings are based on analyses of marijuana samples seized by law enforcement.

So what does this actually mean? For someone new to the drug, it may mean exposure to higher concentrations of THC, with a greater chance of a negative or unpredictable reaction. In fact, increases in potency may account for the rise in emergency room visits involving marijuana use. For those more experienced with marijuana, it may mean a greater risk for addiction if they are exposing themselves to high doses on a regular basis. However, the full range of consequences linked with marijuana's higher potency is not well understood. It is unknown how much people who use marijuana adjust for the increase in potency by using less.

541

Does Using Marijuana Lead to Other Drug Use?

Long-term studies of high school students' patterns of drug use show that most young people who use other drugs have first tried marijuana, alcohol, or tobacco. For example, young people who have used marijuana are at greater risk of using cocaine than those who have not. It is also known from animal studies that rats given repeated doses of THC show heightened behavioral responses and altered brain activation not only when further exposed to THC, but also when exposed to other drugs such as morphine. Researchers are now looking at the possibility that exposure to marijuana as a teen may cause changes in the brain that make a person more likely to get addicted to marijuana or other drugs, such as alcohol, opioids, or cocaine.

It is important to point out, however, that research has not fully explained any of these observations, which are complex and likely to involve a combination of biological, social, and psychological factors. In addition, most people who use marijuana do not go on to use "harder" drugs.

Does Smoking Marijuana Cause Lung Cancer?

Studies have not found an increased risk of lung cancer in marijuana smokers compared with nonsmokers. However, marijuana smoke does irritate the lungs and increases the likelihood of other breathing problems. Repeated exposure to marijuana smoke can lead to daily cough, more frequent chest colds, and a greater risk of lung infections. Moreover, many people who smoke marijuana also smoke cigarettes, which do cause cancer, and quitting tobacco can be harder if the person uses marijuana as well.

Can Marijuana Produce Withdrawal Symptoms When Someone Quits?

Yes. Many people who use the drug long term and then stop have symptoms that are similar to those of nicotine withdrawal—irritability, sleep problems, anxiety, and craving—which may prompt relapse (a return to drug use). Withdrawal symptoms are generally mild and peak a few days after use has stopped. They gradually disappear within about 2 weeks. While these symptoms do not pose an immediate threat to health, they can make it hard for someone to stop using the drug.

How Harmful Is K2/Spice (Or "Synthetic Marijuana")?

Spice, which is sometimes also called K2, herbal incense, or "fake weed," consists of shredded dried plant material that has been sprayed with chemicals designed to act on the same brain cell receptors as THC, but are often much more powerful and unpredictable. Spice products are labeled "not fit for human consumption," and many are now illegal. But their manufacturers are constantly creating new chemical compounds to sidestep legal restrictions. Their effects, like the ingredients, often vary, but emergency rooms report large numbers of young people appearing with rapid heart rates, vomiting, and negative mental responses including hallucinations after using these substances.

Are There Treatments for People Addicted to Marijuana?

Behavioral therapies are available and are similar to those used for treating other substance addictions. These include motivational enhancement to develop people's own motivation to stay in treatment; cognitive behavioral therapies to teach strategies for avoiding drug use and its triggers and for effectively managing stress; and motivational incentives, which provide vouchers or small cash rewards for staying drug free.

However, there are currently no medications approved by the U.S. Food and Drug Administration (FDA) for treating marijuana addiction, although promising research is underway to find medications to treat withdrawal symptoms and ease craving and other effects of marijuana.

What Are Other Risks Related to Marijuana That My Child Should Know?

Many parents and teens may not have thought about some of these risks:

- As with most drugs, marijuana use interferes with judgment, which can lead to risky behaviors. For example, the person may drive under the influence or ride with someone else who is intoxicated and get into a car crash, or engage in risky sexual behavior and contract a sexually transmitted disease.

- In addition to psychosis, regular marijuana use has been linked with increased risk for several mental problems, including depression, anxiety, suicidal thoughts, and personality disturbances. One of the potential effects is *amotivational syndrome*—a diminished or lost drive to engage in formerly rewarding activities. Whether this syndrome is a disorder unto itself or is a subtype of depression associated with marijuana use remains controversial. Furthermore, whether marijuana causes these problems or is a response to them is still unknown. More research is needed to confirm and better understand these links.

- Marijuana use during pregnancy may harm the developing fetus. Research suggests that marijuana use during pregnancy may be linked to subtle neurological changes and, later in childhood, to reduced problem-solving skills, memory, and attention. However, the fact that pregnant women who use marijuana are also more likely to smoke cigarettes or drink alcohol makes it difficult to determine exactly how much of these effects are due to marijuana. In addition, some research suggests that after pregnancy, THC passes into the breast milk of nursing mothers in moderate amounts. Researchers don't yet know how this affects the baby's developing brain.

How Can I Tell If My Child Has Been Using Marijuana?

Parents should be aware of changes in their child's behavior, such as not brushing hair or teeth, skipping showers, mood changes, and loss of relationships with family members and friends. In addition, changes in grades, skipping classes or missing school, loss of interest in sports or other favorite activities, a change in peer group, changes in eating or sleeping habits, and getting in trouble in school or with the law could all be related to drug use—or may indicate other problems. See the list of specific warning signs for marijuana use below.

If your child is using marijuana, he or she might:

- seem unusually giggly and/or uncoordinated

- have very red, bloodshot eyes or use eye drops often

- have a hard time remembering things that just happened

- have drugs or drug paraphernalia—drug-related items including pipes and rolling papers—possibly claiming they belong to a friend if confronted

- have strangely smelling clothes or bedroom

- use incense and other deodorizers

- wear clothing or jewelry or have posters that promote drug use
- have unexplained lack of money or extra cash on hand

Talk to Your Child about Marijuana

Marijuana use can affect the health and well-being of children and teens at a critical point in their lives—when they are growing, learning, maturing, and laying the foundation for their adult years. As a parent, your children look to you for help and guidance in working out problems and in making decisions, including the decision not to use drugs. Even if you have used drugs in the past, you can have an open conversation about the dangers. Whether or not you tell your child about your past drug use is a personal decision. But experience can better equip us to teach others by drawing on the value of past mistakes. You can explain that marijuana is significantly more potent now and that we now know a lot more about the potential harmful effects of marijuana on the developing brain.

Greater acceptance of marijuana use, compared with use of other illegal drugs, continues to be the basis of differing opinions about its dangers, legal status, and potential value. The ongoing public debate about medical marijuana may complicate your discussion. Even so, be certain the discussion focuses on how much you care about your child's health.

Whether or not marijuana becomes legal for adult use or allowed for medical use, it can be harmful for teens and can alter the course of a young life, preventing a person from reaching his or her full potential. That's reason enough to have this sometimes difficult conversation with your children.

Is Marijuana Medicine?

There has been much debate about the possible medical use of marijuana for certain conditions. A growing number of states have legalized marijuana for medical use, but the FDA, which assesses the safety and effectiveness of medications, hasn't approved marijuana as a medicine. There haven't been enough large-scale studies (clinical trials) showing that the benefits of the whole plant outweigh its risks in the patients it's meant to treat. To be approved, medicines need to have well-defined and measurable ingredients that are consistent from one dose (such as a pill or injection) to the next. In addition to THC, the marijuana leaf contains more than 400 other chemical compounds, which may have different effects in the body and which vary from plant to plant. This makes it difficult to consider its use as a medicine even if some of marijuana's specific ingredients may offer benefits.

However, THC itself is an FDA-approved medication. Two medicines in pill form (dronabinol [synthetic THC] and nabilone [a synthetic chemical similar to THC]) are available to treat nausea during cancer chemotherapy and boost appetite in people with acquired immune deficiency syndrome (AIDS). Scientists continue to investigate the medicinal properties of THC and other cannabinoids to better evaluate and harness their ability to help patients suffering from a broad range of conditions.

Chapter 55

Prescription Medicine Abuse

Misuse of prescription drugs means taking a medication in a manner or dose other than prescribed; taking someone else's prescription, even if for a legitimate medical complaint such as pain; or taking a medication to feel euphoria (i.e., to get high). The term nonmedical use of prescription drugs also refers to these categories of misuse. The three classes of medication most commonly misused are:

- opioids—usually prescribed to treat pain

- central nervous system [CNS] depressants (this category includes tranquilizers, sedatives, and hypnotics)—used to treat anxiety and sleep disorders

- stimulants—most often prescribed to treat attention-deficit hyperactivity disorder (ADHD)

Prescription drug misuse can have serious medical consequences. Increases in prescription drug misuse over the last 15 years are reflected in increased emergency room visits, overdose deaths associated with prescription drugs, and treatment admissions for prescription drug use disorders, the most severe form of which is addiction. Among those who reported past-year nonmedical use of a prescription drug, nearly 12 percent met criteria for prescription drug use disorder. Unintentional overdose deaths involving opioid pain relievers

This chapter includes text excerpted from "Misuse of Prescription Drugs," National Institute on Drug Abuse (NIDA), August 2016.

have more than quadrupled since 1999 and have outnumbered those involving heroin and cocaine since 2002.

What Is the Scope of Prescription Drug Misuse?

Misuse of prescription opioids, central nervous system (CNS) depressants, and stimulants is a serious public health problem in the United States. Although most people take prescription medications responsibly, an estimated 54 million people (more than 20 percent of those aged 12 and older) have used such medications for nonmedical reasons at least once in their lifetime. According to results from the 2014 National Survey on Drug Use and Health (NSDUH), an estimated 2.1 million Americans used prescription drugs nonmedically for the first time within the past year, which averages to approximately 5,750 initiates per day. Fifty-four percent were females and about 30 percent were adolescents.

The reasons for the high prevalence of prescription drug misuse vary by age, gender, and other factors, but likely include ease of access. The number of prescriptions for some of these medications has increased dramatically since the early 1990s. Moreover, misinformation about the addictive properties of prescription opioids and the perception that prescription drugs are less harmful than illicit drugs are other possible contributors to the problem.

Although misuse of prescription drugs affects many Americans, certain populations such as youth, older adults, and women may be at particular risk. In addition, while more men than women currently misuse prescription drugs, the rates of misuse and overdose among women are increasing faster than among men.

Among Adolescents and Young Adults

Nonmedical use of prescription drugs is highest among young adults aged 18 to 25, with 4.4 percent reporting nonmedical use in the past month. Among youth aged 12 to 17, 2.6 percent reported past-month nonmedical use of prescription medications.

After alcohol, marijuana, and tobacco, prescription drugs (taken nonmedically) are among the most commonly used drugs by 12th graders. The National Institute on Drug Abuse (NIDA)'s Monitoring the Future survey of substance use and attitudes in teens found that about 1 in 13 high school seniors reported past-year nonmedical use of the prescription stimulant Adderall® in 2015, and nearly 1 in 23 reported misusing the opioid pain reliever Vicodin®.

Although nonmedical use of CNS depressants and opioid pain relievers decreased among 12th graders between 2011 and 2015, this is not the case for the nonmedical use of stimulants. Nonmedical use of Adderall® increased between 2009 and 2013 and has remained elevated. When asked how they obtained prescription stimulants for nonmedical use, more than half of the adolescents and young adults surveyed said they either bought or received the drugs from a friend or relative. Interestingly, the number who purchased these drugs through the Internet was negligible.

Youth who misuse prescription medications are also more likely to report use of other drugs. Multiple studies have revealed associations between prescription drug misuse and higher rates of cigarette smoking; heavy episodic drinking; and marijuana, cocaine, and other illicit drug use among U.S. adolescents, young adults, and college students. In the case of prescription opioids, medical use is also associated with a greater risk of future opioid misuse, particularly in adolescents who disapprove of illegal drug use and have little to no history of drug use.

Is It Safe to Use Prescription Drugs in Combination with Other Medications?

The safety of using prescription drugs in combination with other substances depends on a number of factors including the types of medications, dosages, other substance use (e.g., alcohol), and individual patient health factors. Patients should talk with their healthcare provider about whether they can safely use their prescription drugs with other substances, including prescription and over-the-counter (OTC) medications as well as alcohol, tobacco, and illicit drugs. Specifically, drugs that slow down breathing rate, such as opioids, alcohol, antihistamines, prescription central nervous system depressants (including barbiturates and benzodiazepines), or general anesthetics, should not be taken together because these combinations increase the risk of life-threatening respiratory depression. Stimulants should also not be used with other medications unless recommended by a physician. Patients should be aware of the dangers associated with mixing stimulants and OTC cold medicines that contain decongestants, as combining these substances may cause blood pressure to become dangerously high or lead to irregular heart rhythms.

Which Classes of Prescription Drugs Are Commonly Misused?

Opioids

Opioids are medications that act on opioid receptors in both the spinal cord and brain to reduce the intensity of pain-signal perception. They also affect brain areas that control emotion, which can further diminish the effects of painful stimuli. They have been used for centuries to treat pain, cough, and diarrhea. The most common modern use of opioids is to treat acute pain. However, since the 1990s, they have been increasingly used to treat chronic pain, despite sparse evidence for their effectiveness when used long term. Indeed, some patients experience a worsening of their pain or increased sensitivity to pain as a result of treatment with opioids, a phenomenon known as hyperalgesia. Importantly, in addition to relieving pain, opioids also activate reward regions in the brain causing the euphoria—or high—that underlies the potential for misuse and addiction. Chemically, these medications are very similar to heroin, which was originally synthesized from morphine as a pharmaceutical in the late 19th century. These properties confer an increased risk of addiction and overdose even in patients who take their medication as prescribed.

Prescription opioid medications include hydrocodone (e.g., Vicodin®), oxycodone (e.g., OxyContin®, Percocet®), oxymorphone (e.g., Opana®), morphine (e.g., Kadian®, Avinza®), codeine, fentanyl, and others. Hydrocodone products are the most commonly prescribed in the United States for a variety of indications, including dental- and injury-related pain. Oxycodone and oxymorphone are also prescribed for moderate to severe pain relief. Morphine is often used before and after surgical procedures to alleviate severe pain, and codeine is typically prescribed for milder pain. In addition to their pain-relieving properties, some of these drugs—codeine and diphenoxylate (Lomotil®), for example—are used to relieve coughs and severe diarrhea.

How Do Opioids Affect the Brain and Body?

Opioids act by attaching to and activating opioid receptor proteins, which are found on nerve cells in the brain, spinal cord, gastrointestinal tract, and other organs in the body. When these drugs attach to their receptors, they inhibit the transmission of pain signals. Opioids can also produce drowsiness, mental confusion, nausea, constipation, and respiratory depression, and since these drugs also act on brain regions involved in reward, they can induce euphoria, particularly when they are taken at a higher-than-prescribed dose or administered in other ways than intended. For example, OxyContin® is an oral medication used to treat moderate to severe pain through a slow, steady release of the opioid. Some people who misuse OxyContin® intensify their experience by snorting or injecting it. This is a very dangerous practice, greatly increasing the person's risk for serious medical complications, including overdose.

What Are the Possible Consequences of Prescription Opioid Misuse?

When taken as prescribed, patients can often use opioids to manage pain safely and effectively. However, it is possible to develop a substance use disorder when taking opioid medications as prescribed. This risk and the risk for overdose increase when these medications are misused. Even a single large dose of an opioid can cause severe respiratory depression (slowing or stopping of breathing), which can be fatal; taking opioids with alcohol or sedatives increases this risk.

When properly managed, short-term medical use of opioid pain relievers—taken for a few days following oral surgery, for instance—rarely leads to an opioid use disorder or addiction. But regular (e.g., several times a day, for several weeks or more) or longer-term use of opioids can lead to dependence (physical discomfort when not taking the drug), tolerance (diminished effect from the original dose, leading to increasing the amount taken), and, in some cases, addiction (compulsive drug seeking and use). With both dependence and addiction, withdrawal symptoms may occur if drug use is suddenly reduced or stopped. These symptoms may include restlessness, muscle and bone pain, insomnia, diarrhea, vomiting, cold flashes with goose bumps, and involuntary leg movements. Misuse of prescription opioids is also a risk factor for transitioning to heroin use.

How Is Prescription Opioid Misuse Related to Chronic Pain?

Healthcare providers have long wrestled with how best to treat the more than 100 million Americans who suffer from chronic pain. Opioids have been the most common treatment for chronic pain since the late 1990s, but recent research has cast doubt both on their safety and their efficacy in the treatment of chronic pain when it is not related to cancer or palliative care. The potential risks involved with long-term opioid treatment, such as the development of drug tolerance, hyperalgesia, and addiction, present doctors with a dilemma, as there is limited research on alternative treatments for chronic pain. Patients themselves may even be reluctant to take an opioid medication prescribed to them for fear of becoming addicted.

Estimates of the rate of opioid addiction among chronic pain patients vary from about 3 percent up to 26 percent. This variability is the result of differences in treatment duration, insufficient research on long-term outcomes, and disparate study populations and measures used to assess nonmedical use or addiction.

Before prescribing, physicians should assess pain and functioning, consider if nonopioid treatment options are appropriate, discuss a treatment plan with the patient, evaluate the patient's risk of harm or misuse, and co-prescribe naloxone to mitigate the risk for overdose. When first prescribing opioids, physicians should give the lowest effective dose for the shortest therapeutic duration. As treatment continues, the patient should be monitored at regular intervals, and opioid treatment should be continued only if meaningful clinical improvements in pain and functioning are seen without harm.

CNS Depressants

What Are CNS Depressants?

Central nervous system (CNS) depressants, a category that includes tranquilizers, sedatives, and hypnotics, are substances that can slow brain activity. This property makes them useful for treating anxiety and sleep disorders. The following are among the medications commonly prescribed for these purposes:

- **Benzodiazepines,** such as diazepam (Valium®), clonazepam (Klonopin®), and alprazolam (Xanax®), are sometimes prescribed to treat anxiety, acute stress reactions, and panic attacks. Clonazepam may also be prescribed to treat seizure disorders. The more sedating benzodiazepines, such as triazolam (Halcion®) and estazolam (Prosom®) are prescribed for short-term treatment of sleep disorders. Usually, benzodiazepines are not prescribed for long-term use because of the high risk for developing tolerance, dependence, or addiction.

- **Nonbenzodiazepine** sleep medications, such as zolpidem (Ambien®), eszopiclone (Lunesta®), and zaleplon (Sonata®), known as z-drugs, have a different chemical structure but act on the same GABA type A receptors in the brain as benzodiazepines. They are thought to have fewer side effects and less risk of dependence than benzodiazepines.

- **Barbiturates,** such as mephobarbital (Mebaral®), phenobarbital (Luminal®), and pentobarbital sodium (Nembutal®), are used less frequently to reduce anxiety or to help with sleep problems because of their higher risk of overdose compared to benzodiazepines. However, they are still used in surgical procedures and to treat seizure disorders.

How Do CNS Depressants Affect the Brain and Body?

Most CNS depressants act on the brain by increasing activity at receptors for the inhibitory neurotransmitter gamma-aminobutyric acid (GABA). Although the different classes of depressants work in unique ways, it is through their ability to increase GABA signaling—thereby increasing inhibition of brain activity—that they produce a drowsy or calming effect that is medically beneficial to those suffering from anxiety or sleep disorders.

What Are the Possible Consequences of CNS Depressant Misuse?

Despite their beneficial therapeutic effects, benzodiazepines and barbiturates have the potential for misuse and should be used only as prescribed. The use of nonbenzodiazepine sleep aids, or z-drugs, is less well-studied, but certain indicators have raised concern about their psychoactive properties as well.

During the first few days of taking a depressant, a person usually feels sleepy and uncoordinated, but as the body becomes accustomed to the effects of the drug and tolerance develops, these side effects begin to disappear. If one uses these drugs long term, he or she may need larger doses to achieve the therapeutic effects. Continued use can also lead to dependence and withdrawal when use is abruptly reduced or stopped. Because all sedatives work by slowing the brain's activity, when an individual stops taking them, there can be a rebound effect, resulting in seizures or other harmful consequences.

Although withdrawal from benzodiazepines can be problematic, it is rarely life threatening, whereas withdrawal from prolonged use of barbiturates can have life-threatening complications. Therefore, someone who is thinking about discontinuing a sedative or who is suffering withdrawal from CNS depressants should speak with a physician or seek immediate medical treatment.

Stimulants

Stimulants increase alertness, attention, and energy, as well as elevate blood pressure, heart rate, and respiration. Historically, stimulants were used to treat asthma and other respiratory problems, obesity, neurological disorders, and a variety of other ailments. But as their potential for misuse and addiction became apparent, the number of conditions treated with stimulants has decreased. Now, stimulants are prescribed for the treatment of only a few health conditions, including attention-deficit hyperactivity disorder (ADHD), narcolepsy, and occasionally treatment-resistant depression.

How Do Stimulants Affect the Brain and Body?

Stimulants, such as dextroamphetamine (Dexedrine®, Adderall®) and methylphenidate (Ritalin®, Concerta®), act in the brain on the family of monoamine neurotransmitter systems, which include norepinephrine and dopamine. Stimulants enhance the effects of these chemicals. An increase in dopamine signaling from nonmedical use of stimulants can induce a feeling of euphoria, and these medications' effects on norepinephrine increase blood pressure and heart rate, constrict blood vessels, increase blood glucose, and open up breathing passages.

What Are the Possible Consequences of Stimulant Misuse?

As with other drugs in the stimulant category, such as cocaine, it is possible for people to become dependent on or addicted to prescription stimulants. Withdrawal symptoms associated with discontinuing stimulant use include fatigue, depression, and disturbed sleep patterns. Repeated misuse of some stimulants (sometimes within a short period) can lead to feelings of hostility or paranoia, or even psychosis. Further, taking high doses of a stimulant may result in dangerously high body temperature and an irregular heartbeat. There is also the potential for cardiovascular failure or seizures.

Cognitive Enhancers

The dramatic increases in stimulant prescriptions over the last 2 decades have led to their greater availability and to increased risk for diversion and nonmedical use. When taken to improve properly diagnosed conditions, these medications can greatly enhance a patient's quality of life. However, because many perceive them to be generally safe and effective, prescription stimulants such as Adderall® and Modafinil® are being misused more frequently.

Stimulants increase wakefulness, motivation, and aspects of cognition, learning, and memory. Some people take these drugs in the absence of medical need in an effort to enhance mental performance. Militaries have long used stimulants to increase performance in the face of fatigue, and the United States Armed Forces allow for their use in limited operational settings. The practice is now reported by some professionals to increase their productivity, by older people to offset declining cognition, and by both high school and college students to improve their academic performance.

Nonmedical use of stimulants for cognitive enhancement poses potential health risks, including addiction, cardiovascular events, and psychosis. The use of pharmaceuticals for cognitive enhancement has also sparked debate over the ethical implications of the practice. Issues of fairness arise if those with access and willingness to take these drugs have a performance edge over others, and implicit coercion takes place if a culture of cognitive enhancement gives the impression that a person must take drugs in order to be competitive.

Are Prescription Drugs Safe to Take When Pregnant?

Prescription medications taken by a pregnant woman can cause her baby to develop dependence, which can result in withdrawal symptoms after birth, known as neonatal abstinence syndrome (NAS). This can require a prolonged stay in neonatal intensive care and, in the case of opioids, treatment with medication. Women should consult with their doctors to determine which medications they can continue taking during pregnancy.

Opioid pain medications require particular attention; rising rates of NAS have been associated with increases in the prescription of opioids for pain in pregnant women. NAS associated with opioid use (heroin or prescription opioids) increased fivefold from 2000 to 2012, with a higher rate of increase in more recent years.

How Can Prescription Drug Misuse Be Prevented?

Clinicians, Patients, and Pharmacists

Physicians, their patients, and pharmacists all can play a role in identifying and preventing nonmedical use of prescription drugs.

- **Clinicians.** More than 80 percent of Americans had contact with a healthcare professional in the past year, placing doctors in a unique position to identify nonmedical use of prescription drugs and take measures to prevent the escalation of a patient's misuse to a substance use disorder. By asking about all drugs, physicians can help their patients recognize that a problem exists, provide or refer them to appropriate treatment, and set recovery goals. Evidence-based screening tools for nonmedical use of prescription drugs can be incorporated into routine medical visits. Doctors should also take note of rapid increases in the amount of medication needed or frequent, unscheduled refill requests. Doctors should be alert to the fact that those misusing prescription drugs may engage in "doctor shopping"—moving from provider to provider—in an effort to obtain multiple prescriptions for their drug(s) of choice. Prescription drug monitoring programs (PDMPs), state-run electronic databases used to track the prescribing and dispensing of controlled prescription drugs to patients, are also important tools for preventing and identifying prescription drug misuse. While research regarding the impact of these programs is currently mixed, the use of PDMPs in some states has been associated with lower rates of opioid prescribing and overdose, though issues of best practices, ease of use, and interoperability remain to be resolved. In 2015, the federal government launched an initiative directed toward reducing opioid misuse and overdose, in part by promoting more cautious and responsible prescribing of opioid medications. In line with these efforts, Centers for Disease Control and Prevention (CDC) published its *CDC Guideline for Prescribing Opioids for Chronic Pain* to establish clinical standards for balancing the benefits and risks of chronic opioid treatment. Preventing or stopping nonmedical use of prescription drugs is an important part of patient care. However, certain patients can benefit from prescription stimulants, sedatives, or opioid pain relievers. Therefore, physicians should balance the legitimate medical needs of patients with the potential risk for misuse and related harms.

- **Patients.** Patients can take steps to ensure that they use prescription medications appropriately by:

  - following the directions as explained on the label or by the pharmacist

  - being aware of potential interactions with other drugs as well as alcohol

- never stopping or changing a dosing regimen without first discussing it with the doctor

- never using another person's prescription, and never giving their prescription medications to others

- storing prescription stimulants, sedatives, and opioids safely

Additionally, patients should properly discard unused or expired medications by following U.S. Food and Drug Administration (FDA) guidelines or visiting U.S. Drug Enforcement Administration (DEA) collection sites. In addition to describing their medical problem, patients should always inform their healthcare professionals about all the prescriptions, over-the-counter medicines, and dietary and herbal supplements they are taking before they obtain any other medications.

- **Pharmacists.** Pharmacists can help patients understand instructions for taking their medications. In addition, by being watchful for prescription falsifications or alterations, pharmacists can serve as the first line of defense in recognizing problematic patterns in prescription drug use. Some pharmacies have developed hotlines to alert other pharmacies in the region when they detect a fraudulent prescription. Along with physicians, pharmacists can use PDMPs to help track opioid-prescribing patterns in patients.

Medication Formulation and Regulation

Manufacturers of prescription drugs continue to work on new formulations of opioid medications, known as abuse-deterrent formulations (ADF), which include technologies designed to prevent people from misusing them by snorting or injection. Approaches currently being used or studied for use include:

- **physical or chemical barriers** that prevent the crushing, grinding, or dissolving of drug products

- **agonist/antagonist combinations** that cause an antagonist (which will counteract the drug effect) to be released if the product is manipulated

- **aversive substances** that are added to create unpleasant sensations if the drug is taken in a way other than directed

- **delivery systems** such as long-acting injections or implants that slowly release the drug over time

- **new molecular entities or prodrugs** that attach a chemical extension to a drug that renders it inactive unless it is taken orally

Several ADF opioids are on the market, and the FDA has also called for the development of ADF stimulants. While ADF opioids have been shown to decrease the illicit value of a drug, in the absence of reduced demand, they can shift use to other formulations. Medication regulation has been shown to be effective in decreasing the prescribing of opioid medications. In 2014, the Drug Enforcement Administration moved hydrocodone products from schedule III to the more restrictive schedule II, which resulted in a decrease in hydrocodone prescribing that did not result in any attendant increases in the prescribing of other opioids.

Development of Safer Medications

The development of effective, nonaddicting pain medications is a public health priority. A growing number of older adults and an increasing number of injured military service members add to the urgency of finding new treatments. Researchers are exploring alternative treatment approaches that target other signaling systems in the body such as the endocannabinoid system, which is also involved in pain. More research is also needed to better understand effective chronic pain management, including identifying factors that predispose some patients to substance use disorders and developing measures to prevent the nonmedical use of prescription medications.

How Can Prescription Drug Addiction Be Treated?

Years of research have shown that substance use disorders are brain disorders that can be treated effectively. Treatment must take into account the type of drug used and the needs of the individual. Successful treatment may need to incorporate several components, including detoxification, counseling, and medications, when available. Multiple courses of treatment may be needed for the patient to make a full recovery.

The two main categories of drug addiction treatment are behavioral treatments (such as contingency management and cognitive-behavioral therapy) and medications. Behavioral treatments help patients stop drug use by changing unhealthy patterns of thinking and behavior;

teaching strategies to manage cravings and avoid cues and situations that could lead to relapse; or, in some cases, providing incentives for abstinence. Behavioral treatments, which may take the form of individual, family, or group counseling, also can help patients improve their personal relationships and their ability to function at work and in the community.

Addiction to prescription opioids can additionally be treated with medications including buprenorphine, methadone, and naltrexone. These drugs can counter the effects of opioids on the brain or relieve withdrawal symptoms and cravings, helping the patient avoid relapse. Medications for the treatment of addiction are administered in combination with psychosocial supports or behavioral treatments, known as medication-assisted treatment (MAT).

Medication-Assisted Treatment (MAT)

Naltrexone is an antagonist medication that prevents other opioids from binding to and activating opioid receptors. It is used to treat overdose and addiction. An injectable, long-acting form of naltrexone (Vivitrol®) can be a useful treatment choice for patients who do not have ready access to healthcare or who struggle with taking their medications regularly.

Methadone is a synthetic opioid agonist that prevents withdrawal symptoms and relieves drug cravings by acting on the same brain targets as other opioids such as heroin, morphine, and opioid pain medications. It has been used successfully for more than 40 years to treat heroin addiction but is generally only available through specially licensed opioid treatment programs.

Buprenorphine is a partial opioid agonist—it binds to the opioid receptor but only partially activates it—that can be prescribed by certified physicians in an office setting. Like methadone, it can reduce cravings and is well tolerated by patients. In May 2016, the U.S. Food and Drug Administration (FDA) approved the NIDA-supported development of an implantable formulation of buprenorphine. It provides 6 months of sustained treatment, which will give buprenorphine-stabilized patients greater ease in treatment adherence.

There has been a popular misconception that medications with agonist activity, such as methadone or buprenorphine, replace one addiction with another. This is not the case. Opioid use disorder is associated with imbalances in brain circuits that mediate reward, decision-making, impulse control, learning, and other functions. These medications restore balance to these brain circuits, preventing opioid

559

withdrawal and restoring the patient to a normal affective state to allow for effective psychosocial treatment and social functioning.

While MAT is the standard of care for treating opioid use disorder, far fewer people receive MAT than could potentially benefit from it. Not all people with opioid use disorder seek treatment. Even when they seek treatment, they will not necessarily receive MAT. The most recent treatment admissions data available show that only 18 percent of people admitted for prescription opioid use disorder have a treatment plan that includes MAT. However, even if the nationwide infrastructure were operating at capacity, between 1.3 and 1.4 million more people have opioid use disorder than could currently be treated with MAT due to limited availability of opioid treatment programs that can dispense methadone and the regulatory limit on the number of patients that physicians can treat with buprenorphine. Coordinated efforts are underway nationwide to expand access to MAT, including a recent increase in the buprenorphine patient limit from 100 patients to 275 for qualified physicians who request the higher limit.

The NIDA is supporting research needed to determine the most effective ways to implement MAT. For example, recent work has shown that buprenorphine maintenance treatment is more effective than tapering patients off of buprenorphine. Also, starting buprenorphine treatment when a patient is admitted to the emergency department, such as for an overdose, is a more effective way to engage a patient in treatment than referral or brief intervention. Finally, data have shown that treatment with methadone, buprenorphine, or naltrexone for incarcerated individuals improves post-release outcomes.

Reversing an Opioid Overdose with Naloxone

The opioid overdose-reversal drug naloxone is an opioid antagonist that can rapidly restore normal respiration to a person who has stopped breathing as a result of overdose on prescription opioids or heroin. Naloxone can be used by emergency medical personnel, first responders, and bystanders.

Treating Addiction to CNS Depressants

Patients addicted to central nervous system (CNS) depressants such as tranquilizers, sedatives, and hypnotics should not attempt to stop taking them on their own. Withdrawal symptoms from these drugs can be severe and—in the case of certain medications—potentially life-threatening. Research on treating addiction to CNS depressants is sparse; however, patients who are dependent on these medications should undergo medically supervised detoxification because the dosage they take should be tapered gradually. Inpatient or outpatient counseling can help individuals through this process. Cognitive-behavioral therapy, which focuses on modifying the patient's thinking, expectations, and behaviors while increasing skills for coping with various life stressors, has also been used successfully to help individuals adapt to discontinuing benzodiazepines.

Often CNS depressant misuse occurs in conjunction with the use of other drugs (polydrug use), such as alcohol or opioids. In such cases, the treatment approach should address the multiple addictions.

At this time, there are no FDA-approved medications for treating addiction to CNS depressants, though research is ongoing in this area.

Treating Addiction to Prescription Stimulants

Treatment of addiction to prescription stimulants such as Adderall® and Concerta® is based on behavioral therapies that are effective for treating cocaine and methamphetamine addiction. At this time, there are no FDA-approved medications for treating stimulant addiction.

Depending on the patient, the first steps in treating prescription stimulant addiction may be to taper the drug dosage and attempt to ease withdrawal symptoms. Behavioral treatment may then follow the detoxification process.

Where Can I Get Further Information about Prescription Drug Misuse?

To learn more about prescription drugs and other drugs, visit the NIDA website at drugabuse.gov or contact the DrugPubs Research Dissemination Center at 877-NIDA-NIH (877-643-2644; TTY/TDD: 240-645-0228).

Chapter 56

Inhalants

What Are Inhalants?

Inhalants are chemicals found in ordinary household or workplace products that people inhale on purpose to get "high." Because many inhalants can be found around the house, people often don't realize that inhaling their fumes, even just once, can be very harmful to the brain and body and can lead to death. In fact, the chemicals found in these products can change the way the brain works and cause other problems in the body.

Although different inhalants cause different effects, they generally fall into one of four categories.

Volatile solvents are liquids that become a gas at room temperature. They are found in:

- paint thinner, nail polish remover, degreaser, dry-cleaning fluid, gasoline, and contact cement

- some art or office supplies, such as correction fluid, felt-tip marker fluid, and electronic contact cleaner

Aerosols are sprays that contain propellants and solvents. They include:

- spray paint, hairspray, deodorant spray, vegetable oil sprays, and fabric protector spray

---

This chapter includes text excerpted from "Inhalants," National Institute on Drug Abuse (NIDA) for Teens, March 2017.

Gases may be in household or commercial products, or used in the medical field to provide pain relief. They are found in:

- butane lighters, propane tanks, whipped cream dispensers, and refrigerant gases

- anesthesia, including ether, chloroform, halothane, and nitrous oxide (commonly called "laughing gas")

Nitrites are a class of inhalants used mainly to enhance sexual experiences. Organic nitrites include amyl, butyl, and cyclohexyl nitrites and other related compounds. Amyl nitrite was used in the past by doctors to help with chest pain and is sometimes used today to diagnose heart problems. Nitrites are now banned (prohibited by the Consumer Product Safety Commission) but can still be found, sold in small bottles labeled as "video head cleaner," "room odorizer," "leather cleaner," or "liquid aroma."

How Inhalants Are Used

People who use inhalants breathe in the fumes through their nose or mouth, usually by:

- "sniffing" or "snorting" fumes from container

- spraying aerosols directly into the nose or mouth

- sniffing or inhaling fumes from substances sprayed or placed into a plastic or paper bag ("bagging")

- "huffing" from an inhalant-soaked rag stuffed in the mouth

- inhaling from balloons filled with nitrous oxide

How Many Teens Use Inhalants?

Inhalants are often among the first drugs that young adolescents use. In fact, they are one of the few classes of drugs that are used more by younger adolescents than older ones. Inhalant use can become chronic and continue into adulthood.

Table 56.1. Percentage of Teens Who Use Inhalants

Drug	Time Period	8th Graders	10th Graders	12th Graders
Inhalants	Lifetime	[7.70]	6.6	5
	Past Year	[3.80]	2.4	1.7
	Past Month	1.8	1	0.8

What Happens to Your Brain When You Use Inhalants?

The lungs absorb inhaled chemicals into the bloodstream very quickly, sending them throughout the brain and body. Nearly all inhalants (except nitrites) produce a pleasurable effect by slowing down brain activity. Nitrites, in contrast, expand and relax blood vessels.

Short-Term Effects

Within seconds, users feel intoxicated and experience effects similar to those of alcohol, such as slurred speech, lack of coordination, euphoria (a feeling of intense happiness), and dizziness. Some users also experience lightheadedness, hallucinations (seeing things that are not really there), and delusions (believing something that is not true). If enough of the chemical is inhaled, nearly all solvents and gases produce anesthesia—a loss of sensation—and can lead to unconsciousness.

The high usually lasts only a few minutes, causing people to continue the high by inhaling repeatedly, which is very dangerous. Repeated use in one session can cause a person to lose consciousness and possibly even die.

With repeated inhaling, many users feel less inhibited and less in control. Some may feel drowsy for several hours and have a headache that lasts a while.

Long-Term Effects

Inhalants often contain more than one chemical. Some chemicals leave the body quickly, but others stay for a long time and get absorbed by fatty tissues in the brain and central nervous system. Over the long term, the chemicals can cause serious problems:

- **Damage to nerve fibers.** Long-term inhalant use can break down the protective sheath around certain nerve fibers in the brain and elsewhere in the body. This hurts the ability of nerve cells to send messages, which can cause muscle spasms and tremors or even permanent trouble with basic actions like walking, bending, and talking. These effects are similar to what happens to people with the disease multiple sclerosis.

- **Damage to brain cells.** Inhalants also can damage brain cells by preventing them from getting enough oxygen. The effects of this condition, also known as brain hypoxia, depend on the area of the brain that gets damaged. The hippocampus, for example,

565

is responsible for memory, so someone who repeatedly uses inhalants may be unable to learn new things or may have a hard time carrying on simple conversations. If the cerebral cortex is damaged, it will affect a person's ability to solve complex problems and plan ahead. And, if the cerebellum is affected, it can cause a person to move slowly or be clumsy.

What Happens to Your Body When You Use Inhalants?

Regular use of inhalants can cause serious harm to vital organs and systems besides the brain. Inhalants can cause:

- heart damage
- liver failure
- muscle weakness
- aplastic anemia—the body produces fewer blood cells
- nerve damage, which can lead to chronic pain

Damage to these organs is not reversible even when the person stops abusing inhalants.

Effects of Specific Chemicals

Depending on the type of inhalant used, the harmful health effects will differ.

Table 56.2. Harmful Effects of Inhalants

Inhalant	Examples	Possible Effects
Amyl nitrite, butyl nitrite	poppers, video head cleaner	• sudden sniffing death • weakened immune system • damage to red blood cells (interfering with oxygen supply to vital tissues)
Benzene	gasoline	• bone marrow damage • weakened immune system • increased risk of leukemia (a form of cancer) • reproductive system complications

Table 56.2. Continued

Inhalant	Examples	Possible Effects
Butane, propane	lighter fluid, hair and pain sprays	• sudden sniffing death from heart effects • serious burn injuries
Freon (difluoroethane substitutes)	refrigerant and aerosol propellant	• sudden sniffing death • breathing problems and death (from sudden cooling of airways) • liver damage
Methylenelchloride	paint thinners and removers, degreasers	• reduced ability of blood to carry oxygen to the brain and body • changes to heart muscle and heartbeat
Nitrous oxide, hexane	"laughing gas"	• death from lack of oxygen to the brain • altered perception and motor coordination • loss of sensation • spasms • blackouts caused by blood pressure changes • depression of heart muscle functioning
Toluene	gasoline, paint thinners and removers, correction fluid	• brain damage (loss of brain tissue, impaired thinking, loss of coordination, limb spasms, hearing and vision loss) • liver and kidney damage
Tricholoroethylene	spot removers, degreasers	• sudden sniffing death • liver disease • reproductive problems • hearing and vision loss

Signs of Inhalant Use

Sometimes you can see signs that tell you a person is using inhalants, such as:

• chemical odors on breath or clothing

• paint or other stains on the face, hands, or clothing

• hidden empty spray paint or solvent containers, or rags or clothing soaked with chemicals

- drunk or disoriented actions

- slurred speech

- nausea (feeling sick) or loss of appetite and weight loss

- confusion, inattentiveness, lack of coordination, irritability, and depression

- purchase of excessive amounts of products used as inhalants

Can You Overdose or Die If You Use Inhalants?

Yes, using inhalants can cause death, even after just one use, by:

- sudden sniffing death—heart beats quickly and irregularly, and then suddenly stops (cardiac arrest)

- asphyxiation—toxic fumes replace oxygen in the lungs so that a person stops breathing

- suffocation—air is blocked from entering the lungs when inhaling fumes from a plastic bag placed over the head

- convulsions or seizures—abnormal electrical discharges in the brain

- coma—the brain shuts down all but the most vital functions

- choking—inhaling vomit after inhalant use

- injuries—accidents, including driving, while intoxicated

Are Inhalants Addictive?

It isn't common, but addiction can happen. Some people, particularly those who use inhalants a lot and for a long time, report a strong need to continue using inhalants. Using inhalants over and over again can cause mild withdrawal when stopped. In fact, research in animal models shows that toluene can affect the brain in a way that is similar to other drugs of use (e.g., amphetamines). Toluene increases dopamine activity in reward areas of the brain, and the long-term disruption of the dopamine system is one of the key factors leading to addiction.

Chapter 57

Helping Your Teen Who Has a Problem with Drugs

How Do I Know If My Teen or Young Adult Has a Substance Use Disorder?

Addiction can happen at any age, but it usually starts when a person is young. If your teen continues to use drugs despite harmful consequences, he or she may be addicted.

If an adolescent starts behaving differently for no apparent reason—such as acting withdrawn, frequently tired or depressed, or hostile—it could be a sign he or she is developing a drug-related problem. Parents and others may overlook such signs, believing them to be a normal part of puberty. Other signs include:

- a change in peer group
- carelessness with grooming
- decline in academic performance
- missing classes or skipping school
- loss of interest in favorite activities
- trouble in school or with the law

This chapter includes text excerpted from "What to Do If Your Teen or Young Adult Has a Problem with Drugs," National Institute on Drug Abuse (NIDA), January 2016.

- changes in eating or sleeping habits
- deteriorating relationships with family members and friends

Through scientific advances, it's known more than ever before about how drugs work in the brain. It's also known that addiction can be successfully treated to help young people stop abusing drugs and lead productive lives. Intervening early when you first spot signs of drug use in your teen is critical; don't wait for your teen to become addicted before you seek help. However, if a teen is addicted, treatment is the next step.

Why Can't Some Teens Stop Using Drugs on Their Own?

Repeated drug use changes the brain. Brain imaging studies of people with drug addictions show changes in areas of the brain that are critical to judgment, decision-making, learning and memory, and behavior control. Quitting is difficult, even for those who feel ready.

If I Want Help for My Teen or Young Adult, Where Do I Start?

Asking for help from professionals is the first important step. You can start by bringing your child to a doctor who can screen for signs of drug use and other related health conditions. You might want to ask in advance if he or she is comfortable screening for drug use with standard assessment tools and making a referral to an appropriate treatment provider. If not, ask for a referral to another provider skilled in these issues.

You can also contact an addiction specialist directly. There are 3,500 board-certified physicians who specialize in addiction in the United States.

It takes a lot of courage to seek help for a child with a possible drug problem because there is a lot of hard work ahead for both of you, and it interrupts academic, personal, and possibly athletic milestones expected during the teen years. However, treatment works, and teens can recover from addiction, although it may take time and patience.

Treatment enables young people to counteract addiction's powerful disruptive effects on their brain and behavior so they can regain control of their lives. You want to be sure your teen is healthy before venturing into the world with more independence, and where drugs are more easily available.

What Kind of Screening Will the Doctor Do?

The doctor will ask your child a series of questions about use of alcohol and drugs, and associated risk behaviors (such as driving under the influence or riding with other drivers who have been using drugs or alcohol). The doctor might also give a urine and/or blood test to identify drugs that are being abused. This assessment will help determine the extent of a teen's drug use (if any) and whether a referral to a treatment program is necessary.

If My Child Refuses to Cooperate, Should the Family Conduct an Intervention?

Most teens, and many young adults still being supported by their family, only enter treatment when they are compelled to by the pressure of their family, the juvenile justice, or other court system. However, there is no evidence that confrontational "interventions" like those familiar from TV programs are effective. It is even possible for such confrontational encounters to escalate into violence or backfire in other ways. Instead, parents should focus on creating incentives to get the teen to a doctor. Oftentimes, young people will listen to professionals rather than family members, as the latter encounters can sometimes be driven by fear, accusations, and emotions.

People of all ages with substance use disorders live in fear of what will happen if their drugs are taken away. You can ensure your teen that professional treatment centers will keep him or her safe and as comfortable as possible if a detoxification process is needed. Be sure to let your teen know that family and loved ones will stand by and offer loving support.

How Do I Find the Right Treatment Center?

If you or your medical specialist decides your teen can benefit from substance abuse treatment, there are many options available. You can start by contacting the government's Treatment Locator service at 800-662-HELP (800-662-4357) or go online at (www.findtreatment.samhsa.gov). (This service is supported by the Substance Abuse and Mental Health Administration (SAMHSA) in the U.S. Department of Health and Human Services (HHS).) This Treatment Locator service lets you to search for a provider in your area; it will also tell you information about the treatment center and if it works with teens.

571

What Do I Look for in a Treatment Center for This Age Group?

Treatment approaches must be tailored to address each patient's unique substance abuse patterns and related medical, psychiatric, and social problems. Some treatment centers offer outpatient treatment programs, which would allow your teen to stay in school, at least part time. However, some adolescents do better in inpatient (residential) treatment. An addiction specialist can advise you about your best options.

Who Will Provide Treatment to My Child?

Different kinds of addiction specialists will work together in your teen's care, including doctors, nurses, therapists, social workers, and others.

Is There Medication That Can Help?

There are medications available to treat addictions to alcohol, nicotine, and opioids (heroin and pain relievers). These are generally prescribed for adults but, in some circumstances, doctors may prescribe them for younger patients. When medication is available, it can be combined with behavioral therapy to ensure success for most patients. In addition, nonaddictive medication is sometimes prescribed to help with withdrawal. Other medications are available to treat possible mental health conditions (such as depression) that might be contributing to your child's addiction.

Your treatment provider will advise you about what medications are available for your particular situation. Some treatment centers follow the philosophy that they should not treat a drug addiction with other drugs, but research shows that medication can help in many cases.

If My Teen or Young Adult Confides in His or Her Doctor, Will I Be Able to Find out What's Going On?

If your child talks to a doctor or other medical expert, privacy laws might prevent that expert from sharing the information with you. However, you can speak to the doctor before your child's appointment and express your concerns, so the doctor knows the importance of a drug use screening in your child's situation. In addition, most healthcare providers that specialize in addiction treatment can't share your information with anyone (even other providers) without your written permission.

In certain cases when health professionals believe your child might be a danger to him- or herself or to others, the provider may be able to share relevant information with family members.

What If My Teen or Young Adult Has Been in Rehab Before?

This means your child has already learned many of the skills needed to recover from addiction, and he or she will only benefit from further treatment. Relapse does not mean the first treatment failed. Relapse rates with addiction are similar to rates for other chronic diseases, such as hypertension, diabetes, and asthma. Treatment of chronic diseases involves changing deeply imbedded behaviors, so setbacks are to be expected along the way. A return to substance abuse indicates that treatment needs to be reinstated or adjusted, or that a different treatment might be called for.

How Will I Pay for Treatment?

If your child has health insurance, it may cover substance abuse treatment services. Many insurance plans offer inpatient stays. When setting up appointments with treatment centers, you can ask about payment options and what insurance plans they take. They can also advise you on low-cost options.

Note that the new Mental Health Parity and Addiction Equity Act (MHPAEA) ensures that co-pays, deductibles, and visit limits are generally not more restrictive for mental health and substance abuse disorder benefits than they are for medical and surgical benefits. The Affordable Care Act (ACA) builds on this law and requires coverage of mental health and substance use disorder services as one of ten essential health benefits categories. Under the essential health benefits rule, individual and small group health plans are required to comply with these parity regulations.

What Kind of Counseling Is Best for a Teen or Young Adult?

You child's treatment provider will probably recommend counseling. Behavioral treatment (also known as "talk therapy") can help patients engage in the treatment process, change their attitudes and behaviors related to substance abuse, and increase healthy life skills.

These treatments can also enhance the effectiveness of medications and help people stay in treatment longer.

Treatment for substance abuse and addiction can be delivered in many different settings using a variety of behavioral approaches. With adults, both individual therapy and group counseling settings with peers are used. However, studies suggest group therapy can be risky with a younger age group, as some participants in a group may have negative influence over the others, or even steer conversation toward stories about having fun with drugs. Some research suggests that the most effective treatments for teens are those that involve one or more family members present.

Will a Support Group Help My Teen?

While group counseling is sometimes discouraged for teens, peer support groups for teens can be a useful companion to treatment. Self-help groups and other support services can extend the effects of professional treatment for a teen recovering from an addiction. Such groups can be particularly helpful during recovery, offering an added layer of community-level social support to help teens maintain healthy lifestyle behaviors over the course of a lifetime. If your teen is in treatment, your treatment provider will likely be able to tell you about good support groups.

The most well-known self-help groups are those affiliated with Alcoholics Anonymous (AA), Narcotics Anonymous (NA), Cocaine Anonymous (CA), and Teen-Anon. All of these are based on the 12-step model. Support groups for family members of people with addictions, like Alateen, can also be helpful. You can check the web sites of any of these groups for information about teen programs or meetings in your area. To find other meetings in your area, contact local hospitals, treatment centers, or faith-based organizations.

Other services available for teens include recovery high schools (where teens attend school with others in recovery and apart from potentially harmful peer influences) and peer recovery support services. There are other groups in the private sector that can provide a lot of support.

How Do We Keep Things Stable in Our Home until My Teen Is in Treatment?

First, talk to your teen. There are ways to have a conversation about drugs or other sensitive issues that will prevent escalation into an argument.

Acknowledge your child's opinions but know that many people with substance abuse problems are afraid and ashamed and might not always tell the truth. This is why it is important to involve medical professionals who have experience working with people struggling with substance abuse issues.

Second, if your teen has a driver's license, and you suspect drug use, you should take away your child's driving privileges. This could cause an inconvenience for the family, but could prevent a tragic accident. This could also be used as an incentive to get your child to agree to be evaluated by a medical professional.

Part Seven

Adolescent Safety Concerns

Chapter 58

Youth Risk Behavior Surveillance System (YRBSS)

What Is Youth Risk Behavior Surveillance System (YRBSS)?

The Youth Risk Behavior Surveillance System (YRBSS) was developed in 1990 to monitor priority health risk behaviors that contribute markedly to the leading causes of death, disability, and social problems among youth and adults in the United States. These behaviors, often established during childhood and early adolescence, include:

- Behaviors that contribute to unintentional injuries and violence.

- Sexual behaviors related to unintended pregnancy and sexually transmitted infections, including HIV infection.

- Alcohol and other drug use.

This chapter contains text excerpted from the following sources: Text beginning with the heading "What Is the Youth Risk Behavior Surveillance System (YRBSS)?" is excerpted from "Youth Risk Behavior Surveillance System (YRBSS) Overview," Centers for Disease Control and Prevention (CDC), August 9, 2017; Text under the heading "YRBS Results" is excerpted from "CDC Releases Youth Risk Behaviors Survey Results," Centers for Disease Control and Prevention (CDC), June 9, 2016.

579

- Tobacco use.

- Unhealthy dietary behaviors.

- Inadequate physical activity.

In addition, the YRBSS monitors the prevalence of obesity and asthma and other priority health-related behaviors plus sexual identity and sex of sexual contacts. From 1991 through 2015, the YRBSS has collected data from more than 3.8 million high school students in more than 1,700 separate surveys.

What Are the Purposes of YRBSS?

The YRBSS was designed to:

- Determine the prevalence of health behaviors.

- Assess whether health behaviors increase, decrease, or stay the same over time.

- Examine the co-occurrence of health behaviors.

- Provide comparable national, state, territorial, tribal, and local data.

- Provide comparable data among subpopulations of youth.

- Monitor progress toward achieving the Healthy People objectives and other program indicators.

What Are the Components of YRBSS?

The YRBSS includes national, state, territorial, tribal government, and local school-based surveys of representative samples of 9th through 12th grade students. These surveys are conducted every two years, usually during the spring semester. The national survey, conducted by Centers for Disease Control and Prevention (CDC), provides data representative of 9th through 12th grade students in public and private schools in the United States. The state, territorial, tribal government, and local surveys, conducted by departments of health and education, provide data representative of mostly public high school students in each jurisdiction.

YRBS Results

New results from the 2015 YRBS show that while the prevalence of cigarette smoking among high school students dropped to the lowest levels since the survey began in 1991, the use of e-cigarettes among students is posing new challenges.

Although the prevalence of current cigarette use decreased significantly from 28 percent in 1991 to 11 percent in 2015, new data from the 2015 survey found that 24 percent of high school students reported using e-cigarettes during the past 30 days.

Significant progress has been made in reducing physical fighting among adolescents. Since 1991, the percentage of high school students who had been in a physical fight at least once during the past 12 months decreased from 42 percent to 23 percent. However, nationwide, the percentage of students who had not gone to school because of safety concerns is still too high, with 6 percent of students missing at least 1 day of school during the past month because they felt they would be unsafe.

Survey findings indicate that the use of technology while driving continues to put youth at risk. Among high school students who had driven a car or other vehicle during the past 30 days, the percentage of teens who texted or e-mailed while driving ranged from 26 percent to 63 percent across 35 states, and from 14 percent to 39 percent across 18 large urban school districts. Nationwide, 42 percent of students who had driven a car or other vehicle during the past 30 days texted or e-mailed.

The new YRBS report shows mixed results regarding youth sexual risk behaviors. While teens are having less sex, condom use among currently sexually active students and HIV testing among all students has declined. The percentage of high school students who are currently sexually active (had sexual intercourse during the past three months) has decreased from 38 percent in 1991 to 30 percent in 2015. There is also a significant decrease from 2013 (34%). However, among high school students who are currently sexually active, condom use has declined from 63 percent in 2003 to 57 percent in 2015. This decline follows a period of increased condom use throughout the 1990s and early 2000s.

Further analysis of the 2015 National YRBS results showed changes in obesity and sedentary related behaviors in recent years. The percentage of high school students using a computer 3 or more hours per day (for nonschool related work) nearly doubled from 22 percent in 2003 to 42 percent in 2015. There was a significant decline from 2013 to 2015 in the percentage of high school students drinking soda 1 or more times per day—from 27 percent to 20 percent.

Chapter 59

Driving Safety for Teens

Chapter Contents

Section 59.1—Facts about Teen Drivers.................................... 584

Section 59.2—Teen Driving Risks... 587

Section 59.3—Role of Parents in Guiding Teens
for Safe Driving 591

Section 59.1

Facts about Teen Drivers

This section includes text excerpted from "Teen Drivers:
Get the Facts," Centers for Disease Control and
Prevention (CDC), October 16, 2017.

Motor vehicle crashes are the leading cause of death for U.S. teens. Fortunately, teen motor vehicle crashes are preventable, and proven strategies can improve the safety of young drivers on the road.

How Big Is the Problem?

In 2015, 2,333 teens in the United States ages 16–19 were killed and 221,313 were treated in emergency departments for injuries suffered in motor vehicle crashes in 2014. That means that six teens ages 16–19 died every day from motor vehicle injuries.

In 2013, young people ages 15–19 represented only 7 percent of the U.S. population. However, they accounted for 11 percent ($10 billion) of the total costs of motor vehicle injuries.

Who Is Most at Risk?

The risk of motor vehicle crashes is higher among 16–19-year-olds than among any other age group. In fact, per mile driven, teen drivers ages 16 to 19 are nearly three times more likely than drivers aged 20 and older to be in a fatal crash.

Among teen drivers, those at especially high risk for motor vehicle crashes are:

- **Males:** In 2014, the motor vehicle death rate for male drivers and passengers ages 16 to 19 was two times that of their female counterparts.

- **Teens driving with teen passengers:** The presence of teen passengers increases the crash risk of unsupervised teen drivers. This risk increases with the number of teen passengers.

- **Newly licensed teens:** Crash risk is particularly high during the first months of licensure. The crash rate per mile driven is 3 times higher for 16–17 year olds as compared to 18–19 year olds.

What Factors Put Teen Drivers at Risk?

Teens are more likely than older drivers to underestimate dangerous situations or not be able to recognize hazardous situations. Teens are also more likely than adults to make critical decision errors that lead to serious crashes.

- Teens are more likely than older drivers to speed and allow shorter headways (the distance from the front of one vehicle to the front of the next). The presence of male teenage passengers increases the likelihood of this risky driving behavior.

- In 2014, 50 percent of teen deaths from motor vehicle crashes occurred between 3 p.m. and midnight and 53 percent occurred on Friday, Saturday, or Sunday.

- Compared with other age groups, teens have among the lowest rates of seatbelt use. In 2015, only 61 percent of high school students reported they always wear seat belts when riding with someone else.

- At all levels of blood alcohol concentration (BAC), the risk of involvement in a motor vehicle crash is greater for teens than for older drivers.

- Among male drivers between 15 and 20 years of age who were involved in fatal crashes in 2014, 36 percent were speeding at the time of the crash and 24 percent had been drinking.

- In 2014, 17 percent of drivers aged 16 to 20 involved in fatal motor vehicle crashes had a BAC of .08 percent or higher.

- In a national survey conducted in 2015, 20 percent of teens reported that, within the previous month, they had ridden with a driver who had been drinking alcohol. Among students who drove, 8 percent reported having driven after drinking alcohol within the same one-month period.

- In 2014, 64 percent of drivers aged 15 to 20 who were killed in motor vehicle crashes after drinking and driving were not wearing a seat belt.

How Can Deaths and Injuries Resulting from Crashes Involving Teen Drivers Be Prevented?

The following are proven methods to helping teens become safer drivers.

Eight Danger Zones

Make sure your young driver is aware of the leading causes of teen crashes:

1. Driver inexperience
2. Driving with teen passengers
3. Nighttime driving
4. Not using seat belts
5. Distracted driving
6. Drowsy driving
7. Reckless driving
8. Impaired driving

Learn what research has shown parents can do to keep teen drivers safe from each of these risks.

Seat Belts

Of the teens (aged 16–19) who died in passenger vehicle crashes in 2015 approximately 47 percent were not wearing a seatbelt at the time of the crash. Research shows that seat belts reduce serious crash-related injuries and deaths by about half.

Primary Enforcement of Seat Belt Laws

State seat belt laws vary in enforcement. A primary seat belt law allows police to ticket a driver or passenger exclusively for not wearing a seat belt. A secondary law allows police to ticket motorists for not wearing a seat belt only if the driver has been pulled over for a different violation. Some states that have secondary seat belt laws permit primary enforcement for occupants under the age of 18 years.

Not Drinking and Driving

Enforcing minimum legal drinking age laws and zero blood-alcohol tolerance laws for drivers under age 21 are recommended.

Graduated Driver Licensing Programs (GDL)

Driving is a complex skill, one that must be practiced to be learned well. Teenagers' lack of driving experience, together with risk-taking behavior, puts them at heightened risk for crashes. The need for skill-building and driving supervision for new drivers is the basis for graduated driver licensing programs, which exist in all U.S. states and Washington, DC. Graduated Driver Licensing Programs (GDL) provides longer practice periods, limits driving under high risk conditions for newly licensed drivers, and requires greater participation of parents as their teens learn to drive. Research suggests that the more comprehensive GDL programs are associated with reductions of 26 percent to 41 percent in fatal crashes and reductions of 16 percent to 22 percent in overall crashes, among 16-year-old drivers. When parents know their state's GDL laws, they can help enforce the laws and, in effect, help keep their teen drivers safe.

Section 59.2

Teen Driving Risks

This section includes text excerpted from "Teen Driving," National Highway Traffic Safety Administration (NHTSA), October 18, 2017.

Your teen sees a driver's license as a step toward freedom, but you might not be sure your teen is ready for the road. One thing is certain: teens aren't ready to have the same level of driving responsibility as adults. Teen drivers have a higher rate of fatal crashes, mainly because of their immaturity, lack of skills, and lack of experience. They speed, they make mistakes, and they get distracted easily—especially if their friends are in the car.

Distracted Driving

Teens' inexperience behind the wheel makes them more susceptible to distraction behind the wheel. One in three teens who text, say they have done so while driving. Is your teen one of them? Research has found that dialling a phone number while driving increases your teen's risk of crashing by six times, and texting while driving increases the risk by 23 times. Talking or texting on the phone takes your teen's focus off the task of driving, and significantly reduces their ability to react to a roadway hazard, incident, or inclement weather.

Distracted driving can take on many forms beyond texting and talking on the cell phone. Many teens may try to use their driving time to eat their morning breakfast or drink coffee, to apply makeup, or to change the radio station. Many teens are distracted by the addition of passengers in the vehicle. Any distraction is a dangerous distraction. Taking eyes off the road even for five seconds could cost a life.

Speeding

Speeding is a critical safety issue for teen drivers. In 2015, it was a factor in 29 percent of the fatal crashes that involved teen drivers. A study by the Governors Highway Safety Association (GHSA) found that from 2000–2011, teens were involved in 19,447 speeding-related crashes. There is also evidence from naturalistic driving studies that teens' speeding behavior increases over time, possibly as they gain confidence. Teens should especially be aware of their speed during inclement weather, when they may need to reduce their speed, or with other road conditions, like traffic stops or winding roads.

Drunk Driving and Drugs

Remind your teen that underage drinking is illegal, and driving under the influence of any impairing substance—including illicit, over-the-counter, and prescription drugs—could have deadly consequences. Drinking alcohol under the age of 21 is illegal in every State—inside or outside of a vehicle. Drunk-driving laws are always strictly enforced, and many States have zero-tolerance laws, meaning that there can be no trace of alcohol or illegal drugs in your system at any time. Let your teen know: Law enforcement officers will be able to test for these substances.

Show your teen the grim stats. According to the Centers for Disease Control and Prevention (CDC), teens are more likely than anyone else to be killed in an alcohol-related crash. In 2015, almost one out of five teen drivers involved in fatal crashes had been drinking. Even though the minimum legal drinking age in every State is 21, data shows 16 percent of 15- to 18-year-old drivers involved in fatal crashes in 2015 had been drinking. Drugs other than alcohol—illicit as well as prescribed and over-the-counter—can affect your teen's driving, so be sure you and your teen talk about driving and drug use, too.

If lucky enough to survive a crash as an impaired driver, your teenager will face the consequences of breaking the law. Those include a possible trip to jail, the loss of his or her driver's license, and dozens of other expenses including attorney fees, court costs, other fines, and insurance hikes. Your teen will also stand to lose academic eligibility, college acceptance, and scholarship awards.

Seat Belts

Tragically, seat belt use is lowest among teen drivers. In fact, the majority of teenagers involved in fatal crashes are unbuckled. In 2015, a total of 769 teen (15- to 18-year-old) drivers and 531 passengers died in passenger vehicles driven by teen drivers, and 58 percent of the passengers were NOT wearing their seat belts at the time of the fatal crash. As teens start driving and gradually gain independence, they don't always make the smartest decisions regarding their safety. They may think they are invincible, that they don't need seat belts. They may have a false notion that they have the right to choose whether or not to buckle up.

Drowsy Driving

These days, teens are busier than ever: studying, extracurricular activities, part-time jobs, and spending time with friends are among the long list of things they do to fill their time. However, with all of these activities, teens tend to compromise on something very important—sleep. This is a dangerous habit that can lead to drowsy driving. In fact, in 2015, drowsy driving claimed 824 lives, and some studies even suggest drowsiness may have been involved in more than 10–20 percent of fatal or injury crashes. In 2015, teen drivers (aged 15–18) accounted for almost one out of every 10 fatal drowsy driving crashes.

Drowsy driving includes more than just falling asleep. It affects a driver's alertness, attention, reaction time, judgement, and decision-making capabilities. Those who are at higher risk for a crash caused by drowsy driving include drivers 17–23 years old, and those who sleep less than six hours a night, drive on rural roads, or who

589

drive between midnight and 6 am. Make sure your teen gets a good night's sleep, and strictly monitor and limit their nighttime driving as your State's GDL law stipulates. Your teen's friends, passengers, and other drivers will thank them for driving safely.

What Can You Do?

- **Learn about your State's GDL laws.** Note that the laws and restrictions can vary from State to State. Familiarizing yourself with the restrictions placed on your teen's license can better assist you in enforcing those laws. You have the opportunity to establish some important ground rules for your teen driver. Restrict night driving and passengers, prohibit driving while using the phone or other electronic devices, and require seat belt use at all times.

- **Talk to your teen about the dangers of drug and alcohol use.** Remind them that it is illegal to drink under the age of 21, and it is illegal—and deadly—to drink and drive. If a teen is under 21, his or her blood alcohol concentration (BAC) should always be at .00, not just under .08, which is the legal limit for drivers over age 21.

- **Be a good role model.** Remember that your child looks to you as a driver, so practice safe driving yourself. Set aside time to take your teen on practice driving sessions. It can be a great way to spend time together and to allow your teen to improve some basic driving skills. Your teen's learning starts at home.

- **Don't rely solely on a driver's education class to teach your teen to drive.** Remember that driver's education should be used as just part of a GDL system.

You have more influence on your teen than you may think. Be a good example and get involved in their driving habits from the beginning, and stay involved for the duration of their teen years.

Section 59.3

Role of Parents in Guiding Teens for Safe Driving

This section includes text excerpted from "Parents Are the Key to Safe Teen Drivers," Centers for Disease Control and Prevention (CDC), April 20, 2017.

Many parents don't realize it, but the #1 threat to their teen's safety is driving or riding in a car with a teen driver.

The fact is, more than 2,300 teens lost their lives in car crashes in 2015. That's six teens a day too many. The main cause? Driver inexperience.

One of the most important safety features for your teen driver is YOU.

Parents Are the Key, a campaign from the Centers for Disease Control and Prevention (CDC), helps parents, pediatricians, and communities keep teen drivers safe on the road.

Did you know that new drivers are more likely to be involved in a fatal crash simply due to inexperience? Explore the options given below to learn how you can encourage safe driving behavior by your teen.

Eight Danger Zones

Six teens a day are killed in car crashes. But injuries and deaths are preventable. Make sure your young driver is aware of the leading causes of teen crashes. Then use a parent-teen driving agreement to put rules in place that will help your teen stay safe.

Danger Zone One: Driver Inexperience

Crash risk is highest in the first year a teen has their license. What parents can do:

- Provide at least 30 to 50 hours of supervised driving practice over at least six months.

591

- Practice on a variety of roads, at different times of day, and in varied weather and traffic conditions.

- Stress the importance of continually scanning for potential hazards including other vehicles, bicyclists, and pedestrians.

Danger Zone Two: Driving with Teen Passengers

Crash risk goes up when teens drive with other teens in the car. What parents can do:

- Follow your state's Graduated Driver Licensing (GDL) system for passenger restrictions. If your state doesn't have such a rule, limit the number of teen passengers your teen can have to zero or one.

- Keep this rule for at least the first six months that your teen is driving.

Danger Zone Three: Nighttime Driving

For all ages, fatal crashes are more likely to occur at night; but the risk is higher for teens.
What parents can do:

- Make sure your teen is off the road by 9 or 10 p.m. for at least the first six months of licensed driving.

- Practice nighttime driving with your teen when you think they are ready.

Danger Zone Four: Not Using Seat Belts

The simplest way to prevent car crash deaths is to buckle up. What parents can do:

- Require your teen to wear a seat belt on every trip. This simple step can reduce your teen's risk of dying or being badly injured in a crash by about half.

Danger Zone Five: Distracted Driving

Distractions increase your teen's risk of being in a crash. What parents can do:

- Don't allow activities that may take your teen's attention away from driving, such as talking on a cell phone, texting, eating, or playing with the radio.

Danger Zone Six: Drowsy Driving

Young drivers are at high risk for drowsy driving, which causes thousands of crashes every year. Teens are most tired and at risk when driving in the early morning or late at night.

What parents can do:

- Know your teen's schedule so you can be sure he or she is well rested before getting behind the wheel.

Danger Zone Seven: Reckless Driving

Research shows that teens lack the experience, judgment, and maturity to assess risky situations.
What parents can do:

- Make sure your teen knows to follow the speed limit and adjust their speed to match road conditions.

- Remind your teen to maintain enough space behind the vehicle ahead to avoid a crash in case of a sudden stop.

Danger Zone Eight: Impaired Driving

Even one drink will impair your teen's driving ability and increase their risk of a crash.

What parents can do:

- Be a good role model: never drink and drive.

- Reinforce this message with a Parent-Teen Driving Agreement.

- Learn more about impaired driving.

- Get the stats on teen drinking and driving.

Graduated Driver Licensing

Graduated Driver Licensing (GDL) systems help new drivers gain skills under lower-risk conditions. As drivers move through the three stages of GDL, they are given more driving privileges. These privileges may include driving at night or with passengers. GDL systems are proven to reduce teen crashes and deaths.

All states have three-stage GDL systems, though laws vary.

- Stage One: learner's permit

- Stage Two: intermediate license (sometimes called a provisional license)

- Stage Three: unrestricted license

Parent-Teen Driving Agreement

Having regular conversations about safety, practicing driving together, and leading by example go a long way in ensuring your teen makes smart decisions when they get behind the wheel.

But there's another simple step you can take to get on the same page about your family's rules of the road. Create a Parent-Teen Driving Agreement that puts your rules in writing to clearly set expectations and limits. Work with your teen to outline hazards to avoid and consequences for breaking rules. Keep it on the fridge and update it as your teen gains experience and more driving privileges.

Parents: Share What You've Learned

Even though you've been driving for longer than you'd like to admit, having a teen driver in the family is unfamiliar territory for many parents.

Share these resources with other parents of teen drivers and start a safe teen driving conversation:

Through Social Networks and Blogs

Whether you're on Facebook, Twitter, or have your own blog, social networks make it simple to spread the word about safe teen driving. Post a link to Parents Are the Key (www.cdc.gov/parentsarethekey/index.html), share tips from our Pinterest board, or even create an online group so parents can talk with each other about safe teen driving.

At Work

Talk with coworkers who are also parents of teen drivers or soon-to-be teen drivers. Ask your human resources department to place materials on everyone's desk or share them via email or newsletters.

At Parent-Teacher Association (PTA) Meetings

Work with your PTA chapter to plan a safe teen driving event. National safety organizations, such as National Safety Council (NSC) and National Organizations for Youth Safety (NOYS), may have local chapters that could provide speakers. Staff from local law enforcement, highway safety, public health, and medical groups can also participate.

At Faith-Based Organizations

Ask your religious leaders to address the importance of safe teen driving.

Through Parent Social Groups

From bowling to book clubs, your friends may want to compare notes on the ways in which they enforce the rules of the road with their teens. Suggest using a Parent-Teen Driving Agreement to put the rules in writing.

At Health Clubs

Your fitness center can be a good place to display materials and talk with other parents. You can reach both parents and teens, as some families make physical fitness a family outing.

At School Events

Going to your child's track meet, baseball game, or concert? Strike up a safe teen driving conversation with other parents in the stands. Occasions like homecoming, spring break, prom season, and graduation provide even more reasons to talk about safe teen driving.

Chapter 60

Internet Safety

Chapter Contents

Section 60.1—Electronic Aggression.. 598

Section 60.2—Sextortion 600

Section 60.3—Social Networking Sites:
        Safety Tips for Teens 603

Section 60.1

Electronic Aggression

This section includes text excerpted from "Technology and Youth: Protecting Your Child from Electronic Aggression," Centers for Disease Control and Prevention (CDC), August 5, 2008. Reviewed November 2017.

Technology and youth seem destined for each other. They are both young, fast paced, and ever changing. In the last 20 years there has been an explosion in new technology. This new technology has been eagerly embraced by young people and has led to expanding knowledge, social networks, and vocabulary that includes instant messaging ("IMing"), blogging, and text messaging.

New technology has many potential benefits for youth. With the help of new technology, young people can interact with others across the United States and throughout the world on a regular basis. Social networking sites like Facebook and MySpace also allow youth to develop new relationships with others, some of whom they have never even met in person.

New technology also provides opportunities to make rewarding social connections for those youth who have difficulty developing friendships in traditional social settings or because of limited contact with same-aged peers. In addition, regular Internet access allows teens and pre-teens to quickly increase their knowledge on a wide variety of topics.

However, the recent explosion in technology does not come without possible risks. Youth can use electronic media to embarrass, harass, or threaten their peers. Increasing numbers of adolescents are becoming victims of this new form of violence—electronic aggression. Research suggests that 9 percent to 35 percent of young people report being victims of this type of violence. Like traditional forms of youth violence, electronic aggression is associated with emotional distress and conduct problems at school.

Electronic aggression is any type of harassment or bullying that occurs through e-mail, a chat room, instant messaging, a website (including blogs), or text messaging.

Examples of Electronic Aggression

- Disclosing someone else's personal information in a public area (e.g., website) in order to cause embarrassment.

- Posting rumors or lies about someone in a public area (e.g., discussion board).

- Distributing embarrassing pictures of someone by posting them in a public area (e.g., website) or sending them via e-mail.

- Assuming another person's electronic identity to post or send messages about others with the intent of causing the other person harm.

- Sending mean, embarrassing, or threatening text messages, instant messages, or e-mails.

Tips for Parents and Caregivers

- **Talk to your child.**

  Parents and caregivers often ask children where they are going and who they are going with when they leave the house. You should ask these same questions when your child goes on the Internet. Because children are reluctant to disclose victimization for fear of having their Internet and cellular phone privileges revoked; develop solutions to prevent or address victimization that do not punish the child.

- **Develop rules.**

  Together with your child, develop rules about acceptable and safe behaviors for all electronic media. Make plans for what they should do if they become a victim of electronic aggression or know someone who is being victimized. The rules should focus on ways to maximize the benefits of technology and decrease its risks.

- **Explore the Internet.**

  Visit the websites your child frequents, and assess the pros and cons. Remember, most websites and online activities are beneficial. They help young people learn new information, interact with others, and connect with people who have similar interests.

- **Talk with other parents and caregivers.**

  Talk to other parents and caregivers about how they have discussed technology use with their children. Ask about the rules they have developed and how they stay informed about their child's technology use.

- **Connect with the school.**

  Parents and caregivers are encouraged to work with their child's school and school district to develop a class for parents and caregivers that educates them about school policies on electronic aggression, recent incidents in the community involving electronic aggression, and resources available to parents and caregivers who have concerns. Work with the school and other partners to develop a collaborative approach to preventing electronic aggression.

- **Educate yourself.**

  Stay informed about the new devices and websites your child is using. Technology changes rapidly, and many developers offer information to keep people aware of advances. Continually talk with your child about "where they are going" and explore the technology yourself. Technology is not going away, and forbidding young people to access electronic media may not be a good long-term solution. Together, parents and children can come up with ways to maximize the benefits of technology and decrease its risks.

Section 60.2

Sextortion

This section includes text excerpted from "Sextortion Affecting Thousands of U.S. Children," Federal Bureau of Investigation (FBI), April 4, 2016.

Sextortion is a type of online sexual exploitation in which individuals coerce victims into providing sexually explicit images or videos of themselves, often in compliance with offenders' threats to post the images publicly or send the images to victims' friends and family. The FBI (Federal Bureau of Investigation) has seen a significant increase in sextortion activity against children who use the Internet, typically ages 10 to 17, but any age child can become a victim of sextortion.

Technical Details

The FBI is seeking to warn parents, educators, caregivers, and children about the dangers of sextortion. Sending just one inappropriate image to another person online could become the catalyst for sextortion if that image, shared publicly or with their family and friends, is considered compromising to the victim. Offenders easily misrepresent themselves online to appear to be friendly and age appropriate or simply an adult who will listen to a child. This relationship can be manipulated to groom the child to eventually send inappropriate images or video to the offender.

Furthermore, children may send images or videos to a known individual on purpose, but an offender may come into possession of those images or videos through the sextortion of the original recipient or if the original recipient puts the image on the Internet and the offender comes across it. Younger children can become victims when their friend or sibling is being sextorted and the offender threatens to make images or videos public if their requests to include the sexual abuse of younger children in the images or videos are not satisfied.

Threat

Children tend to be trusting online and will befriend people of any age or sex they may not know. Offenders take advantage of this naivety and target children who openly engage others online or have a strong social networking presence. In most instances, they openly post pictures or videos of themselves. Offenders can gain information from the online presence of potential victims by reviewing posts and "friends lists" and pose as an acquaintance, another teen from the same or a different school, or a stranger with similar interests. "Friends lists" may serve as a source to identify additional victims once the sextortion process starts. Once a child becomes a victim of sextortion, the victimization may last for years. Victims have reported having to meet demands for sexually explicit images and videos multiple times per day. The FBI has identified cases in which children committed suicide, attempted suicide, or engaged in other acts of self-harm due to their sextortion victimization. In one instance, the victim purposely engaged in activity that put them in the hospital to get a break from their offender's demands. As soon as the victim was released from the hospital, the victimization continued.

Defense

Sextortion is a crime. The coercion of a child by an adult to produce what is considered child pornography carries heavy penalties, which can include up to life sentences for the offender. The FBI does not treat a child as an offender in the production of child pornography as a result of their sextortion or coercion. In order for the victimization to stop, children typically have to come forward to someone—normally a parent, teacher, caregiver, or law enforcement. The embarrassment of the activity a child was forced to engage in is what typically prevents them from coming forward. Sextortion offenders may have hundreds of victims around the world, so coming forward to help law enforcement identify the offender may prevent countless other incidents of sexual exploitation to that victim and others.

The following measures may help educate and prevent children from becoming victims of this type of sexual exploitation:

- Make children aware that anything done online may be available to others;

- Make sure children's apps and social networking sites' privacy settings are set to the strictest level possible;

- Anyone who asks a child to engage in sexually explicit activity online should be reported to a parent, guardian, or law enforcement;

- It is not a crime for a child to send sexually explicit images to someone if they are compelled to do so, so victims should not be afraid to tell law enforcement if they are being sexually exploited;

- Parents should put personal computers in a central location in the home;

- Parents should review and approve apps downloaded to smart phones and mobile devices and monitor activity on those devices;

- Ensure an adult is present and engaged when children communicate via webcam; and

- Discuss Internet safety with children before they engage in any online activity and maintain those discussions as children become teenagers.

What to do if you believe you are or someone you know is the victim of sextortion:

- Contact your local law enforcement agency, your local FBI field office (contact information can be found at www.fbi.gov), or the National Center for Missing and Exploited Children (1-800-the-lost or Cybertipline.org);

- Do not delete anything before law enforcement is able to review it; and

- Tell law enforcement everything about the encounters you had online-it may be embarrassing, but it is necessary to find the offender.

Section 60.3

Social Networking Sites: Safety Tips for Teens

This section includes text excerpted from "Teens' Social Media Use:
How They Connect and What It Means for Health," U.S. Department
of Health and Human Services (HHS), May 13, 2016.

In this digital age, technology and the Internet are part of everyday life. Social media platforms such as Instagram, Twitter, and Facebook are especially prominent in the lives of adolescents, and they're not just for talking with friends: adolescents use social media to express themselves and find information. This section takes a look at their habits, the risks and benefits of social media use, and resources to keep youth safe online.

How Teens Are Connected

The Pew Research Center regularly conducts surveys on technology use in the United States, and collects data on adolescents' social media use.

- **Teens connect via mobile.** Widespread and improved mobile technology means teens can access social media more easily. According to a Pew survey conducted during 2014 and 2015, 94 percent of teens who go online using a mobile device do so daily.

- **Teens use multiple social platforms.** Facebook, Instagram, and Snapchat are the most popular, and 71 percent of teens say they use more than one social media site.

- **Teens' social media use differs by gender.** Boys report going on Facebook most often; while girls are more likely than boys to use visually-oriented platforms such as Tumblr, Pinterest, and Instagram.

- **Teens share a lot of their personal information.** A survey of over 600 teens from 2012 found that nearly all shared their real name and photos of themselves, and most shared their school name, birthdate, and the city or town where they lived.

- **Teens use social media for romance too.** Another 2015 Pew report—on the role of technology in teen romantic relationships notes that half of teens say they've used Facebook or other social networking sites to express romantic interest in someone, and many use these sites to display their romantic relationships.

Social Media: Health Resource or Health Risk?

As with most technology, there are potential benefits and risks to teens' social media use. These platforms can help teens socialize and communicate with peers; find learning opportunities; and become engaged in causes important to them. Social media also provide a wealth of information and resources that teens can use to maintain their own health and relationships.

On the other hand, teens on social media are at risk of cyberbullying and other aggression online; inappropriate content or exposure to predators; and having their private information available publicly. There is also some evidence that frequent social media use may be linked to depression and other mental health problems.

Ultimately, social media becomes a tool or risk for teen's health based on how they use it, which is in turn shaped by the guidance they get from caring adults. To support teens' healthy social media use, parents, and youth-serving professionals can use these resources:

- Help teens protect their information online with Onguardonline. gov, a federal resource sponsored by the Department of Homeland Security (DHS).

- Talk to teens about being responsible digital citizens and how to prevent and handle issues such as sexting and cyberbullying with additional resources from the DHS's "Stop. Think. Connect." campaign, including a rap video by youth on online safety.

- Set healthy boundaries for social media use (and technology in general) with this family media contract example from the American Academy of Pediatrics (AAP) site for parents, HealthyChildren.org.

- Check out social media resources from the U.S. Department of Health and Human Services (HHS) and many of its offices; including Office of Adolescent Health (OAH), the Centers for Disease Control and Prevention (CDC) and the National Institutes of Health (NIH), for reliable information on adolescent health.

- Direct teens toward sites that are designed to help them directly, including the National Runaway Safeline, National Institute on Drug Abuse (NIDA) for Teens, Smokefree Teen, and the National Suicide Prevention Lifeline. The OAH website also has a page for teens to find action steps and resources they can use to care for their health as well as a list of service locators.

Safety Tips

- **Limit the amount of personal information you post.** Do not post information that would make you vulnerable, such as your address or information about your schedule or routine. If your connections post information about you, make sure the combined information is not more than you would be comfortable with strangers knowing. Also, be considerate when posting information, including photos, about your connections.

605

- **Remember that the Internet is a public resource.** Only post information you are comfortable with anyone seeing. This includes information and photos in your profile and in blogs and other forums. Also, once you post information online, you can't retract it. Even if you remove the information from a site, saved or cached versions may still exist on other people's machines.

- **Be wary of strangers.** The Internet makes it easy for people to misrepresent their identities and motives. Consider limiting the people who are allowed to contact you on these sites. If you interact with people you do not know, be cautious about the amount of information you reveal or agreeing to meet them in person.

- **Be skeptical.** Don't believe everything you read online. People may post false or misleading information about various topics, including their own identities. This is not necessarily done with malicious intent; it could be unintentional, an exaggeration, or a joke. Take appropriate precautions, though, and try to verify the authenticity of any information before taking any action.

- **Evaluate your settings.** Take advantage of a site's privacy settings. The default settings for some sites may allow anyone to see your profile, but you can customize your settings to restrict access to only certain people. There is still a risk that private information could be exposed despite these restrictions, so don't post anything that you wouldn't want the public to see. Sites may change their options periodically, so review your security and privacy settings regularly to make sure that your choices are still appropriate.

- **Be wary of third-party applications.** Third-party applications may provide entertainment or functionality, but use caution when deciding which applications to enable. Avoid applications that seem suspicious, and modify your settings to limit the amount of information the applications can access.

- **Use strong passwords**. Protect your account with passwords that cannot easily be guessed. If your password is compromised, someone else may be able to access your account and pretend to be you.

- **Check privacy policies.** Some sites may share information such as email addresses or user preferences with other companies. This may lead to an increase in spam. Also, try to locate the policy for handling referrals to make sure that you do not unintentionally sign your friends up for spam. Some sites will continue to send email messages to anyone you refer until they join.

- **Keep software, particularly your web browser, up to date.** Install software updates so that attackers cannot take advantage of known problems or vulnerabilities. Many operating systems offer automatic updates. If this option is available, you should enable it.

- **Use and maintain anti-virus software.** Anti-virus software helps protect your computer against known viruses, so you may be able to detect and remove the virus before it can do any damage. Because attackers are continually writing new viruses, it is important to keep your definitions up to date.

Children are especially susceptible to the threats that social networking sites present. Although many of these sites have age restrictions, children may misrepresent their ages so that they can join. By teaching children about Internet safety, being aware of their online habits, and guiding them to appropriate sites, parents can make sure that the children become safe and responsible users.

Chapter 61

Skin Safety Concerns

Chapter Contents

Section 61.1—Cosmetics 610

Section 61.2—Safe Hair Removal 614

Section 61.3—The Risks of Tanning 616

Section 61.4—Tattoos and Teens 622

Section 61.5—Tinea Infections: Ringworm,
    Athlete's Foot, and Jock Itch 625

609

Section 61.1

Cosmetics

This section contains text excerpted from the following sources:
Text in this section begins with excerpts from "Cosmetics: Tips for
Women," U.S. Food and Drug Administration (FDA), October 5,
2016; Text under the heading "FAQs about Cosmetics" is excerpted
from "Cosmetics Safety Q&A: Shelf Life," U.S. Food and Drug
Administration (FDA), March 24, 2014. Reviewed November 2017.

People use cosmetics to enhance their beauty. These products range
from lipstick and nail polish to deodorant, perfume, and hairspray. Get
the facts before using cosmetics.

General Tips

- Read the label. Follow all directions.
- Wash your hands before you use the product.
- Do not share makeup.
- Keep the containers clean and closed tight when not in use.
- Throw away cosmetics if the color or smell changes.
- Do not use spray cans while you are smoking or near an open flame. It could start a fire.
- Use aerosols or sprays in a place with good air flow.

Eye Make-Up Tips

1. Do not add saliva or water to mascara. You could add germs.
2. Throw away your eye makeup if you get an eye infection.
3. Do not use cosmetics near your eyes unless they are meant for your eyes. For example, do not use lip liner on your eyes.
4. Do not dye or tint your eyelashes. U.S. Food And Drug Administration (FDA) has not approved any color additives for permanent dyeing or tinting of your eyelashes or eyebrows.

5. Hold still! Even a slight scratch with the mascara wand or other applicator can result in a serious infection. Do not apply makeup in the car or on the bus.

Bad Reaction to Cosmetics?

FDA does not test cosmetics before they are sold in stores. However, FDA does monitor the safety of cosmetic products. Tell FDA if you have a rash, redness, burns, or other serious problems after using cosmetics.

What Should You Do?

- Stop using the product.

- Call your healthcare provider to find out how to take care of the problem.

Understanding Cosmetic Labels

Read the label including the list of ingredients, warnings, and tips on how to use it safely.

- **Hypoallergenic:** Do not assume that the product will not cause allergic reactions. FDA does not define what it means to be labeled 'hypoallergenic'.

- **Organic or Natural:** The source of the ingredients does not determine how safe it is. Do not assume that these products are safer than products made with ingredients from other sources. FDA does not define what it means to be labeled 'organic' or 'natural'.

- **Expiration Dates:** Cosmetics are not required to have an expiration date. A cosmetic product may go bad if you store it the wrong way like if it is unsealed or in a place that is too warm or too moist.

FAQs about Cosmetics

What Is the Shelf Life of Cosmetics?

The shelf life for eye-area cosmetics is more limited than for other products. Because of repeated microbial exposure during use by the consumer and the risk of eye infections, some industry experts recommend replacing mascara 3 months after purchase.

Among other cosmetics that are likely to have an unusually short shelf life are certain "all natural" products that may contain plant-derived substances conducive to microbial growth. It also is important for consumers and manufacturers to consider the increased risk of contamination in products that contain nontraditional preservatives, or no preservatives at all.

Consumers should be aware that expiration dates are simply "rules of thumb," and that a product's safety may expire long before the expiration date if the product has not been properly stored. Cosmetics that have been improperly stored—for example, exposed to high temperatures or sunlight, or opened and examined by consumers prior to final sale—may deteriorate substantially before the expiration date. On the other hand, products stored under ideal conditions may be acceptable long after the expiration date has been reached.

What Should I Do If I Have a Reaction (Side Effect) to a Cosmetic Product?

If you have a reaction (side effect) to a cosmetic product, you should:

- tell your doctor or other healthcare provider,
- report it to the cosmetic manufacturer, and
- submit a complaint by reporting the problem to the U.S. Food and Drug Administration (FDA)

What Are "Hypoallergenic" Cosmetics?

Hypoallergenic cosmetics are products that manufacturers claim produce fewer allergic reactions than other cosmetic products. Consumers with hypersensitive skin, and even those with "normal" skin, may be led to believe that these products will be gentler to their skin than nonhypoallergenic cosmetics.

What Precautions Should You Take If You Dye Your Hair?

People who dye their hair should follow these safety precautions:

- Follow the directions in the package. Pay attention to all "Caution" and "Warning" statements.
- Do a patch test before using dye on your hair. Here's how: Rub a tiny bit of the dye on the inside of your elbow or behind your ear. Leave it there for two days. If you get a rash, don't use the dye on your hair. You should do the test each time you dye your hair.

- Never dye your eyebrows or eyelashes. This can hurt your eyes. You might even go blind. FDA does not allow using hair dyes on eyelashes and eyebrows.

- Don't leave the dye on longer than the directions say you should.

- Rinse your scalp well with water after dyeing.

- Wear gloves when you apply the hair dye.

- Never mix different hair dye products. This can hurt your hair and scalp.

What Precautions Should You Take When Using Eye Cosmetics?

- If you use eye cosmetics, FDA urges you to follow these safety tips:

- If any eye cosmetic causes irritation, stop using it immediately. If irritation persists, see a doctor.

- Avoid using eye cosmetics if you have an eye infection or the skin around the eye is inflamed. Wait until the area is healed. Discard any eye cosmetics you were using when you got the infection.

- Be aware that there are bacteria on your hands that, if placed in the eye, could cause infections. Wash your hands before applying eye cosmetics.

- Make sure that any instrument you place in the eye area is clean.

- Don't share your cosmetics. Another person's bacteria may be hazardous to you.

- Don't allow cosmetics to become covered with dust or contaminated with dirt or soil. Keep containers clean.

- Don't use old containers of eye cosmetics. Discard mascara three months after purchase.

- Don't store cosmetics at temperatures above 85°F. Cosmetics held for long periods in hot cars, for example, are more susceptible to deterioration of the preservative.

- When applying or removing eye cosmetics, be careful not to scratch the eyeball or other sensitive area. Never apply or remove eye cosmetics in a moving vehicle.

- Don't use any cosmetics near your eyes unless they are intended specifically for that use. For instance, don't use a lip liner as an eye liner. You may be exposing your eyes to contamination from your mouth, or to color additives that are not approved for use in the area of the eye.

- Avoid color additives that are not approved for use in the area of the eye, such as "permanent" eyelash tints and kohl.

Section 61.2

Safe Hair Removal

This section includes text excerpted from "Removing Hair Safely," U.S. Food And Drug Administration (FDA), August 28, 2015.

Laser Hair Removal

In this method, a laser destroys hair follicles with heat. Sometimes it is recommended that a topical anesthetic product be used before a laser hair removal procedure, to minimize pain. In these cases, U.S. Food and Drug Administration (FDA) recommends that consumers discuss with a medical professional the circumstances under which the cream should be used and whether the use is appropriate.

Those who decide to use a skin-numbing product should follow the directions of a healthcare provider and consider using a product that contains the lowest amount of anesthetic drugs possible. FDA's Center for Drug Evaluation and Research (CDER) has received reports of serious and life-threatening side effects after use of large amounts of skin-numbing products for laser hair removal.

Side effects of laser hair removal can include blistering, discoloration after treatment, swelling, redness, and scarring. Sunlight should be avoided during healing after the procedure.

Epilators: Needle, Electrolysis, and Tweezers

Needle epilators introduce a fine wire close to the hair shaft, under the skin, and into the hair follicle. An electric current travels down the wire and destroys the hair root at the bottom of the follicle, and the loosened hair is removed with tweezers.

Medical electrolysis devices destroy hair growth with a shortwave radio frequency after a thin probe is placed in the hair follicle. Risks from these methods include infection from an unsterile needle and scarring from improper technique. Electrolysis is considered a permanent hair removal method since it destroys the hair follicle. It requires a series of appointments over a period of time.

Tweezer epilators also use electric current to remove hair. The tweezers grasp the hair close to the skin, and energy is applied at the tip of the tweezer. There is no body of significant information establishing the effectiveness of the tweezer epilator to permanently remove hair.

Depilatories

Available in gel, cream, lotion, aerosol, and roll-on forms, depilatories are highly alkaline (or, in some cases, acidic) formulations that affect the protein structure of the hair, causing it to dissolve into a jelly like mass that the user can easily wipe from the skin. Consumers should carefully follow instructions and heed all warnings on the product label.

For example, manufacturers typically recommend conducting a preliminary skin test for allergic reaction and irritation. Depilatories should not be used for eyebrows or around eyes or on inflamed or broken skin.

FDA's Office of Cosmetics and Colors has received reports of burns, blisters, stinging, itchy rashes, and skin peeling associated with depilatories and other types of cosmetic hair removers.

Waxing, Sugaring, and Threading

Unlike chemical depilatories that remove hair at the skin's surface, these methods pluck hairs out of the follicle, below the surface.

With waxing, a layer of melted wax is applied to the skin and allowed to harden. (Cold waxes, which are soft at room temperature, allow the user to skip the steps of melting and hardening.) It is then pulled off quickly in the opposite direction of the hair growth, taking the uprooted hair with it. Labeling of waxes may caution that these products should not be used by people with diabetes and circulatory problems. Waxes should not be used over varicose veins, moles, or warts. Waxes also shouldn't be used on eyelashes, the nose, ears, or on nipples, genital areas, or on irritated, chapped, or sunburned skin.

As with chemical depilatories, it can be a good idea to do a preliminary test on a small area for allergic reaction or irritation.

Sugaring is similar to waxing. A heated sugar mixture is spread on the skin, sometimes covered with a strip of fabric, and then lifted off to remove hair. Threading is an ancient technique in which a loop of thread is rotated across the skin to pluck the hair. All of these techniques may cause skin irritation and infection.

Shaving

Shaving hair only when it's wet, and shaving in the direction in which the hairs lie can help lessen skin irritation and cuts. It's important to use a clean razor with a sharp blade. Contrary to popular belief, shaving does not change the texture, color, or growth rate of hair. Razors and electric shavers are under the jurisdiction of the Consumer Product Safety Commission (CPSC).

Section 61.3

The Risks of Tanning

This section includes text excerpted from "The Risks of Tanning," U.S. Food and Drug Administration (FDA), October 14, 2015.

Sunburn

Sunburn, also called erythema, is one of the most obvious signs of ultraviolet (UV) exposure and skin damage. Often marked by redness and peeling (usually after a few days), sunburn is a form of short-term skin damage.

Why It Happens

When UV rays reach your skin, they damage cells in the epidermis. In response, your immune system increases blood flow to the affected areas. The increased blood flow is what gives sunburn its characteristic redness and makes the skin feel warm to the touch. At the same time, the damaged skin cells release chemicals that send messages through the body until they are translated as a painful burning sensation by the brain.

White blood cells, which help protect you from infection and disease, attack and remove the damaged skin cells. It is this process of removing damaged cells that can cause sunburned skin to itch and peel.

Symptoms

The earliest signs of sunburn are skin that looks flushed, is tender or painful, or gives off more heat than normal. Unfortunately, if your skin tone is medium to dark you may not notice any obvious physical signs until several hours later. It can take 6–48 hours for the full effects of sunburn to appear.

Treatment

The American Academy of Dermatology (AAD) recommends treating mild sunburn with cool baths, over-the-counter (OTC) hydrocortisone creams, and aspirin to ease pain and swelling.

Severe sunburn should be treated as a medical emergency and examined by a doctor right away. Severe sunburn is often characterized by a large area of red, blistered skin with a headache, fever, or chills.

The Bottom Line

Sunburn can be a very painful effect of UV exposure. Studies have shown a link between severe sunburn and melanoma, the deadliest form of skin cancer. Pay careful attention to protecting yourself from UV rays.

Sun Tan

There is no such thing as a safe tan. The increase in skin pigment, called melanin, which causes the tan color change in your skin is a sign of damage.

Why It Happens

Once skin is exposed to UV radiation, it increases the production of melanin in an attempt to protect the skin from further damage. Melanin is the same pigment that colors your hair, eyes, and skin.

The increase in melanin may cause your skin tone to darken over the next 48 hours.

Symptoms

Skin tones that are capable of developing a tan, typically skin types II through V, will probably darken in tone within two days.

The Bottom Line

Evidence suggests that tanning greatly increases your risk of developing skin cancer. And, contrary to popular belief, getting a tan will not protect your skin from sunburn or other skin damage. The extra melanin in tanned skin provides a sun-protection factor (SPF) of about 2 to 4; far below the minimum recommended SPF of 15.

Premature Aging

Sometimes referred to as "photoaging," premature aging is the result of unprotected UV exposure. It takes the form of leathery, wrinkled skin, and dark spots.

Why It Happens

Although the causes of premature aging are not always clear, unprotected exposure to harmful UV rays break down the collagen and elastin fibers in healthy young skin, and cause wrinkles and loosened folds. Frequent sunburns or hours spent tanning can result in a permanent darkening of the skin, dark spots, and a leathery texture.

Symptoms

- Wrinkles

- Dark spots

- Leathery skin

Treatment

A dermatologist or plastic surgeon can develop a treatment plan based on your needs. Treatments can include chemical peels, dermabrasion, and skin fillers.

The Bottom Line

Premature aging is a long-term side effect of UV exposure, meaning it may not show on your skin until many years after you have had a sunburn or suntan. Avoiding UV exposure is essential to maintaining healthy skin.

Skin Cancer

There are two main types of skin cancer:

• Melanoma

• Nonmelanoma

Melanoma is the less common, but more dangerous form of skin cancer, and accounts for most of the deaths due to skin cancer each year. Melanoma is cancer that begins in the epidermal cells that produce melanin (melanocytes). According to the American Cancer Society (ACS) melanoma is almost always curable when detected in its early stages.

Nonmelanomas (basal cell and squamous cell carcinomas) occur in the basal or squamous cells located at the base of the epidermis, both inside and outside the body. Nonmelanomas often develop in sun-exposed areas of the body, including the face, ears, neck, lips, and the backs of the hands.

Why It Happens

Predisposition to skin cancer can be hereditary, meaning it is passed through the generations of a family through genes. There is also strong evidence suggesting that exposure to UV rays, both UVA and UVB, can cause skin cancer.

UV radiation may promote skin cancer in two different ways:

• By damaging the DNA in skin cells, causing the skin to grow abnormally and develop benign or malignant growths.

• By weakening the immune system and compromising the body's natural defenses against aggressive cancer cells.

Symptoms

Performing regular self-skin-cancer exams is a good way to protect yourself against skin cancer. The following are possible signs of skin cancer, and should be checked by a doctor.

619

- Any changes on the skin, especially in the size or color of a mole, birthmark, or other dark pigmentation

- Unexplained scaliness, oozing, or bleeding on the skin's surface

- A spot on the skin that suddenly feels itchy, tender, or painful

Treatment

Skin cancer treatment varies depending on the type and severity of the cancer. Your doctor will develop a treatment plan based on your needs.

The Bottom Line

According to the American Cancer Society (ACS), most of the more than one million skin cancers diagnosed each year in the United States are considered sun-related. Skin cancer occurs in people of all skin tones, though it is less common in those with darker skin tones. Assessing your risk with the help of your doctor, protecting your skin, and performing regular skin cancer checks are the best methods of prevention.

Actinic or Solar Keratoses

A fourth type of growth, actinic or solar keratoses, is a concern because it can progress into cancer. Actinic keratoses are considered the earliest stage in the development of skin cancer, and are caused by long-term exposure to sunlight. They are the most common premalignant skin condition, occurring in more than 5 million Americans each year.

Symptoms

Actinic or solar keratoses share some of the symptoms of skin cancer. Look for raised, rough-textured, or scaly bumps that occur in areas that have been sunburned or tanned.

Treatment

Most cases of actinic keratoses are easily treated in a dermatologist's office by removing them with liquid nitrogen or chemical peels.

The Bottom Line

Actinic or solar keratoses are the most common premalignant skin condition. Check with your doctor if you find any suspicious-looking bumps.

Eye Damage: Photokeratitis

Photokeratitis can be thought of as a sunburn of the cornea. It is caused by intense UVC/UVB exposure of the eye. Photokeratitis is also called "snow blindness" because many people develop this condition at high altitudes in a snowy environment where the reflections of UVB are high. This condition can also be produced by exposure to intense artificial sources of UVC/UVB, like broken mercury vapor lamps, or certain types of tanning lamps.

Symptoms

- Tearing

- Pain

- Swollen eyelids

- A feeling of sand in the eye

- Hazy or decreased vision

Treatment

Consult your doctor if you have any of these symptoms. Your doctor can prescribe a topical solution which will aid your cornea in healing. Since the cornea usually heals in 24 to 48 hours, the symptoms are not long-lasting.

Eye Damage: Cataracts

Cataracts are one form of eye damage that research has shown may increase with UV exposure. Clouding of the natural lens of the eye causing decreased vision and possible blindness are all effects of cataracts.

Other types of eye damage include cancer around the eyes, macular degeneration, and irregular tissue growth that can block vision (pterygium).

Symptoms

Consult your doctor if you experience any of the following symptoms.

- Clouded or spotty vision

- Pain or soreness in and around the eyes

Treatment

Cataracts can be surgically removed.

The Bottom Line

Wearing sun protection gear such as a wide-brimmed hat and sunglasses with 100 percent UV protection can help decrease the risks of eye damage.

Immune System Suppression

According to the World Health Organization (WHO), all people, regardless of skin color, are vulnerable to the effects of immune suppression. Overexposure to UV radiation may suppress proper functioning of the body's immune system and the skin's natural defenses, increasing sensitivity to sunlight, diminishing the effects of immunizations or causing reactions to certain medications.

In people who have been treated for an infection of the Herpes simplex virus, sun exposure can weaken the immune system so that it can no longer keep the virus under control. This results in reactivation of the infection and recurring cold sores.

Section 61.4

Tattoos and Teens

This section includes text excerpted from "Consumer Updates—
Think before You Ink: Are Tattoos Safe?" U.S. Food and Drug
Administration (FDA), November 6, 2017.

Popularity of Tattoos among Teens

Tattoos are more popular than ever. According to a 2015 Harris Poll, about 3 in 10 (or 29%) people surveyed have at least one tattoo. The U.S. Food and Drug Administration (FDA) is also seeing reports of people developing infections from contaminated tattoo inks, as well as adverse reactions to the inks themselves.

Over the years, the FDA has received hundreds of adverse event reports involving tattoos: 363 from 2004–2016.

Before you get a tattoo, consider the following key questions.

Should I Be Concerned about Unsafe Practices, or the Tattoo Ink Itself?

Both. While you can get serious infections from unhygienic practices and equipment that isn't sterile, infections can also result from ink that was contaminated with bacteria or mold. Using nonsterile water to dilute the pigments (ingredients that add color) is a common culprit, although not the only one.

There's no sure-fire way to tell if the ink is safe. An ink can be contaminated even if the container is sealed or the label says the product is sterile.

What Is in Tattoo Ink?

Published research has reported that some inks contain pigments used in printer toner or in car paint. FDA has not approved any pigments for injection into the skin for cosmetic purposes.

FDA reviews reports of adverse reactions or infections from consumers and healthcare providers. We may learn about outbreaks from the state authorities who oversee tattoo parlors.

What Kinds of Reactions May Happen after Getting a Tattoo?

You might notice a rash—redness or bumps—in the area of your tattoo, and you could develop a fever.

More aggressive infections may cause high fever, shaking, chills, and sweats. Treating such infections might require a variety of antibiotics—possibly for months—or even hospitalization and/or surgery. A rash may also mean you're having an allergic reaction. And because the inks are permanent, the reaction may persist. Contact your healthcare professional if you have any concerns.

Can Scar Tissue Build Up after Getting a Tattoo?

Scar tissue may form when you get a tattoo, or you could develop "granulomas," small knots or bumps that may form around material that the body perceives as foreign. If you tend to get keloids—scars that grow beyond normal boundaries—you may develop the same kind of reaction to the tattoo.

What Do I Need to Know about MRIs If I Get a Tattoo?

Some people may have swelling or burning in the tattoo when they have magnetic resonance imaging (MRI), although this happens rarely and does not last long. Let your healthcare professional know that you have a tattoo before an MRI is ordered.

What about Do-It-Yourself Tattoo Inks and Kits?

Inks and kits sold as "do-it-yourself" to consumers have been associated with infections and allergic reactions. FDA is also concerned that consumers may not know how to control and avoid all sources of contamination.

Could Other Problems Occur Later On?

Although research is ongoing at FDA and elsewhere, there are still a lot of questions about the long-term effects of the pigments, other ingredients, and possible contaminants in tattoo inks. FDA has received reports of bad reactions to tattoo inks right after tattooing and even years later. You also might become allergic to other products, such as hair dyes, if your tattoo contains p-Phenylenediamene (PPD).

Then there's tattoo removal. We don't know the short- or long-term consequences of how pigments break down after laser treatment. However, we do know some tattoo removal procedures may leave permanent scarring.

If I Get a Tattoo and Develop an Infection or Other Reaction, What Should I Do?

First, contact your healthcare professional.

Second, notify the tattoo artist so he or she can identify the ink and avoid using it again. Ask for the brand, color, and any lot or batch number of the ink or diluent to help determine the source of the problem and how to treat it.

Third, whether you're a consumer, tattoo artist, or healthcare professional, tell FDA. Provide as much detail as possible about the ink and your reaction and outcome.

Removing Tattoos May Be Harder Than You Think

So think before you ink. Consider the risks. Remember, too, that removing a tattoo is a painstaking process, and complete removal without scarring may be impossible. If you do decide to get a tattoo, make sure the tattoo parlor and artist comply with state and local laws.

Section 61.5

Tinea Infections: Ringworm, Athlete's Foot, and Jock Itch

This section contains text excerpted from the following sources: Text under the heading "Ringworm" is excerpted from "Fungal Diseases—Ringworm," Centers for Disease Control and Prevention (CDC), December 4, 2015; Text under the heading "Athlete's Foot (Tinea Pedis)" is excerpted from "Water, Sanitation and Environmentally-Related Hygiene—Hygiene-Related Diseases," Centers for Disease Control and Prevention (CDC), February 6, 2017; Text under the heading "Jock Itch" is © 2017 Omnigraphics. Reviewed November 2017.

Ringworm

Ringworm is a common infection of the skin and nails that is caused by fungus. The infection is called "ringworm" because it can cause an itchy, red, circular rash. Ringworm is also called "tinea" or "dermatophytosis." The different types of ringworm are usually named for the location of the infection on the body.

Areas of the body that can be affected by ringworm include:

- Feet (*tinea pedis*, commonly called "athlete's foot")

- Groin, inner thighs, or buttocks (tinea cruris, commonly called "jock itch")

- Scalp (tinea capitis)

- Beard (tinea barbae)

- Hands (tinea manuum)

- Toenails or fingernails (tinea unguium, also called "onychomycosis") Click here for more information about fungal nail infections. Note: please link this last sentence to the new nail infections page.

- Other parts of the body such as arms or legs (tinea corporis)

Approximately 40 different species of fungi can cause ringworm; the scientific names for the types of fungi that cause ringworm are Trichophyton, Microsporum, and Epidermophyton.

Symptoms

Ringworm can affect skin on almost any part of the body as well as fingernails and toenails. The symptoms of ringworm often depend on which part of the body is infected, but they generally include:

- Itchy skin

- Ring-shaped rash

- Red, scaly, cracked skin

- Hair loss

Symptoms typically appear between 4 and 14 days after the skin comes in contact with the fungi that cause ringworm.

Symptoms of Ringworm by Location on the Body

- **Feet (*tinea pedis* or "athlete's foot"):** The symptoms of ringworm on the feet include red, swollen, peeling, itchy skin between the toes (especially between the pinky toe and the one next to it). The sole and heel of the foot may also be affected. In severe cases, the skin on the feet can blister.

- **Scalp (*tinea capitis*):** Ringworm on the scalp usually looks like a scaly, itchy, red, circular bald spot. The bald spot can grow in size and multiple spots might develop if the infection spreads. Ringworm on the scalp is more common in children than it is in adults.

- **Groin (*tinea cruris* or "jock itch"):** Ringworm on the groin looks like scaly, itchy, red spots, usually on the inner sides of the skin folds of the thigh.

- **Beard (*tinea barbae*):** Symptoms of ringworm on the beard include scaly, itchy, red spots on the cheeks, chin, and upper neck. The spots might become crusted over or filled with pus, and the affected hair might fall out.

Ringworm Risk and Prevention

Who Gets Ringworm?

Ringworm is very common. Anyone can get ringworm, but people who have weakened immune systems may be especially at risk for infection and may have problems fighting off a ringworm infection. People who use public showers or locker rooms, athletes (particularly those who are involved in contact sports such as wrestling), people who wear tight shoes and have excessive sweating, and people who have close contact with animals may also be more likely to come in contact with the fungi that cause ringworm.

How Can I Prevent Ringworm?

- Keep your skin clean and dry.

- Wear shoes that allow air to circulate freely around your feet.

- Don't walk barefoot in areas like locker rooms or public showers.

- Clip your fingernails and toenails short and keep them clean.

- Change your socks and underwear at least once a day.

- Don't share clothing, towels, sheets, or other personal items with someone who has ringworm.

- Wash your hands with soap and running water after playing with pets. If you suspect that your pet has ringworm, take it to see a veterinarian. If your pet has ringworm, follow the steps below to prevent spreading the infection.

- If you're an athlete involved in close contact sports, shower immediately after your practice session or match, and keep all of your sports gear and uniform clean. Don't share sports gear (helmet, etc.) with other players.

Sources of Infection

The fungi that cause ringworm can live on skin and in the environment. There are three main ways that ringworm can spread:

1. From a person who has ringworm.

   People can get ringworm after contact with someone who has the infection. To avoid spreading the infection, people with ringworm shouldn't share clothing, towels, combs, or other personal items with other people.

2. From an animal that has ringworm.

    People can get ringworm after touching an animal that has ringworm. Many different kinds of animals can spread ringworm to people, including dogs and cats, especially kittens and puppies. Other animals, like cows, goats, pigs, and horses can also spread ringworm to people.

3. From the environment.

    The fungi that cause ringworm can live on surfaces, particularly in damp areas like locker rooms and public showers. For that reason, it's a good idea not to walk barefoot in these places

Diagnosis

Your healthcare provider can usually diagnose ringworm by looking at the affected skin and asking questions about your symptoms. He or she may also take a small skin scraping to be examined under a microscope or sent to a laboratory for a fungal culture.

Physical examination. A thorough history and physical examination is often sufficient to diagnose tinea. The classic lesion is an erythematous, raised, scaly ring with central clearing. Multiple lesions may be present. The severity of the infection can range from mild, scaly lesions, to erythematous, exudative lesions characteristic of superimposed bacterial infections.

Microscopy. Potassium hydroxide (KOH) stain a commonly-used method for diagnosing tinea because it is inexpensive, easy to perform, and has high sensitivity. Scrapings from the lesion(s) are placed in a drop of KOH and examined under a microscope for the presence of fungal hyphae.

Ultraviolet light (Wood's lamp). Normally, ultraviolet light is not useful in the diagnosis of tinea with the exception of two species—*Microsporum canis* and *audouinii*. Although both species fluoresce blue-green under a Wood's lamp, both species are uncommon causes of tinea infections. A Wood's lamp may be useful to differentiate between erythrasma caused by *Corynebacterium minutissimum* (which fluoresces coal-red) from tinea cruris, which is nonfluorescent.

Culture. Fungal culture can be performed as a confirmatory test if results from a KOH stain are inconclusive. Hair and/or scrapings extracted from affected areas are placed on Sabouraud's medium. Fungal culture is more specific than KOH stain, but it can take up to three weeks to become positive.

Treatment

The treatment for ringworm depends on its location on the body and how serious the infection is. Some forms of ringworm can be treated with nonprescription ("over-the-counter") medications, but other forms of ringworm need treatment with prescription antifungal medication.

- Ringworm on the skin like athlete's foot (*tinea pedis*) and jock itch (tinea cruris) can usually be treated with nonprescription antifungal creams, lotions, or powders applied to the skin for 2 to 4 weeks. There are many nonprescription products available to treat ringworm, including:

  - Clotrimazole (Lotrimin, Mycelex)

  - Miconazole (Aloe Vesta Antifungal, Azolen, Baza Antifungal, Carrington Antifungal, Critic Aid Clear, Cruex Prescription Strength, DermaFungal, Desenex, Fungoid Tincture, Micaderm, Micatin, Micro-Guard, Miranel, Mitrazol, Podactin, Remedy Antifungal, Secura Antifungal)

  - Terbinafine (Lamisil)

  - Ketoconazole (Xolegel)

For nonprescription creams, lotions, or powders, follow the directions on the package label. Contact your healthcare provider if your infection doesn't go away or gets worse.

- Ringworm on the scalp (tinea capitis) usually needs to be treated with prescription antifungal medication taken by mouth for 1 to 3 months. Creams, lotions, or powders don't work for ringworm on the scalp. Prescription antifungal medications used to treat ringworm on the scalp include:

  - Griseofulvin (Grifulvin V, Gris-PEG)

  - Terbinafine

  - Itraconazole (Onmel, Sporanox)

- Fluconazole (Diflucan)

You should contact your healthcare provider if:

- Your infection gets worse or doesn't go away after using nonprescription medications.

- You or your child has ringworm on the scalp. Ringworm on the scalp needs to be treated with prescription antifungal medication.

Athlete's Foot (Tinea Pedis)

Athlete's foot, or *tinea pedis*, is an infection of the skin and feet that can be caused by a variety of different fungi. Although *tinea pedis* can affect any portion of the foot, the infection most often affects the space between the toes. Athlete's foot is typically characterized by skin fissures or scales that can be red and itchy.

Tinea pedis is spread through contact with infected skin scales or contact with fungi in damp areas (for example, showers, locker rooms, swimming pools). *Tinea pedis* can be a chronic infection that recurs frequently. Treatment may include topical creams (applied to the surface of the skin) or oral medications.

Appropriate hygiene techniques may help to prevent or control *tinea pedis*. The following hygiene techniques should be followed:

Prevention of athlete's foot:

- Nails should be clipped short and kept clean. Nails can house and spread the infection.

- Avoid walking barefoot in locker rooms or public showers (wear sandals).

For control of athlete's foot infection, persons with active *tinea pedis* infection should:

- Keep feet clean, dry, and cool.

- Avoid using swimming pools, public showers, or foot baths.

- Wear sandals when possible or air shoes out by alternating them every 2–3 days.

- Avoid wearing closed shoes and wearing socks made from fabric that doesn't dry easily (for example, nylon).

- Treat the infection with recommended medication.

Jock Itch

Jock itch (tinea cruris) is a fungal skin infection affecting the genital area, inner thighs, and buttocks. It is characterized by an itchy, ring-shaped rash in moist areas of the skin. It is caused by the same fungus that causes athlete's foot. The fungus spreads from the foot to the groin by touch or through contaminated towels or clothing from person to person.

Jock itch is named so because it is seen in people who sweat a lot, which is common in athletes. It is also seen in people who are overweight.

Jock itch is usually diagnosed with a physical examination or with a laboratory culture test in unclear cases. Though uncomfortable, jock itch is not a serious complaint and it can be treated with the application of topical antifungal medications for one to two weeks.

Jock itch can be prevented by staying dry, wearing clean and fitting clothes, and avoiding sharing personal items such as towels, clothes, etc.

Reference

"Jock Itch," Mayo Foundation for Medical Education and Research (MFMER), July 26, 2016.

Chapter 62

Work Safety for Teens

Fast Stats on Young Workers' Health

Young workers have high rates of job-related injury. These injuries are often the result of the many hazards present in the places they typically work, such as sharp knives and slippery floors in restaurants. Limited or no prior work experience and a lack of safety training also contribute to high injury rates. Middle and high school workers may be at increased risk for injury since they may not have the strength or cognitive ability needed to perform certain job duties.

- In 2016, there were about 19.3 million workers under the age of 24. These workers represented 13 percent of the total workforce.

- In 2015, 403 workers under the age of 24 died from work-related injuries.

- In 2015, there were 24 deaths to workers under 18 years of age.

- In 2015, the incidence rate for nonfatal injuries for workers, ages 16–19, was 110.5 per 10,000 full-time employees (FTE) and 98.3 per 10,000 FTE for workers, ages 20–243.

This chapter contains text excerpted from the following sources: Text under the heading "Fast Stats on Young Workers' Health" is excerpted from "Young Worker Safety and Health," Centers for Disease Control and Prevention (CDC), April 11, 2017; Text under the heading "What You Should Know about Safety and Health on the Job" is excerpted from "Are You a Working Teen," Centers for Disease Control and Prevention (CDC), June 6, 2014. Reviewed November 2017.

- In 2014, the rate of work-related injuries treated in emergency departments for workers, ages 15–19, was 2.18 times greater than the rate for workers 25 years of age and older. In the same year, the rate of work-related injuries treated in emergency departments for workers, ages 20–24, was 1.76 times greater than the rate for workers 25 years of age and older.

What You Should Know about Safety and Health on the Job

Could I Get Hurt or Sick on the Job?

Every year about 70 teens die from work injuries in the United States. Another 70,000 get hurt badly enough that they go to a hospital emergency room.

Why do injuries like these occur? Teens are often injured on the job due to unsafe equipment, stressful conditions, and speedup. Also teens may not receive adequate safety training and supervision. As a teen, you are much more likely to be injured when working on jobs that you are not allowed to do by law.

What Are My Rights on the Job?

By law, your employer must provide:

- A safe and healthful workplace.

- Safety and health training, in many situations, including providing information on chemicals that could be harmful to your health.

- For many jobs, payment for medical care if you get hurt or sick because of your job. You may also be entitled to lost wages.

- At least the Federal minimum wage of $4.75 (increases to $5.15 on 9/1/97) to most teens, after their first 90 days on the job. Many states have minimum wages which may be higher than the Federal wage, and lower wages may be allowed when workers receive tips from customers.

You also have a right to:

- Report safety problems to the Occupational Safety and Health Administration (OSHA).

- Work without racial or sexual harassment.

- Refuse to work if the job is immediately dangerous to your life or health.

- Join or organize a union.

Table 62.1. Hazards to Be Watched Out For

Type of Work	Examples of Hazards
Janitor/Clean-up	Toxic chemicals in cleaning products
	Blood on discarded needles
Food Service	Slippery floors
	Hot cooking equipment
	Sharp objects
Retail/Sales	Violent crimes
	Heavy lifting
Office/Clerical	Stress
	Harassment
	Poor computer work station design

Is It OK to Do Any Kind of Work?

NO! There are laws that protect teens from doing dangerous work. No worker under 18 may:

- Drive a motor vehicle as a regular part of the job or operate a forklift at any time.

- Operate many types of powered equipment like a circular saw, box crusher, meat slicer, or bakery machine.

- Work in wrecking, demolition, excavation, or roofing.

- Work in mining, logging, or a sawmill.

- Work in meat packing or slaughtering.

- Work where there is exposure to radiation.

- Work where explosives are manufactured or stored.

Also, no one 14 or 15 years old may:

- Bake or cook on the job (except at a serving counter).

- Operate power driven machinery, except certain types which pose little hazard such as those used in offices.

- Work on a ladder or scaffold.

- Work in warehouses.

- Work in construction, building, or manufacturing.

- Load or unload a truck, railroad car, or conveyor.

Are There Other Things I Can't Do?

YES! There are many other restrictions regarding the type of work you can and cannot do. If you are under 14, there are even stricter laws to protect your health and safety. States have their own child labor laws which may be stricter than the federal laws. Check with your school counselor, job placement coordinator, or state Department of Labor to make sure the job you are doing is allowed.

What Are My Safety Responsibilities on the Job?

To work safely you should:

- Follow all safety rules and instructions.

- Use safety equipment and protective clothing when needed.

- Look out for co-workers.

- Keep work areas clean and neat.

- Know what to do in an emergency.

- Report any health and safety hazard to your supervisor.

Should I Be Working This Late or This Long?

Federal child labor laws protect younger teens from working too long, too late, or too early. Some states have laws on the hours that older teens may work.

Table 62.2. Work Hours for Teens—Ages 14 and 15

Hours	Periods
Work Hours	not before 7 a.m. or after 7 p.m. between Labor Day and June 1
	Not during school hours
	7 a.m. – 9 p.m. between June 1 and Labor Day

Table 62.2. Continued

Maximum Hours When School Is in Session	18 hours a week, but not over: 3 hours a day on school days 8 hours a day Saturday, Sunday, and holidays
Maximum Hours When School Is not in Session	40 hours a week 8 hours a day

What If I Need Help?

- Talk to your boss about the problem.

- Talk to your parents or teachers.

- For a Hazard Alert on preventing injuries and deaths of adolescent workers or for information on specific workplace hazards, contact:

  - NIOSH at 800-35-NIOSH (800-356-4674) and ask for Report #95–125

Chapter 63

Other Teen Safety Concerns

Chapter Contents

Section 63.1—Concussion.. 640

Section 63.2—Noise and Hearing Damage............................... 643

Section 63.3—Repetitive Stress Injuries in Teens.................... 648

Section 63.1

Concussion

This section includes text excerpted from "Concussion Information Sheet," Centers for Disease Control and Prevention (CDC), May 2015.

What Is a Concussion?

A concussion is a type of traumatic brain injury—or TBI—caused by a bump, blow, or jolt to the head or by a hit to the body that causes the head and brain to move quickly back and forth. This fast movement can cause the brain to bounce around or twist in the skull, creating chemical changes in the brain and sometimes stretching and damaging the brain cells.

How Can I Help Keep My Children or Teens Safe?

Sports are a great way for children and teens to stay healthy and can help them do well in school. To help lower your children's or teens' chances of getting a concussion or other serious brain injury, you should:

- Help create a culture of safety for the team.
  - Work with their coach to teach ways to lower the chances of getting a concussion.
  - Talk with your children or teens about concussion and ask if they have concerns about reporting a concussion. Talk with them about their concerns; emphasize the importance of reporting concussions and taking time to recover from one.
  - Ensure that they follow their coach's rules for safety and the rules of the sport.
  - Tell your children or teens that you expect them to practice good sportsmanship at all times.
- When appropriate for the sport or activity, teach your children or teens that they must wear a helmet to lower the chances of

the most serious types of brain or head injury. However, there is no "concussion-proof" helmet. So, even with a helmet, it is important for children and teens to avoid hits to the head.

How Can I Spot a Possible Concussion?

Children and teens who show or report one or more of the signs and symptoms listed below—or simply say they just "don't feel right" after a bump, blow, or jolt to the head or body—may have a concussion or other serious brain injury.

Signs Observed by Parents or Coaches

- Appears dazed or stunned.
- Forgets an instruction, is confused about an assignment or position, or is unsure of the game, score, or opponent.
- Moves clumsily.
- Answers questions slowly.
- Loses consciousness (even briefly).
- Shows mood, behavior, or personality changes.
- Can't recall events prior to or after a hit or fall.

Symptoms Reported by Children and Teens

- Headache or "pressure" in head.
- Nausea or vomiting.
- Balance problems or dizziness, or double or blurry vision.
- Bothered by light or noise.
- Feeling sluggish, hazy, foggy, or groggy.
- Confusion, or concentration or memory problems.
- Just not "feeling right," or "feeling down."

Talk with your children and teens about concussion. Tell them to report their concussion symptoms to you and their coach right away. Some children and teens think concussions aren't serious or worry that if they report a concussion they will lose their position on the team or look weak. Be sure to remind them that it's better to miss one game than the whole season.

Concussions affect each child and teen differently. While most children and teens with a concussion feel better within a couple of weeks, some will have symptoms for months or longer. Talk with your children's or teens' healthcare provider if their concussion symptoms do not go away or if they get worse after they return to their regular activities.

What Are Some More Serious Danger Signs to Look Out For?

In rare cases, a dangerous collection of blood (hematoma) may form on the brain after a bump, blow, or jolt to the head or body and can squeeze the brain against the skull. Call 9-1-1 or take your child or teen to the emergency department right away if, after a bump, blow, or jolt to the head or body, he or she has one or more of these danger signs:

- One pupil larger than the other.

- Drowsiness or inability to wake up.

- A headache that gets worse and does not go away.

- Slurred speech, weakness, numbness, or decreased coordination. Repeated vomiting or nausea, convulsions or seizures (shaking or twitching).

- Unusual behavior, increased confusion, restlessness, or agitation.

- Loss of consciousness (passed out/knocked out). Even a brief loss of consciousness should be taken seriously.

What Should I Do If My Child or Teen Has a Possible Concussion?

As a parent, if you think your child or teen may have a concussion, you should:

1. Remove your child or teen from play.

2. Keep your child or teen out of play the day of the injury. Your child or teen should be seen by a healthcare provider and only return to play with permission from a healthcare provider who is experienced in evaluating for concussion.

3. Ask your child's or teen's healthcare provider for written instructions on helping your child or teen return to school. You can give the instructions to your child's or teen's school nurse and teacher(s) and return-to-play instructions to the coach and/or athletic trainer.

Do not try to judge the severity of the injury yourself. Only a healthcare provider should assess a child or teen for a possible concussion. Concussion signs and symptoms often show up soon after the injury. But you may not know how serious the concussion is at first, and some symptoms may not show up for hours or days.

The brain needs time to heal after a concussion. A child's or teen's return to school and sports should be a gradual process that is carefully managed and monitored by a healthcare provider.

Section 63.2

Noise and Hearing Damage

This section includes text excerpted from "Noise Induced Hearing Loss," National Institute on Deafness and Other Communication Disorders (NIDCD), February 7, 2017.

What Is Noise Induced Hearing Loss (NIHL)?

Every day, we experience sound in our environment, such as the sounds from television and radio, household appliances, and traffic. Normally, these sounds are at safe levels that don't damage our hearing. But sounds can be harmful when they are too loud, even for a brief time, or when they are both loud and long-lasting. These sounds can damage sensitive structures in the inner ear and cause noise induced hearing loss (NIHL).

NIHL can be immediate or it can take a long time to be noticeable. It can be temporary or permanent, and it can affect one ear or both ears. Even if you can't tell that you are damaging your hearing, you could have trouble hearing in the future, such as not being able to understand other people when they talk, especially on the phone or in a noisy room. Regardless of how it might affect you, one thing is certain: noise induced hearing loss is something you can prevent.

Who Is Affected by NIHL?

Exposure to harmful noise can happen at any age. People of all ages, including children, teens, young adults, and older people, can develop NIHL. Based on a 2011–2012 the Centers for Disease Control and Prevention (CDC) study involving hearing tests and interviews with participants, at least 10 million adults (6 percent) in the United States under age 70—and perhaps as many as 40 million adults (24 percent)—have features of their hearing test that suggest hearing loss in one or both ears from exposure to loud noise. Researchers have also estimated that as many as 17 percent of teens (ages 12 to 19) have features of their hearing test suggestive of NIHL in one or both ears, based on data from 2005–2006.

What Causes NIHL?

NIHL can be caused by a one-time exposure to an intense "impulse" sound, such as an explosion, or by continuous exposure to loud sounds over an extended period of time, such as noise generated in a wood-working shop.

Recreational activities that can put you at risk for NIHL include target shooting and hunting, snowmobile riding, listening to MP3 players at high volume through earbuds or headphones, playing in a band, and attending loud concerts. Harmful noises at home may come from sources including lawnmowers, leaf blowers, and woodworking tools.

Sound is measured in units called decibels (dB). Sounds of less than 75 decibels, even after long exposure, are unlikely to cause hearing loss. However, long or repeated exposure to sounds at or above 85 decibels can cause hearing loss. The louder the sound, the shorter the amount of time it takes for NIHL to happen.

Here are the average decibel ratings of some familiar sounds:

- The humming of a refrigerator: 45 decibels

- Normal conversation: 60 decibels

- Noise from heavy city traffic: 85 decibels

- Motorcyle: 95 decibels

- An MP3 player at maximum volume: 105 decibels

- Sirens: 120 decibels

- Firecrackers and firearms: 150 decibels

Your distance from the source of the sound and the length of time you are exposed to the sound are also important factors in protecting your hearing. A good rule of thumb is to avoid noises that are too loud, too close, or last too long.

How Can Noise Damage Our Hearing?

To understand how loud noises can damage our hearing, we have to understand how we hear. Hearing depends on a series of events that change sound waves in the air into electrical signals. Our auditory nerve then carries these signals to the brain through a complex series of steps.

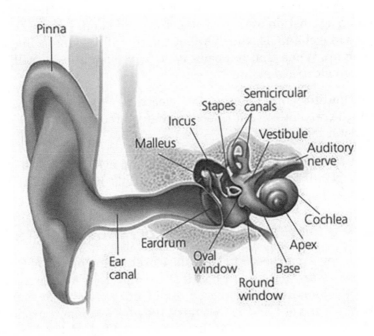

Figure 63.1. *Parts of the Inner Ear*

- Sound waves enter the outer ear and travel through a narrow passage way called the ear canal, which leads to the eardrum.

- The eardrum vibrates from the incoming sound waves and sends these vibrations to three tiny bones in the middle ear. These bones are called the malleus, incus, and stapes.

- The bones in the middle ear couple the sound vibrations from the air to fluid vibrations in the cochlea of the inner ear, which is shaped like a snail and filled with fluid. An elastic partition runs from the beginning to the end of the cochlea, splitting it into an upper and lower part. This partition is called the basilar membrane because it serves as the base, or ground floor, on which key hearing structures sit.

- Once the vibrations cause the fluid inside the cochlea to ripple, a traveling wave forms along the basilar membrane. Hair cells—sensory cells sitting on top of the basilar membrane—ride the wave.

- As the hair cells move up and down, microscopic hair like projections (known as stereocilia) that perch on top of the hair cells bump against an overlying structure and bend. Bending causes pore like channels, which are at the tips of the stereocilia, to open up. When that happens, chemicals rush into the cell, creating an electrical signal.

- The auditory nerve carries this electrical signal to the brain, which translates it into a sound that we recognize and understand.

Most NIHL is caused by the damage and eventual death of these hair cells. Unlike bird and amphibian hair cells, human hair cells don't grow back. They are gone for good.

What Are the Effects and Signs of NIHL?

When you are exposed to loud noise over a long period of time, you may slowly start to lose your hearing. Because the damage from noise exposure is usually gradual, you might not notice it, or you might ignore the signs of hearing loss until they become more pronounced. Over time, sounds may become distorted or muffled, and you might find it difficult to understand other people when they talk or have to turn up the volume on the television. The damage from NIHL, combined with aging, can lead to hearing loss severe enough that you need hearing aids to magnify the sounds around you to help you hear, communicate, and participate more fully in daily activities.

NIHL can also be caused by extremely loud bursts of sound, such as gunshots or explosions, which can rupture the eardrum or damage the bones in the middle ear. This kind of NIHL can be immediate and permanent. Loud noise exposure can also cause tinnitus—a ringing, buzzing, or roaring in the ears or head. Tinnitus may subside over time, but can sometimes continue constantly or occasionally throughout a person's life. Hearing loss and tinnitus can occur in one or both ears.

Sometimes exposure to impulse or continuous loud noise causes a temporary hearing loss that disappears 16 to 48 hours later. Research suggests, however, that although the loss of hearing seems to disappear, there may be residual long-term damage to your hearing.

Can NIHL Be Prevented?

NIHL is the only type of hearing loss that is completely preventable. If you understand the hazards of noise and how to practice good hearing health, you can protect your hearing for life. Here's how:

- Know which noises can cause damage (those at or above 85 decibels).

- Wear earplugs or other protective devices when involved in a loud activity (activity specific earplugs and earmuffs are available at hardware and sporting goods stores).

- If you can't reduce the noise or protect yourself from it, move away from it.

- Be alert to hazardous noises in the environment.

- Protect the ears of children who are too young to protect their own.

- Make family, friends, and colleagues aware of the hazards of noise.

- Have your hearing tested if you think you might have hearing loss.

What Research Is Being Done on NIHL?

The National Institute on Deafness and Other Communication Disorders (NIDCD) supports research on the causes, diagnosis, treatment, and prevention of hearing loss. NIDCD supported researchers have helped to identify some of the many genes important for hair cell development and function and are using this knowledge to explore new treatments for hearing loss.

Researchers are also looking at the protective properties of supporting cells in the inner ear, which appear to be capable of lessening the damage to sensory hair cells upon exposure to noise.

The NIDCD sponsors It's a Noisy Planet. Protect Their Hearing®, a national public education campaign to increase awareness among parents of preteens about the causes and prevention of NIHL. Armed with this information, parents, teachers, school nurses, and other adults can encourage children to adopt healthy hearing habits.

Section 63.3

Repetitive Stress Injuries in Teens

"Repetitive Stress Injuries in Teens," © 2017 Omnigraphics.
Reviewed November 2017.

What Are Repetitive Stress Injuries (RSIs)?

Repetitive stress injuries (RSIs) happen when undue pressure is placed on a part of the body repeatedly over an extended period of time. RSIs can cause pain, swelling, inflammation, muscle strains, spinal discs problems, and tendon or nerve damages. Sometimes, an RSI is also known as cumulative trauma disorder (CTD). These injuries are most often linked to work-related activities; however, in teens, they tend to occur while playing sports or during the regular use of computers, phones, and tablets.

Sports-related injuries may be referred to as overuse injuries, which frequently happen at growth plates—the area at the end of bones—as the bone cells multiply rapidly. When there is repeated stress for a long time in a particular area of the body, the joints and surrounding tissues get inflamed leading to an injury. The elbows, knees, shoulders, and heels are areas that are often affected by RSIs.

Causes of RSI

Many activities can result in RSIs; however, some of the most common causes in teens can include:

- Typing, holding a mouse, or using a keyboard for a long period of time.
- Sports, such as tennis or football, that involve repetitive, forceful motions.
- Playing video games and texting frequently.
- Playing a musical instrument.
- Working in cold temperatures.
- Poorly designed equipment or tools.
- Awkward posture.
- Heavy lifting.

Symptoms of RSI

An RSI is caused by physical stress; however, mental stress can worsen the condition. Some typical symptoms of RSI include:

- Weakness or tiredness in the hands or arms.
- Stiffness or soreness in the neck and back area.
- Pulsating or throbbing sensation in the muscles or joints.
- Numbness, pain, or tingling in the affected area.

If these symptoms are present, a healthcare provider needs to be consulted immediately. Even though these symptoms may tend to be intermittent, ignoring them can lead to even more serious issues.

Types of RSIs That Affect Teens

There are more than 100 different types of RSIs. Some of them affect teens most often include:

- **Stress fractures.** When a bone undergoes repeated strain from walking, running, or jumping, tiny cracks can develop on the surface of the bone due to rhythmic and repetitive overloading. These are called stress fractures.

- **Tendonitis.** Tendons are bands that connect muscles to bones. When the tendons become inflamed, the condition is known as tendonitis.

- **Bursitis.** A bursa is a sac filled with fluid that acts as a cushion for the joints. An inflammation or swelling of the bursa is known as bursitis.

- **Carpal tunnel syndrome.** The median nerve and a number of ligaments run through a space in the wrist called the carpal tunnel. When swelling occurs in this area, the result is a disorder called carpal tunnel syndrome.

Some other RSIs that can affect teens include **Osgood-Schlatter disease in childhood, shin splints, patellofemoral syndrome**, and **epicondylitis.**

Diagnosis and Treatment of RSI

In order to diagnose RSI, a healthcare provider will generally begin by asking a series of questions about daily activities, repeated tasks, types of discomfort, and when and how pain is experienced. A doctor may order blood tests and X-rays to aid in the diagnosis. If RSI is not treated, it can become severe and possibly have permanent consequences.

Treatment is based on the type of RSI diagnosed; but in all cases, it's important to stop the repetitive motion and rest the affected area. Some types of commonly used treatments include:

- **Physical therapy.** Exercises or manual therapy under the direction of trained professional can help improve joint movement.

- **Bracing or splinting**. These can help protect the injury by immobilizing it and giving it time to heal.

- **Heat or cold treatment.** Warm or cold packs on the affected area can help bring relief.

- **Medications.** Anti-inflammatory painkillers and muscle relaxers may be prescribed by healthcare providers. In some cases, antidepressants or sleep aids might also be recommended.

- **Steroid injections.** These may be required to reduce inflammation, but only if it is severe, as adverse effects are possible.

- **Surgery**. If the condition is extremely serious and can't be treated by other means, surgery may be necessary.

Prevention of RSI

Growing bodies are more prone to RSIs because of their rapid growth spurts. And modern teens tend to spend a lot of time on computers and phones, as well as engaging in sports and other physical activities, which make them particularly susceptible to RSIs. Below are some ways to help minimize the risk.

For computer-related injuries:

- Make sure the top of the computer screen is aligned to the forehead of the user.

- Sit upright in the chair with feet touching the ground and back resting on the back of the seat.

- Avoid slouching, since this can cause unnecessary strain on the neck, back, and spine.

- Ensure that fingers and wrists are aligned at the same level while typing.

- Avoid excessive texting.

- Take a break about every 30 minutes.

  For sports-related injuries:

- Warm up and cool down before and after a workout or playing a game.

- Uses properly fitted sports gear.

- Alternate between different activities to avoid repetitive stress.

References

1. Gavin, Mary L., MD. "Repetitive Stress Injuries," KidsHealth, January 2014.

2. Newman, Tim. "Repetitive Strain Injury (RSI): Diagnosis, Symptoms, and Treatment," Medical News Today, September 8, 2017.

3. Pitchford, Keith, MD. "Your Teenager and Repetitive Stress Injuries," Great Lakes Orthopedics & Sports Medicine, December 16, 2016.

4. "Repetitive Stress Injuries Handbook," National Education Association (NEA), October 2004.

5. "Teen RSI—Repetitive Stress Injuries," Parentingteens.com, October 30, 2010.

Part Eight

Violence against Adolescents

Chapter 64

Youth Violence: A Public Health Problem

Chapter Contents

Section 64.1—Understanding Youth Violence 656

Section 64.2—Statistics on Youth Violence............................. 658

Section 64.3—Youth Violence Risk and Protective
Factors 661

Section 64.1

Understanding Youth Violence

This section includes text excerpted from "Understanding Youth
Violence," Centers for Disease Control and Prevention (CDC), 2015.

Youth violence refers to harmful behaviors that can start early and
continue into young adulthood. The young person can be a victim, an
offender, or a witness to the violence. Youth violence includes various
behaviors. Some violent acts—such as bullying, slapping, or hitting—
can cause more emotional harm than physical harm. Others, such as
robbery and assault (with or without weapons), can lead to serious
injury or even death.

Why Is Youth Violence a Public Health Problem?

Youth violence is widespread in the United States. It is the third
leading cause of death for young people between the ages of 15 and 24.

- In 2012, 4,787 young people aged 10 to 24 years were victims of
  homicide—an average of 13 each day

- Over 599,000 young people aged 10 to 24 years had physical
  assault injuries treated in U.S. emergency departments—an
  average of 1642 each day.

- In a 2013 nationwide survey, about 24.7 percent of high school
  students reported being in a physical fight in the 12 months
  before the survey.

- About 17.9 percent of high school students in 2013 reported taking a weapon to school in the 30 days before the survey.

- In 2013, 19.6 percent of high school students reported being bullied on school property and 14.8 percent reported being bullied
  electronically

- Each year, youth homicides and assault-related injuries result
  in an estimated $16 billion in combined medical and work loss
  costs.

How Does Youth Violence Affect Health?

Deaths resulting from youth violence are only part of the problem. Many young people need medical care for violence-related injuries. These injuries can include cuts, bruises, broken bones, and gunshot wounds. Some injuries, like gunshot wounds, can lead to lasting disabilities. Violence can also affect the health of communities. It can increase healthcare costs, decrease property values, and disrupt social services.

Who Is at Risk for Youth Violence?

A number of factors can increase the risk of a youth engaging in violence. However, the presence of these factors does not always mean that a young person will become an offender.

Risk factors for youth violence include:

- Prior history of violence
- Drug, alcohol, or tobacco use
- Association with delinquent peers
- Poor family functioning
- Poor grades in school
- Poverty in the community

How Can We Prevent Youth Violence?

The ultimate goal is to stop youth violence before it starts. Several prevention strategies have been identified.

- Parent- and family-based programs improve family relations. Parents receive training on child development. They also learn skills for talking with their kids and solving problems in nonviolent ways.

- Social-development strategies teach children how to handle tough social situations. They learn how to resolve problems without using violence.

- Mentoring programs pair an adult with a young person. The adult serves as a positive role model and helps guide the young person's behavior.

- Changes can be made to the physical and social environment. These changes address the social and economic causes of violence.

Section 64.2

Statistics on Youth Violence

This section includes text excerpted from "Youth Violence—
Facts at a Glance," Centers for Disease Control and
Prevention (CDC), November 8, 2016.

Youth Violence

- In 2014, 4,300 young people ages 10 to 24 were victims of homicide—an average of 12 each day.

- Homicide is the 3rd leading cause of death for young people ages 10 to 24 years old.

- Among homicide victims 10 to 24 years old in 2014, 86 percent (3,703) were male and 14 percent (597) were female.

- Among homicide victims ages 10 to 24 years old in 2014, 86 percent were killed with a firearm.

- Youth homicides and assault-related injuries result in an estimated $18.2 billion in combined medical and work loss costs.

Violence-Related Behaviors

In a 2015 nationally-representative sample of youth in grades 9–12:

- 22.6 percent reported being in a physical fight in the 12 months preceding the survey; the prevalence was higher among males (28.4%) than females (16.5%).

- 16.2 percent reported carrying a weapon (gun, knife, or club) on one or more days in the 30 days preceding the survey; the prevalence was higher among males (24.3%) than females (7.5%).

- 5.3 percent reported carrying a gun on one or more days in the 30 days preceding the survey; the prevalence was higher among males (8.7%) than females (1.6%).

Health Disparities

- Among 10 to 24 year-olds, homicide is the leading cause of death for African Americans; the second leading cause of death for Hispanics; and the third leading cause of death American Indians and Alaska Natives.

- Homicide rates in 2014 among non-Hispanic, African-American males 10–24 years of age (48.2 per 100,000) exceeded those of Hispanic males (9.6 per 100,000) and non-Hispanic, White males in the same age group (2.6 per 100,000).

School Violence

In a 2015 nationally representative sample of youth in grades 9–12:

- 7.8 percent reported being in a physical fight on school property in the 12 months preceding the survey.

- 10.3 percent of male students and 5 percent of female students reported being in a physical fight on school property in the 12 months preceding the survey.

- 5.6 percent did not go to school on one or more days in the 30 days preceding the survey because they felt unsafe at school or on their way to or from school.

- 4.1 percent reported carrying a weapon (gun, knife, or club) on school property on one or more days in the 30 days preceding the survey.

- 6 percent reported being threatened or injured with a weapon (gun, knife, or club) on school property one or more times in the 12 months preceding the survey.

Nonfatal Injuries due to Violence

- In 2014, 501,581 young people ages 10 to 24 were treated in emergency departments for injuries sustained from physical assaults.

- In 2015, of a nationally-representative sample of students in grades 9–12, 2.9 percent reported being in a physical fight one or more times in the previous 12 months that resulted in injuries that had to be treated by a doctor or nurse.

Juvenile Arrests

- Juveniles (<18 years) accounted for 10.2 percent of all violent crime arrests and 14.3 percent of all property crime arrests in 2015.

- In 2015, 605 juveniles (<18 years) were arrested for murder, 2,745 for forcible rape, and 21,993 for aggravated assault.

Bullying

In a 2015 nationally-representative sample of youth in grades 9–12:

- 20.2 percent reported being bullied on school property in the 12 months preceding the survey; the prevalence was higher among females (24.8%) than males (15.8%).

- 15.5 percent reported being bullied electronically (email, chat room, instant messaging, website, texting) in the 12 months preceding the survey; the prevalence was higher among females (21.7%) than males (9.7%).

School-Associated Violent Deaths

- During the 2012–2013 school year, 31 homicides of school-age youth ages 5 to 18 years occurred at school.

- Approximately 2.6 percent of all youth homicides in 2012–2013 occurred at school, and the percentage of all youth homicides occurring at school has been less than 3 percent since the 1992–1993 school year.

- There was approximately one homicide or suicide of a school-age youth at school per 1.5 million students enrolled during the 2012–2013 school year.

Section 64.3

Youth Violence Risk and Protective Factors

This section includes text excerpted from "Risk and
Protective Factors—Youth Violence," Centers for
Disease Control and Prevention (CDC), June 23, 2017.

Risk Factors for the Perpetration of Youth Violence

Research on youth violence has increased our understanding of
factors that make some populations more vulnerable to victimization
and perpetration. Risk factors increase the likelihood that a young
person will become violent. However, risk factors are not direct causes
of youth violence; instead, risk factors contribute to the likelihood of
youth violence occurring.

Research associates the following risk factors with perpetration of
youth violence:

Individual risk factors:

- History of violent victimization
- Attention deficits, hyperactivity, or learning disorders
- History of early aggressive behavior
- Involvement with drugs, alcohol, or tobacco
- Low IQ
- Poor behavioral control
- Deficits in social cognitive or information-processing abilities
- High emotional distress
- History of treatment for emotional problems
- Antisocial beliefs and attitudes
- Exposure to violence and conflict in the family

Family risk factors:

- Authoritarian childrearing attitudes
- Harsh, lax, or inconsistent disciplinary practices

- Low parental involvement
- Low emotional attachment to parents or caregivers
- Low parental education and income
- Parental substance abuse or criminality
- Poor family functioning
- Poor monitoring and supervision of children

Peer and social risk factors:

- Association with delinquent peers
- Involvement in gangs
- Social rejection by peers
- Lack of involvement in conventional activities
- Poor academic performance
- Low commitment to school and school failure

Community risk factors:

- Diminished economic opportunities
- High concentrations of poor residents
- High level of transiency
- High level of family disruption
- Low levels of community participation
- Socially disorganized neighborhoods

Protective Factors for the Perpetration of Youth Violence

Protective factors buffer young people from the risks of becoming violent. These factors exist at various levels. To date, protective factors have not been studied as extensively or rigorously as risk factors. However, identifying and understanding protective factors are equally as important as researching risk factors. Studies suggest the following protective factors.

Individual protective factors:

- Intolerant attitude toward deviance
- High IQ

- High grade point average (as an indicator of high academic achievement)

- High educational aspirations

- Positive social orientation

- Popularity acknowledged by peers

- Highly developed social skills/competencies

- Highly developed skills for realistic planning

- Religiosity

Family protective factors:

- Connectedness to family or adults outside the family

- Ability to discuss problems with parents

- Perceived parental expectations about school performance are high

- Frequent shared activities with parents

- Consistent presence of parent during at least one of the following: when awakening, when arriving home from school, at evening mealtime or going to bed

- Involvement in social activities

- Parental/family use of constructive strategies for coping with problems (provision of models of constructive coping)

Peer and social protective factors:

- Possession of affective relationships with those at school that are strong, close, and prosocially oriented

- Commitment to school (an investment in school and in doing well at school)

- Close relationships with nondeviant peers

- Membership in peer groups that do not condone antisocial behavior

- Involvement in prosocial activities

Exposure to school climates that characterized by:

- Intensive supervision

- Clear behavior rules
- Consistent negative reinforcement of aggression
- Engagement of parents and teachers

Chapter 65

Bullying and Other Types of Aggressive Behavior

Chapter Contents

Section 65.1—Understanding Bullying 666

Section 65.2—Facts and Statistics on Bullying 671

Section 65.3—Stalking and Hazing 673

Section 65.4—Hazing 677

Section 65.1

Understanding Bullying

This section includes text excerpted from "About Bullying,"
Eunice Kennedy Shriver National Institute of Child Health and
Human Development (NICHD), March 13, 2017.

Bullying is when a person or a group shows unwanted aggression toward another person. To be considered bullying, the behavior in question must be aggressive. The behavior must also involve an imbalance of power (e.g., physical strength, popularity, access to embarrassing details about a person) and be repetitive, meaning that it happens more than once or is highly likely to be repeated.

Bullying can be:

- **Physical:** punching, beating, kicking, or pushing; stealing, hiding, or damaging another person's belongings; forcing someone to do things against his or her will

- **Verbal:** teasing, calling names, or insulting another person; threatening another person with physical harm; spreading rumors or untrue statements about another person

- **Relational:** refusing to talk to someone or making them feel left out; encouraging other individuals to bully someone

Bullying also includes cyberbullying and workplace bullying.

- **Cyberbullying** has increased with the increased use of the social media sites, the Internet, email, and mobile devices. Unlike more traditional bullying, cyberbullying can be more anonymous and can occur nearly constantly. A person can be cyberbullied day or night, such as when they are checking their email, using Facebook or another social network site, or even when they are using a mobile phone.

- **Workplace bullying** refers to adult behavior that is repeatedly aggressive and involves the use of power over another person at the workplace. Certain laws apply to adults in the workplace to help prevent such violence.

Who Is Affected and How Many Are at Risk for Bullying?

People of all ages can be bullied. Bullying may take place at home, school, or work.

- A 2013 survey from the National Center for Education Statistics (NCES) found that bullying continues to affect many school-aged children: Slightly more than 1 out of 5 students in middle and high school experienced "traditional" bullying at school during the 2012–2013 school year. Six percent of students ages 12 to 18 reported that they had been pushed, shoved, tripped, or spit on during the school year. Of these students, 22 percent reported being injured in the event.

- The 2013 survey found that, during the same school year, 7 percent of students reported being cyberbullied.

- Data from the 2015 Youth Risk Behavior Surveillance System (YRBSS) from the Centers for Disease Control and Prevention (CDC) indicate that about 20 percent of U.S. students in grades 9 through 12 experienced bullying on school property within the last year.

What Are Common Signs of Being Bullied?

Signs of bullying include:

- Depression, loneliness, or anxiety
- Low self-esteem
- Headaches, stomach aches, tiredness, or poor eating habits
- Missing school, disliking school, or having poorer school performance than previously
- Self-destructive behaviors, such as running away from home or inflicting harm on oneself
- Thinking about suicide or attempting to commit suicide
- Unexplained injuries
- Lost or destroyed clothing, books, electronics, or jewelry
- Difficulty sleeping or frequent nightmares
- Sudden loss of friends or avoidance of social situations

How Does Bullying Affect Health and Well-Being?

Bullying can affect physical and emotional health, both in the short term and later in life. It can lead to physical injury, social problems, emotional problems, and even death. Those who are bullied are at increased risk for mental health problems, headaches, and problems adjusting to school. Bullying also can cause long-term damage to self-esteem.

Children and adolescents who are bullies are at increased risk for substance use, academic problems, and violence to others later in life.

Those who are both bullies and victims of bullying suffer the most serious effects of bullying and are at greater risk for mental and behavioral problems than those who are only bullied or who are only bullies.

Eunice Kennedy Shriver National Institute of Child Health and Human Development (NICHD) research studies show that anyone involved with bullying—those who bully others, those who are bullied, and those who bully and are bullied—are at increased risk for depression.

NICHD-funded research studies also found that unlike traditional forms of bullying, youth who are bullied electronically—such as by computer or cell phone—are at higher risk for depression than the youth who bully them. Even more surprising, the same studies found that cyber victims were at higher risk for depression than were cyberbullies or bully-victims (i.e., those who both bully others and are bullied themselves), which was not found in any other form of bullying.

What Are Risk Factors for Being Bullied?

Those who are at risk of being bullied may have one or more risk factors:

- Are seen as different from their peers (e.g., overweight, underweight, wear their hair differently, wear different clothing or wear glasses, or come from a different race/ethnicity)

- Are seen as weak or not able to defend themselves

- Are depressed, anxious, or have low self-esteem

- Have few friends or are less popular

- Do not socialize well with others

- Suffer from an intellectual or developmental disability

What Can Be Done to Help Someone Who Is Being Bullied?

To help someone who is being bullied, support the person and address the bullying behavior. Other ways to help—including what to do if a person is in immediate danger—are listed below.

Support a child who is being bullied:

- You can listen to the child and let him or her know you are available to talk or even help. A child who is being bullied may struggle talking about it. Consider letting the child know there are other people who can talk with him or her about bullying. In addition, you might consider referring the child to a school counselor, psychologist, or other mental health specialist.

- Give the child advice about what he or she can do. You might want to include role-playing and acting out a bullying incident as you guide the child so that the child knows what to do in a real situation.

- Follow up with the child to show that you are committed to helping put a stop to the bullying.

Address the bullying behavior:

- Make sure a child whom you suspect or know is bullying knows what the problem behavior is and why it is not acceptable.

- Show kids that bullying is taken seriously. If you know someone is being a bully to someone else, tell the bully that bullying will not be tolerated. It is important, however, to demonstrate good behavior when speaking with a bully so that you serve as a role model of good interpersonal behavior.

The "Bullying: Be More Than a Bystander" resource (www.nichd. nih.gov/publications/Pages/pubs_details.aspx?pubs_id=5878), which includes a presentation and facilitator's guide, seeks to educate people about taking action against bullying. It suggests you can help someone who is being bullied in the following ways:

- Be a friend to the person who is being bullied, so they do not feel alone.
- Tell a trusted adult if you see someone being bullied.
- Help the person get away from the bullying without putting yourself at risk.

- Don't enable bullying by providing an audience.
- Set a good example by not bullying.

If you feel that you have taken all possible steps to prevent bullying and nothing has worked, or someone is in immediate danger, there are other ways for you to help.

Table 65.1. Help Someone Who Is Being Bullied

The Problem	What You Can Do
A crime has occurred or someone is at immediate risk of harm.	Call 911.
Someone is feeling hopeless, helpless, or thinking of suicide.	Contact the National Suicide Prevention Lifeline online or at 800-273-TALK (800-273-8255). This toll-free call goes to the nearest crisis center in a national network. These centers provide crisis counseling and mental health referrals.
Someone is acting differently, such as sad or anxious, having trouble completing tasks, or not taking care of themselves.	Find a local counselor or other mental health services.
A child is being bullied in school.	Contact the: • Teacher • School counselor • School coach • School principal • School superintendent • Board of Education
Child is being bullied after school on the playground or in the neighborhood	• Neighborhood watch • Playground security • Team coach • Local precinct/community police
The child's school is not addressing the bullying	Contact the: • School superintendent • Local Board of Education • State Department of Education

Section 65.2

Facts and Statistics on Bullying

This section includes text excerpted from "Facts about
Bullying," StopBullying.gov, U.S. Department of Health and
Human Services (HHS), September 28, 2017.

Prevalence

- Between 1 in 4 and 1 in 3 U.S. students say they have been
  bullied at school. Many fewer have been cyberbullied. See more
  prevalence statistics.

- Most bullying happens in middle school. The most common types
  are verbal and social bullying.

- There is growing awareness of the problem of bullying, which
  may lead some to believe that bullying is increasing. However,
  studies suggest that rates of bullying may be declining. It still
  remains a prevalent and serious problem in today's schools.

National Statistics

Been Bullied

- 28 percent of U.S. students in grades 6–12 experienced
  bullying.

- 20 percent of U.S. students in grades 9–12 experienced bullying.

Bullied Others

- Approximately 30 percent of young people admit to bullying others in surveys.

Seen Bullying

- 70.6 percent of young people say they have seen bullying in their
  schools.

- 70.4 percent of school staff have seen bullying. 62 percent witnessed bullying two or more times in the last month and 41 percent witness bullying once a week or more.

- When bystanders intervene, bullying stops within 10 seconds 57 percent of the time.

Been Cyberbullied

- 9 percent of students in grades 6–12 experienced cyberbullying.

  - 15 percent of high school students (grades 9–12) were electronically bullied in the past year.

  - However, 55.2 percent of LGBTQ students experienced cyberbullying.

How Often Bullied

- In one large study, about 49 percent of children in grades 4–12 reported being bullied by other students at school at least once during the past month, whereas 30.8 percent reported bullying others during that time.

- Defining "frequent" involvement in bullying as occurring two or more times within the past month, 40.6 percent of students reported some type of frequent involvement in bullying, with 23.2 percent being the youth frequently bullied, 8.0 percent being the youth who frequently bullied others, and 9.4 percent playing both roles frequently.

Types of Bullying

- The most common types of bullying are verbal and social. Physical bullying happens less often. Cyberbullying happens the least frequently.

- According to one large study, the following percentages of middle schools' students had experienced these various types of bullying: name calling (44.2%); teasing (43.3%); spreading rumors or lies (36.3%); pushing or shoving (32.4%); hitting, slapping, or kicking (29.2%); leaving out (28.5%); threatening (27.4%); stealing belongings (27.3%); sexual comments or gestures (23.7%); e-mail or blogging (9.9%).

Where Bullying Occurs

- Most bullying takes place in school, outside on school grounds, and on the school bus. Bullying also happens wherever kids gather in the community. And of course, cyberbullying occurs on cell phones and online.

- According to one large study, the following percentages of middle schools' students had experienced bullying in these various places at school: classroom (29.3%); hallway or lockers (29.0%); cafeteria (23.4%); gym or PE class (19.5%); bathroom (12.2%); playground or recess (6.2%).

How Often Adult Notified

- Only about 20 to 30 percent of students who are bullied notify adults about the bullying.

Section 65.3

Stalking

This section includes text excerpted from "Stalking," Office on Women's Health (OWH), U.S. Department of Health and Human Services (HHS), November 14, 2017.

Stalking is repeated contact that makes you feel afraid or harassed. Someone may stalk you by following you or calling you often. Stalkers may also use technology to stalk you by sending unwanted emails or social media messages. About one in six women has experienced stalking in her lifetime. Women are twice as likely to be stalked as men are. Stalking is a crime.

What Is Stalking?

Stalking is any repeated and unwanted contact with you that makes you feel unsafe. You can be stalked by a stranger, but most stalkers are people you know—even an intimate partner. Stalking may get worse or become violent over time. Stalking may also be a sign of an abusive relationship.

Someone who is stalking you may threaten your safety by clearly saying they want to harm you. Some stalkers harass you with less threatening but still unwanted contact. The use of technology to stalk, sometimes called "cyberstalking," involves using the Internet, email, or other electronic communications to stalk someone. Stalking is against the law.

Stalking and cyberstalking can lead to sleeping problems or problems at work or school.

What Are Some Examples of Stalking?

Examples of stalking may include:

- Following you around or spying on you
- Sending you unwanted emails or letters
- Calling you often
- Showing up uninvited at your house, school, or work
- Leaving you unwanted gifts
- Damaging your home, car, or other property
- Threatening you, your family, or pets with violence

What Are Some Examples of Cyberstalking?

Examples of cyberstalking include:

- Sending unwanted, frightening, or obscene emails, text messages, or instant messages (IMs)
- Harassing or threatening you on social media
- Tracking your computer and Internet use
- Using technology such as GPS to track where you are

Are There Laws against Stalking?

Yes. Stalking is a crime. Learn more about the laws against stalking in your state at the Stalking Resource Center (victimsofcrime.org/our-programs/stalking-resource-center/stalking-laws). If you are in immediate danger, call 911.

You can file a complaint with the police and get a restraining order (court order of protection) against the stalker. Federal law says that you can get a restraining order for free. Do not be afraid to take steps to stop your stalker.

What Can I Do If I Think I'm Being Stalked?

If you are in immediate danger, call 911. Find a safe place to go if you are being followed or worry that you will be followed. Go to a police station, friend's house, domestic violence shelter, fire station, or public area.

You can also take the following steps if you are being stalked:

- File a complaint with the police. Make sure to tell them about all threats and incidents.

- Get a restraining order. A restraining order requires the stalker to stay away from you and not contact you. You can learn how to get a restraining order from a domestic violence shelter, the police, or an attorney in your area.

- Write down every incident. Include the time, date, and other important information. If the incidents occurred online, take screenshots as records.

- Keep evidence such as videotapes, voicemail messages, photos of property damage, and letters.

- Get names of witnesses.

- Get help from domestic violence hotlines (www.thehotline.org), domestic violence shelters, counseling services, and support groups. Put these numbers in your phone in case you need them.

- Tell people about the stalking, including the police, your employer, family, friends, and neighbors.

- Always have your phone with you so you can call for help.

- Consider changing your phone number (although some people leave their number active so they can collect evidence). You can also ask your service provider about call blocking and other safety features.

- Secure your home with alarms, locks, and motion-sensitive lights.

For more information or emotional support, call the Stalking Resource Center National Center for Victims of Crime Helpline (victimsofcrime.org/our-programs/stalking-resource-center) at 800-FYI-CALL (800-394-2255), Monday through Friday, 10 a.m. to 6 p.m. ET.

What Can I Do If Someone Is Cyberstalking Me?

If you are being cyberstalked:

- Send the person one clear, written warning not to contact you again.

- If they contact you again after you've told them not to, do not respond.

- Print out copies of evidence such as emails or screenshots of your phone. Keep a record of the stalking and any contact with police.

- Report the stalker to the authority in charge of the site or service where the stalker contacted you. For example, if someone is stalking you through Facebook, report them to Facebook.

- If the stalking continues, get help from the police. You also can contact a domestic violence shelter and the National Center for Victims of Crime Helpline (victimsofcrime.org) for support and suggestions.

- Consider blocking messages from the harasser.

- Change your email address or screen name.

- Never post online profiles or messages with details that someone could use to identify or locate you (such as your age, sex, address, workplace, phone number, school, or places you hang out).

Section 65.4

Hazing

This section includes text excerpted from "Hazing vs. Bullying," girlshealth.gov, Office on Women's Health (OWH), August 25, 2014. Reviewed November 2017.

Hazing is when a person who wants to join a group is expected to do things that are very embarrassing, dangerous, or illegal. The group might be a club, sorority, or team, for example.

People sometimes think hazing is a just a harmless part of joining a group. But hazing can really hurt someone physically and emotionally.

What Is Hazing?

Hazing can take many forms. Examples of hazing can include the following:

- Making someone stay awake for many hours
- Yelling, swearing, or insulting someone
- Forcing someone to wear very embarrassing clothes
- Telling someone they have to eat disgusting things
- Physical beatings
- Pressuring someone to drink a lot of alcohol
- Making someone get a tattoo

What Are Warning Signs of Hazing?

Here are some possible signs of hazing:

- You have heard from friends about a group using hazing.
- You feel a knot in your stomach—trust your instincts!
- You have been warned by teachers or other adults that the group is dangerous.

677

- You have seen the group push others to do things that you believe are wrong or dangerous.

- You feel afraid to break away from the group.

- The group leaders are very mean.

- The group leaders do things that don't seem right and then make you promise not to tell anyone.

What Can I Do to Stay Safe from Hazing?

If you are concerned about hazing, try to find out if a group is known for having mean rituals. If you think you are going a place where you might be hazed, have a plan to stay safe. Stick together with friends you trust, and make sure you have a way to get home safely.

If you are being hazed, tell an adult. Some states have laws against hazing. Remember, no one has a right to hurt you or pressure you to do something that feels wrong!

Chapter 66

Dating Violence and Abusive Relationships

Dating violence is a type of intimate partner violence. It occurs between two people in a close relationship. The nature of dating violence can be physical, emotional, or sexual.

- **Physical**—This occurs when a partner is pinched, hit, shoved, slapped, punched, or kicked.

- **Psychological/Emotional**—This means threatening a partner or harming his or her sense of self-worth. Examples include name calling, shaming, bullying, embarrassing on purpose, or keeping him/her away from friends and family.

- **Sexual**—This is forcing a partner to engage in a sex act when he or she does not or cannot consent. This can be physical or nonphysical, like threatening to spread rumors if a partner refuses to have sex.

- **Stalking**—This refers to a pattern of harassing or threatening tactics that are unwanted and cause fear in the victim.

This chapter contains text excerpted from the following sources: Text in this section begins with excerpts from "Understanding Teen Dating Violence," Centers for Disease Control and Prevention (CDC), 2016; Text beginning with the heading "Leaving an Abusive Dating Relationship" is excerpted from "Dating Violence," Office on Women's Health (OWH), U.S. Department of Health and Human Services (HHS), September 30, 2015.

Dating violence can take place in person or electronically, such as repeated texting or posting sexual pictures of a partner online.

Unhealthy relationships can start early and last a lifetime. Teens often think some behaviors, like teasing and name calling, are a "normal" part of a relationship. However, these behaviors can become abusive and develop into more serious forms of violence.

Why Is Dating Violence a Public Health Problem?

Dating violence is a widespread issue that has serious long-term and short-term effects. Many teens do not report it because they are afraid to tell friends and family.

- Among high school students who dated, 21 percent of females and 10 percent of males experienced physical and/or sexual dating violence.

How Does Dating Violence Affect Health?

Dating violence can have a negative effect on health throughout life. Youth who are victims are more likely to experience symptoms of depression and anxiety, engage in unhealthy behaviors, like using tobacco, drugs, and alcohol, or exhibit antisocial behaviors and think about suicide. Youth who are victims of dating violence in high school are at higher risk for victimization during college.

Who Is at Risk for Dating Violence?

Factors that increase risk for harming a dating partner include the following:

- Belief that dating violence is acceptable

- Depression, anxiety, and other trauma symptoms

- Aggression towards peers and other aggressive behavior

- Substance use

- Early sexual activity and having multiple sexual partners

- Having a friend involved in dating violence

- Conflict with partner

- Witnessing or experiencing violence in the home

Leaving an Abusive Dating Relationship

If you think you are in an abusive relationship, learn more about getting help. See a doctor or nurse to take care of any physical problems. And reach out for support for your emotional pain. Friends, family, and mental health professionals all can help. If you're in immediate danger, dial 911.

If you are thinking about ending an abusive dating relationship, keep some tips in mind:

- Create a safety plan, like where you can go if you are in danger.

- Make sure you have a working cell phone handy in case you need to call for help.

- Create a secret code with people you trust. That way, if you are with your partner, you can get help without having to say you need help.

- If you're breaking up with someone you see at your high school or college, you can get help from a guidance counselor, advisor, teacher, school nurse, dean's office, or principal. You also might be able to change your class schedules or even transfer to another school.

- If you have a job, talk to someone you trust at work. Your human resources department or employee assistance program (EAP) may be able to help.

- Try to avoid walking or riding alone.

- Be smart about technology. Don't share your passwords. Don't post your schedule on Facebook, and keep your settings private.

Staying Safe When Meeting Someone New

If you are meeting someone you don't know or don't know well, you can take steps to stay safe. Try to:

- Meet your date in a public place

- Tell a friend or family member your date's name and where you are going

- Avoid parties where a lot of alcohol may be served

- Make sure you have a way to get home if you need to leave

- Have a cell phone handy in case you need to call for help

Avoiding Date Rape Drugs

Date rape drugs are drugs that are sometimes put into a drink to prevent a person from being able to fight back during a rape. These drugs have no color, taste, or smell, so you would not know if someone put them in your drink. They also make it hard to remember what happened while you were under their influence.

If you go to a club, bar, or party, here are some steps to take to avoid date rape drugs:

- Don't accept drinks from other people.

- Keep your drink with you at all times, even when you go to the bathroom.

- Don't drink from punch bowls or other open containers.

- If you lose track of your drink, dump it out.

And keep in mind that drinking a lot of alcohol can make it hard to fight off an attacker, too.

Chapter 67

Sexual Assault

What Is Sexual Assault?

Sexual assault is any type of sexual activity, including rape, that you do not agree to. Also called sexual violence or abuse, sexual assault is never your fault.

What Is Rape?

The U.S. Department of Justice (DOJ) defines rape as "The penetration, no matter how slight, of the vagina or anus with any body part or object, or oral penetration by a sex organ of another person, without the consent of the victim." This legal definition is used by the federal government to collect information from local police about rape. The definition of rape may be slightly different in your community.

Rape also can happen when you cannot physically give consent, such as while you were drunk, passed out, or high. Rape can also happen when you cannot legally give consent, such as when you are underage.

This chapter includes text excerpted from "Sexual Assault," Office on Women's Health (OWH), U.S. Department of Health and Human Services (HHS), May 21, 2015.

What Does Sexual Assault Include?

Sexual assault can include:

- Any type of sexual contact with someone who cannot consent, such as someone who is underage, has an intellectual disability, or is passed out

- Rape

- Attempted rape

- Sexual coercion

- Sexual contact with a child

- Incest (sexual contact between family members)

- Fondling or unwanted touching above or under clothes

Sexual assault can also be verbal or visual. It is anything that forces a person to join in unwanted sexual contact or attention. Examples can include:

- Voyeurism, or peeping (when someone watches private sexual acts without consent)

- Exhibitionism (when someone exposes himself or herself in public)

- Sexual harassment or threats

- Forcing someone to pose for sexual pictures

What Does "Consent" Mean in Sexual Assault?

Consent is a clear "yes" to sexual activity. Not saying "no" does not mean you have given consent.

Your consent means:

- You know and understand what is going on (you are not unconscious or blacked out or intellectually disabled).

- You know what you want to do.

- You are able to say what you want to do.

- You are sober (not under the influence of alcohol or drugs).

Sometimes you *cannot* give legal consent to sexual activity or contact. For example, if you are:

- Threatened, forced, coerced, or manipulated into agreeing

- Not physically able to (you are drunk, high, drugged, passed out, or asleep)

- Not mentally able to (due to illness or disability)

- Younger than 16 (in most states) or 18 (in other states)

Remember:

- **Consent is an ongoing process,** not a one-time question. If you consent to sexual activity, you can change your mind and choose to stop, even after sexual activity has started.

- **Past consent does not mean future consent.** Giving consent in the past to sexual activity does not mean you have to give consent now or in the future.

- **Saying yes to a sexual activity is not consent for all types of sexual activity.** If you consent to sexual activity, it is only for types of sexual activities that you are comfortable with at that time with that partner.

What Is NOT Considered Consent in Sexual Assault?

- **Silence.** Just because someone does not say "no" it doesn't mean she is saying "yes."

- **Having consented before.** Just because someone said "yes" in the past does not mean she is saying "yes" now. Consent must be part of every sexual activity, every time.

- **Being in a relationship.** Being married, dating, or having sexual contact with someone before does not mean that there is consent now.

- **Being drunk or high.**

- **Not fighting back.** Not putting up a physical fight does not mean that there is consent.

- **Sexy clothing, dancing, or flirting.** Only "yes" means "yes."

What Is Sexual Coercion?

Not all sexual assault involves a physical attack. Sexual coercion is unwanted sexual activity that happens after someone is pressured, tricked, or forced in a nonphysical way.

Anyone can use coercion—for example, husbands, partners, boyfriends, friends, coworkers, bosses, or dates.

What Are Some Examples of Sexual Coercion?

Sexual coercion can be social or emotional pressure to force you into sexual activity that you do not want or agree to. See the table below for ways someone might use sexual coercion:

Table 67.1. Examples of Sexual Coercion

Ways Someone Might Use Sexual Coercion	What He or She May Say
Wearing you down by asking for sex again and again, or making you feel bad, guilty, or obligated	• "If you really loved me, you'd do it." • "Come on, it's my birthday." • "You don't know what you do to me."
Making you feel like it's too late to say no	• "But you've already gotten me all worked up." • "You can't just make a guy stop."
Telling you that not having sex will hurt your relationship	• "Everything's perfect. Why do you have to ruin it?" • "I'll break up with you if you don't have sex with me."
Lying or threatening to spread rumors about you	• "Everyone thinks we already have, so you might as well." • "I'll just tell everyone you did it anyway."
Making promises	• "I'll make it worth your while." • "You know I have a lot of connections."
Threatening your children or other family members	• "I'll do this to your daughter if you don't do it with me."
Threatening your job, home, or school career	• "I really respect your work here. I'd hate for something to change that." • "I haven't decided yet who's getting bonuses this year." • "Don't worry about the rent. There are other things you can do." "You work so hard; it'd be a shame for you not to get an A."

How Can I Respond in the Moment to Sexual Coercion?

Sexual coercion is not your fault. If you are feeling pressured to do something you don't want to do, speak up or leave the situation. It is better to risk a relationship ending or hurting someone's feelings than to do something you aren't ready or willing to do.

Some possible responses include:

- "I do like you, but I'm not ready for sex."
- "If you really care for me, you'll respect that I don't want to have sex."
- "I don't owe you an explanation or anything at all."

Be clear and direct with the person coercing you. Tell him or her how you feel and what you do not want to do. If the other person is not listening to you, leave the situation. If you or your family is in physical danger, try to get away from the person as quickly as possible. Call 911 if you are in immediate danger.

How Can I Get Help after Being Sexually Coerced?

Sexual coercion is a type of sexual assault. Call the National Sexual Assault Hotline at 800-656-HOPE (800-656-4673) or chat online with a trained hotline worker on the National Sexual Assault Online Hotline at any time to get help.

Some sexual coercion is against the law or violates school or workplace policies. If you are younger than 18, tell a trusted adult about what happened. If you are an adult, consider talking to someone about getting help and reporting the person to the local authorities. You could talk to a counselor, the human resources department, or the local police.

Who Is Sexually Assaulted?

Sexual assault can happen to anyone of any age, race or ethnicity, religion, ability, appearance, sexual orientation, or gender identity. However, women have higher rates of sexual assault than men.

- **Women.** More than 23 million women in the United States have been raped. More than one in five African-American and white women and one in eight Hispanic women have been raped.
- **Young women.** Most women who have been raped were younger than 25 when the rape happened. Almost half of female rape victims were under 18.
- **Men.** Almost 2 million men in the United States have been raped. Almost 6 percent of men have experienced sexual

coercion, and almost 11 percent of men have experienced unwanted sexual contact.

- **Lesbians, gays, and bisexual and transgender (LGBT) people.** Bisexual women have higher rates of sexual assault than lesbians and heterosexual women. Nearly half of all bisexual women have been raped. Lesbians and bisexual women also have higher rates of sexual violence by a partner than heterosexual women. More than half of transgender people have been sexually assaulted.

Who Commits Sexual Assault?

Sometimes, sexual assault is committed by a stranger. Most often, though, it is by someone you know, including a friend, acquaintance, relative, date, or your partner.

Both women and men commit sexual assault, but nearly 99 percent of all people who are reported for sexual assault are men. Six in 10 of those are white. The majority of sexual assault victims know the person who assaulted them.

Can I Be Sexually Assaulted by My Partner or Spouse?

Yes. Sexual assault is unwanted sexual activity—no matter whom it is with. Sexual assault by an intimate partner is common. More than half of female rape victims were raped by their partner.

What Do I Do If I've Been Sexually Assaulted?

If you are in danger or need medical care, call 911. If you can, get away from the person who assaulted you and get to a safe place as fast as you can.

If you have been physically assaulted or raped, there are other important steps you can take right away:

- **Save everything that might have the attacker's DNA on it.** As hard as it may be to not wash up, you might wash away important evidence if you do. Don't brush, comb, or clean any part of your body. Don't change clothes, if possible. Don't touch or change anything at the scene of the assault. That way the local police will have physical evidence from the person who assaulted you.

- **Go to your nearest hospital emergency room as soon as possible.** You need to be examined and treated for injuries. You can be given medicine to prevent HIV and other sexually transmitted infections (STIs) and emergency contraception to prevent pregnancy. The National Sexual Assault Hotline at 800-656-HOPE (800-656-4673) can help you find a hospital able to collect evidence of sexual assault. Ask for a sexual assault forensic examiner (SAFE). A doctor or nurse will use a rape kit to collect evidence. This might be fibers, hairs, saliva, semen, or clothing left behind by the attacker. **You do not have to decide whether to press charges while at the hospital.**

- If you think you were drugged, talk to the hospital staff about being tested for date rape drugs, such as Rohypnol and Gamma Hydroxybutyrate (GHB), and other drugs.

- The hospital staff can also connect you with the local rape crisis center. Staff there can help you make choices about reporting the sexual assault and getting help through counseling and support groups.

- **Reach out for help.** Call a friend or family member you trust, or call a crisis center or hotline. Crisis centers and hotlines have trained volunteers and counselors who can help you find support and resources near you. One hotline is the National Sexual Assault Hotline at 800-656-HOPE (4673). If you are in the military, you may also call the DoD Safe Helpline at 877-995-5246.

- **Report the sexual assault to the police:** Call 911. If you want to talk to someone first about reporting the assault, you can also call the National Sexual Assault Hotline at 800-656-HOPE (800-656-4673). A counselor can help you understand how to report the crime. Even though these calls are free, they may appear on your phone bill. If you think that the person who sexually assaulted you may check your phone bill, try to call from a friend's phone or a public phone.

- **Write down the details** about the person who sexually assaulted you and what happened.

How Can I Get Help after a Sexual Assault?

After a sexual assault, you may feel fear, shame, guilt, or shock. These feelings are normal. But sexual assault is never your fault. It may be frightening to think about talking about the assault, but it is important to get help. You can call these organizations any time, day or night. The calls are free and confidential:

- **National Sexual Assault Hotline, 800-656-HOPE (800-656-4673).** You can also chat with a trained hotline worker on the National Sexual Assault Online Hotline.

- **National Domestic Violence Hotline, 800-799-SAFE (800-799-7233)** or **800-787-3224 (TTY)**

Each state and territory has organizations and hotlines to help people who have been sexually assaulted.

How Can I Lower My Risk of Sexual Assault?

You cannot always prevent sexual assault. If you are assaulted, or if you find yourself in a situation that feels unsafe, it is not your fault. But you can take steps to help stay safe in general:

- **Go to parties or gatherings with friends.** Arrive together, check in with each other, and leave together. Talk about your plans for the evening so that everyone knows what to expect.

- **Look out for your friends, and ask them to look out for you.** If a friend seems out of it, is way too drunk for the amount of alcohol she's had, is acting out of character, or seems too drunk to stay safe in general, get her to a safe place. Ask your friends to do the same for you.

- **Have a code word with your family and friends** that means "Come get me, I need help" or "Call me with a fake emergency." Call or text them and use the code word to let them know you need help.

- **Download an app on your phone.** You can download free apps you can use if you feel unsafe or are threatened. Some apps share your location with your friends or the police if you need help. You can also set up an app to send you texts throughout the night to make sure you're safe. If you don't respond, the app will notify police.

- **Avoid drinks in punch bowls or other containers that can be easily "spiked"** (when alcohol is added to a drink without permission). If you think that you or one of your friends has been drugged, call the police. Tell them what happened so that you can be tested for the right drugs.

- **Know your limits when using alcohol or drugs.** Don't let anyone pressure you into drinking or doing more than you want to.

- **Trust your instincts.** If you find yourself alone with someone you don't know or trust, leave. If you feel uncomfortable in any situation for any reason, leave. You are the only person who gets to say whether you feel safe.

- **Be aware of your surroundings.** Especially if walking alone, avoid talking on your phone or listening to music with headphones. Stay in busy, well-lit areas, especially at night.

Is There a Link between Alcohol and Drugs and Sexual Assault?

Yes. Sexual assault and alcohol often go together. Research shows that up to three out of four attackers had been drinking when the attack happened.

Research also shows that about half of sexual assault victims had been drinking. However, this does not mean that drinking causes sexual assault. Many perpetrators use alcohol as a tool to lower a person's ability to give consent, resist, understand what is happening, or remember the assault. They may take advantage of a victim who has already been drinking or encourage her to drink more than she might normally drink.

Some perpetrators also use drugs called "date rape drugs." These drugs are slipped into drinks—even nonalcoholic drinks—or food without the victim's knowledge. The drugs can cause memory loss, so victims may not know what happened. Some attackers also use other drugs, such as ecstasy, marijuana, or prescription pills. They may give drugs to someone who takes them willingly or may drug her without her knowledge.

Someone who is drunk, drugged, or high on drugs cannot give consent. Without consent, sexual activity is sexual assault.

Does Sexual Assault Have Long-Term Health Effects?

Yes, sexual assault can have long-term health effects. People who have been sexually assaulted are more likely to report:

- Frequent headaches
- Long-term pain

- Trouble sleeping
- Poor physical and mental health

  Other health effects can include:

- Severe anxiety, stress, or fear
- Abuse of alcohol or drugs
- Depression
- Eating disorders
- Sexually transmitted infections (STIs)
- Pregnancy
- Self-injury or suicide

How Can I Help Someone Who Has Been Sexually Assaulted?

You can help a friend or family member who has been sexually assaulted by listening, offering comfort, and not judging. Reinforce the message that she or he is not at fault and that it is natural to feel angry, confused, or ashamed—or any combination of feelings.

Ask your loved one if she would like you to go with her to the hospital or to counseling. If she decides to report the crime to the police, ask if she would like you to go with her. Let her know that professional help is available.

Chapter 68

Youth Gangs and Violence

What Is a Gang?

There is no universally agreed upon definition of "gang" in the United States. Gang, youth gang and street gang are terms widely and often interchangeably used in mainstream coverage. Reference to gangs often implies youth gangs. In some cases, youth gangs are distinguished from other types of gangs; how youth is defined may vary as well.

Motorcycle gangs, prison gangs, hate groups, adult organized crime groups, terrorist organizations, and other types of security threat groups are frequently but not always treated separately from gangs in both practice and research.

"Youth Gangs"

The National Gang Center (NGC) (which is cosponsored by the Bureau of Justice Assistance (BJA) and the Office of Juvenile Justice and Delinquency Prevention (OJJDP)) conducts the National Youth

This chapter contains text excerpted from the following sources: Text beginning with the heading "What Is a Gang?" is excerpted from "Gangs and Gang Crime—What Is a Gang?" National Institute of Justice (NIJ), U.S. Department of Justice (DOJ), October 28, 2011. Reviewed November 2017; Text beginning with the heading "Girls, Juvenile Delinquency, and Gangs" is excerpted from "Gang Involvement Prevention—Girls, Juvenile Delinquency, and Gangs," Youth.gov, March 6, 2013. Reviewed November 2017.

Gang Survey. The survey reports solely on youth gangs, which the National Gang Center describes as "a group of youths or young adults [the responding agency is] willing to identify as a 'gang.'"

When they report to the National Youth Gang Survey, law enforcement agencies indicate that group criminality is of greatest importance in how they define a gang. The presence of leadership is of least importance.

Much of the research literature about gangs focuses primarily on youth gangs, as opposed to adult gangs. Researchers accept the following criteria for classifying groups as gangs:

- The group has three or more members, generally aged 12–24.

- Members share an identity, typically linked to a name, and often other symbols.

- Members view themselves as a gang, and they are recognized by others as a gang.

- The group has some permanence and a degree of organization.

- The group is involved in an elevated level of criminal activity.

"Types" of Gangs

The National Gang Intelligence Center (NGIC) and the National Drug Intelligence Center (NDIC) collaborated to produce the National Gang Threat Assessment (NGTA) in 2009. The book discusses street gangs, prison gangs and outlaw motorcycle gangs. Each gang type merits its own definition and discussion of the characteristics that differ at national, regional, and local levels.

"Gang Member" and "Gang Crime"

Localities interested in pursuing antigang policies, strategies and programs face the challenge of developing operational definitions for the terms "gang," "gang member" and "gang crime" (or "gang-related offense"). Many criminal justice policymakers and practitioners operate under practical definitions unique to their locality and its explicit gang-related challenges.

Some localities fail to address the need for definition or to consider elements of definitions already in use. Failing to define the terms "gang" and "gang crime" as the terms are commonly used in a community undermines the community's ability to reliably measure progress and outcomes related to gangs and gang activity.

California and other states and localities have instituted various criteria and threshold levels an offender must meet to be classified as a gang member. Multiple criteria may need to be documented. For example, 1) a reliable source must identify the offender as a gang member, and 2) the offender must display gang symbols or use hand signs and display gang tattoos.

Girls, Juvenile Delinquency, and Gangs

While females make up a little less than ten percent of the overall gang population, research suggests that girls may account for between one-fourth and one-half of the gang members in younger adolescent gangs. Overall, female gang members appear to be more heavily represented in gangs located outside of large cities, with half of gangs located in these areas reporting female members, compared to large cities, where about a quarter of gangs located in larger cities report female members.

While the types of delinquent acts that girls in gangs commit are often less severe than boys, their involvement with gangs is still a concern and demands unique prevention, response, incarceration, and rehabilitation efforts. Research on this topic has identified several key factors that are significantly correlated with girls' delinquency including gang involvement:

- As girls mature through adolescence they face an increased chance of experiencing risk factors for gang involvement and delinquency, such as physical and sexual abuse and assault, and have higher rates of diagnosed depression, anxiety, and post-traumatic stress disorder.

- A lack of family supervision and monitoring has been shown to have a causal link to delinquency for both boys and girls, but ineffective parenting practices (harsh or inconsistent discipline), family conflict, growing up in poverty, a lack of a consistent caregiver, and frequent family moves are more likely to affect the chance that girls will be involved in gangs and conduct delinquent acts.

- A strong attachment or connection with school has been found to act as a protective factor for girls, while a lack of connection or engagement with school is connected with increased rates of delinquency for girls.

As a result, it is important to ensure services targeted at young women include trauma-informed approaches, provide adequate mental health services, focus on school connectedness, and address family relationships.

Risk and Protective Factors

The risk and protective factors of youth gang involvement can span multiple domains from the individual level (aggressiveness) to the peer (delinquent siblings), school (academic failure), and community levels (poverty). Risk factors encourage or increase the likelihood of youth participating in gangs; whereas a protective factor acts as a buffer in the presence of risk factors. Proper assessment of risk and protective factors for youth and gang involvement helps to inform the development and implementation of prevention and intervention strategies.

Most youth who become affiliated with gangs lack positive supports from parents, schools, peers, and community. Research also indicates a close link between gang involvement and delinquent activity such as substance use. Findings indicate that youth who engage in delinquent activities, specifically illicit alcohol and drug use, are more likely to join gangs and that, as a result of gang involvement, youth are more likely to use illicit drugs and alcohol.

Risk factors that significantly affect a youth's chance for gang-involvement include the following:

- Aggressiveness,

- Early initiation of violent behavior,

- Parental criminality,

- Child maltreatment,

- Low levels of parental involvement,

- Parent-child separation,

- Academic failure,

- Lack of school connectedness,

- Truancy and school dropout,

- Frequent school transitions,

- Delinquent siblings and peers,

- Peer gang membership,

- Poverty,

- Substance use (e.g., illicit drugs and alcohol),

- Community disorganization,

- Availability of drugs and firearms, and

- Exposure to violence and racial prejudice.

Research suggests that the greater the number of risk factors that a youth experiences, the more likely he or she is to join a gang. It also shows that a youth's risk for gang involvement significantly increases as he or she accrues more than two risk factors. Therefore, prevention programs that target risk factors can help mitigate youth gang involvement. Additionally, efforts to minimize youth gang involvement can be addressed through promoting protective factors. Research suggests that as youth accumulate more protective factors it lowers the risk of gang involvement.

Protective factors that have been identified as influential to youth gang involvement include:

- Parental involvement and monitoring,

- Family support,

- Coping skills (interpersonal skills),

- Positive social connections,

- Peer support,

- Academic achievement, and

- Reducing delinquency, alcohol, and drug use.

Adverse Effects

Youth gang involvement impacts the health and welfare of the individual, as well as that of his or her family, peers, and community.

Youth Involved in Gangs

The numerous consequences stemming from gang involvement can have varying degrees of short and long-term negative outcomes. Youth who become involved in gangs face the increased risk of:

- dropping out of school;

- teen parenthood;

- unemployment;

- victimization;

- drug and alcohol abuse;

- committing petty and violent crimes; and

- juvenile conviction and incarceration.

Further, a youth's involvement with a gang (or gangs) also leads to an increased likelihood of economic hardship and family problems in adulthood, which in turn, contribute to involvement in street crime and/or arrest in adulthood. Research has suggested that the longer an adolescent stays in a gang the more disruption he or she will experience while transitioning into adulthood and in adulthood itself.

Impact on Communities

Large communities, those with a population over 50,000, are at the greatest risk of significant gang activity, and community members face heightened fear that they, their families, schools, or businesses, will become victims of theft and/or violence. Further, communities with gang activity are disproportionately affected by theft, negative economic impact, vandalism, assault, gun violence, illegal drug trade, and homicide.

Impact on Society

On the societal level, youth gang involvement costs local, state, and federal governments a substantial amount of money in prevention, response, incarceration, and rehabilitation efforts. It has been estimated that overall crime in the U.S. costs taxpayers $655 billion annually with a substantial amount of this crime attributed to gang activity.

Prevention Efforts

The prevention efforts targeted at limiting youth involvement in gangs is integral to promoting optimal individual and community well-being, specifically in those areas that are susceptible to gang activity. In recent years there has been an emphasis placed on evaluating gang prevention programs to discern effective approaches and providing a more comprehensive approach.

The Comprehensive Gang Model

The Comprehensive Gang Model developed by the Office of Juvenile Justice and Delinquency Prevention (OJJDP) focuses on community prevention and intervention in balance with law enforcement suppression activities. The model involves five strategies for responding to gang-involved youth and their families. These include:

- **Community mobilization,** the involvement of local citizens, including former gang members and community groups and agencies, and the coordination of programs and staff functions within and across agencies.

- **Opportunities provision,** the development of a variety of specific education, training, and employment programs targeting gang-involved youth.

- **Social intervention,** youth-serving agencies, schools, street outreach workers, grassroots groups, faith-based organizations, law enforcement agencies, and other criminal justice organizations reaching out and acting as links between gang-involved youth and their families, the conventional world, and needed services.

- **Suppression,** formal and informal social control procedures, including close supervision or monitoring of gang youth by agencies of the criminal justice system and also by community-based agencies, schools, and grassroots groups.

- **Organizational change and development,** development and implementation of policies and procedures that result in the most effective use of available and potential resources to better address the gang problem.

An important facet to implementing the Comprehensive Gang Model in a community is to first assess the youth gang problem. This assessment includes collecting quantitative and qualitative data from community representatives such as law enforcement, school faculty, youth, parents, community leaders, probation officers, gang members, grassroots organizations, and local government. Data collected includes the perception of the gang problem as well as what the community considers as priority needs such as tutoring, jobs training, increased police presence, and mentoring for youth.

Properly assessing a community's gang problem significantly improves the development of an implementation plan. The plan should include goals and objectives based on the assessment findings and should address the five core strategies previously described. The OJJDP Comprehensive Gang Model Guide details the steps required for assessment and provides the necessary data collection tools.

Mentoring

An example of a gang prevention effort that has been widely utilized in the United States to promote positive youth development and help rehabilitate youth involved with a gang(s) is mentoring. Mentoring works on the foundation that youth benefit from close, enduring, caring relationships with adults. By providing adult support and guidance through adolescence, mentoring has been found to provide a range of benefits to both youth and mentors, including the prevention of juvenile delinquency and youth gang involvement. Mentoring is popularly used in school and after school programs, as well as in the broader community.

While mentoring is a strategy that can be used to enhance positive youth development for all youth, it has also been utilized for rehabilitating youth who are already involved with gangs or the juvenile justice system.

National Forum on Youth Violence Prevention

The National Forum on Youth Violence Prevention (Forum) provides an example of the comprehensive ways communities are addressing gang prevention through larger youth violence prevention efforts. The Forum is a network of communities from across the United States that collaborate, share information, and build local capacity to prevent and reduce youth violence. In many cases these violence prevention plans include a focus on gang prevention.

Chapter 69

Coping with Violence and Trauma

Each year, children experience violence and disaster and face other traumas. Young people are injured, they see others harmed by violence, they suffer sexual abuse, and they lose loved ones or witness other tragic and shocking events. Parents and caregivers can help children overcome these experiences and start the process of recovery.

What Is Trauma?

"Trauma" is often thought of as physical injuries. Psychological trauma is an emotionally painful, shocking, stressful, and sometimes life-threatening experience. It may or may not involve physical injuries, and can result from witnessing distressing events. Examples include a natural disaster, physical or sexual abuse, and terrorism.

Disasters such as hurricanes, earthquakes, and floods can claim lives, destroy homes or whole communities, and cause serious physical and psychological injuries. Trauma can also be caused by acts of violence. The September 11, 2001 terrorist attack is one example. Mass shootings in schools or communities and physical or sexual assault are other examples. Traumatic events threaten our sense of safety.

This chapter includes text excerpted from "Helping Children and Adolescents Cope with Violence and Disasters: What Parents Can Do," National Institute of Mental Health (NIMH), 2015.

Reactions (responses) to trauma can be immediate or delayed. Reactions to trauma differ in severity and cover a wide range of behaviors and responses. Children with existing mental health problems, past traumatic experiences, and/or limited family and social supports may be more reactive to trauma. Frequently experienced responses among children after trauma are loss of trust and a fear of the event happening again.

It's important to remember:

- Children's reactions to trauma are strongly influenced by adults' responses to trauma.

- People from different cultures may have their own ways of reacting to trauma.

Commonly Experienced Responses to Trauma among Adolescents

Children age 6 to 11 may react by:

- Isolating themselves
- Becoming quiet around friends, family, and teachers
- Having nightmares or other sleep problems
- Refusing to go to bed
- Becoming irritable or disruptive
- Having outbursts of anger
- Starting fights
- Being unable to concentrate
- Refusing to go to school
- Complaining of physical problems
- Developing unfounded fears
- Becoming depressed
- Expressing guilt over what happened
- Feeling numb emotionally
- Doing poorly with school and homework
- Losing interest in fun activities

Adolescents age 12 to 17 may react by:

- Having flashbacks to the event (flashbacks are the mind reliving the event)
- Having nightmares or other sleep problems
- Avoiding reminders of the event
- Using or abusing drugs, alcohol, or tobacco
- Being disruptive, disrespectful, or behaving destructively
- Having physical complaints
- Feeling isolated or confused
- Being depressed
- Being angry
- Losing interest in fun activities
- Having suicidal thoughts

Adolescents may feel guilty. They may feel guilt for not preventing injury or deaths. They also may have thoughts of revenge.

What Can Parents Do to Help?

After violence or disaster, parents and family members should identify and address their own feelings—this will allow them to help others. Explain to children what happened and let them know:

- You love them
- The event was not their fault
- You will do your best to take care of them
- It's okay for them to feel upset

Do:

- Allow children to cry
- Allow sadness
- Let children talk about feelings
- Let them write about feelings
- Let them draw pictures about the event or their feelings

Don't:

- Expect children to be brave or tough

- Make children discuss the event before they are ready

- Get angry if children show strong emotions

- Get upset if they begin bedwetting, acting out, or thumbsucking

Other tips:

- If children have trouble sleeping give them extra attention, let them sleep with a light on, or let them sleep in your room (for a short time).

- Try to keep normal routines, for example, reading bedtime stories, eating dinner together, watching TV together, reading books, exercising, or playing games. If you can't keep normal routines, make new ones together.

- Help children feel in control when possible by letting them choose meals, pick out clothes, or make some decisions for themselves.

How Can I Help Young Children Who Experienced Trauma?

Helping children can start immediately, even at the scene of the event. Most children recover within a few weeks of a traumatic experience, while some may need help longer. Grief, a deep emotional response to loss, may take months to resolve. Children may experience grief over the loss of a loved one, teacher, friend, or pet. Grief may be re-experienced or worsened by news reports or the event's anniversary.

Some children may need help from a mental health professional. Some people may seek other kinds of help from community leaders. Identify children who need support and help them obtain it.

Examples of problematic behaviors could be:

- Refusing to go to places that remind them of the event

- Emotional numbness

- Behaving dangerously

- Unexplained anger/rage

- Sleep problems including nightmares

Adult helpers should:

- Pay attention to children
  - Listen to them
  - Accept/do not argue about their feelings
  - Help them cope with the reality of their experiences
- Reduce effects of other stressors, such as:
  - Frequent moving or changes in place of residence
  - Long periods away from family and friends
  - Pressures to perform well in school
  - Transportation problems
  - Fighting within the family
  - Being hungry
- Monitor healing
  - It takes time
  - Do not ignore severe reactions
  - Pay attention to sudden changes in behaviors, speech, language use, or strong emotions
- Remind children that adults
  - Love them
  - Support them
  - Will be with them when possible

Help for All People in the First Days and Weeks

There are steps adults can take following a disaster that can help them cope, making it easier for them to provide better care for children. These include creating safe conditions, remaining calm and friendly, and connecting with others. Being sensitive to people under stress and respecting their decisions is important.

When possible, help people:

- Get food
- Get a safe place to live

- Get help from a doctor or nurse if hurt

- Contact loved ones or friends

- Keep children with parents or relatives

- Understand what happened

- Understand what is being done

- Know where to get help

  Don't:

- Force people to tell their stories

- Probe for personal details

- Say things like "everything will be OK," or "at least you survived"

- Say what you think people should feel or how people should have acted

- Say people suffered because they deserved it

- Be negative about available help

- Make promises that you can't keep such as "you will go home soon."

More about Trauma Stress

Some children will have prolonged mental health problems after a traumatic event. These may include grief, depression, anxiety, and posttraumatic stress disorder (PTSD). Some trauma survivors get better with some support. Others may need prolonged care from a mental health professional. If after a month in a safe environment children are not able to perform normal routines or new behavioral or emotional problems develop, then contact a health professional.

Factors influencing how someone may respond include:

- Being directly involved in the trauma, especially as a victim

- Severe and/or prolonged exposure to the event

- Personal history of prior trauma

- Family or personal history of mental illness and severe behavioral problems

- Limited social support; lack of caring family and friends
- Ongoing life stressors such as moving to a new home or new school, divorce, job change, or financial troubles

Some symptoms may require immediate attention. Contact a mental health professional if these symptoms occur:

- Flashbacks
- Racing heart and sweating
- Being easily startled
- Being emotionally numb
- Being very sad or depressed
- Thoughts or actions to end one's life

Part Nine

Additional Help and Information

Chapter 70

Glossary of Terms about Adolescent Health

abstinence: Not having sex of any kind.

acne: Pimples on the skin often caused by hormone changes during puberty.

addiction: A chronic, relapsing disease characterized by compulsive drug-seeking and abuse and by long-lasting chemical changes in the brain.

adolescence: The period of life from puberty to adulthood when a young person grows up.

aggression: Behavior, physical or verbal, that is intended to harm another person.

alcoholic: Someone who is addicted to alcohol.

alcoholism: Alcoholism means that someone often drinks too much alcohol (such as beer, wine, or liquor) and can't stop.

allergy: A sensitivity to things that are usually not harmful, such as certain foods or animals.

This glossary contains terms excerpted from documents produced by several sources deemed reliable.

amenorrhea: When a woman does not have periods either ever (after age 16) or when periods stop as a result of pregnancy, too much exercise, extreme obesity or not enough body fat, or emotional distress.

anal sex: Sex that involves putting the penis in the anus, or butt.

anemia: When the total amount of red blood cells or hemoglobin is below normal. Anemia can cause severe fatigue and other health problems. There are many different types of anemia.

anorexia nervosa: An illness in which people don't eat enough and therefore can't stay at a healthy body weight.

anxiety disorder: Any of a group of illnesses that fill people's lives with overwhelming anxieties and fears that are chronic and unremitting.

asthma: A lung disorder that affects your airways. When the airways are inflamed, a person may wheeze, feel short of breath, cough, and feel tightness in the chest.

attention deficit hyperactivity disorder (ADHD): A mental illness characterized by an impaired ability to regulate activity level (hyperactivity), attend to tasks (inattention), and inhibit behavior (impulsivity).

behavioral therapy: A kind of therapy used by a psychologist or a psychiatrist that helps people to change the way they behave and act.

binge eating disorder (BED): A condition marked by periods of out-of-control eating. Unlike bulimia nervosa, binge-eating disorder usually does not involve purging (throwing up or doing other things to get rid of the food).

bipolar disorder: A depressive disorder in which a person alternates between episodes of major depression and mania (periods of abnormally and persistently elevated mood). Also referred to as manic-depression.

birth control pill: A kind of medicine that women can take daily to prevent pregnancy. It is sometimes called the pill or oral contraception.

body mass index (BMI): A mathematical formula to assess relative body weight. The measure correlates highly with body fat. Calculated as weight in kilograms divided by the square of the height in meters (kg/m2).

bulimia nervosa: An illness defined by uncontrollable overeating, usually followed by making oneself throw up or purge (get rid of food) in other ways.

clitoris: A female sex organ located near the top of the vagina.

condom: A type of birth control used to prevent pregnancy and the spread of some sexually transmitted diseases (STDs). The male condom is a thin rubber-like sheath put on the penis before sex. The female condom is a pouch put into the vagina before sex to prevent pregnancy.

conduct disorder: A personality disorder of children and adolescents involving persistent antisocial behavior. Individuals with conduct disorder frequently participate in activities such as stealing, lying, truancy, vandalism, and substance abuse.

date rape: When you are forced to have sex by someone you know.

depression: An illness that involves the body, mood, and thoughts. It affects the way a person functions, eats and sleeps, feels about herself, and thinks about things. It is more than just feeling "down in the dumps" or "blue" for a short time.

diabetes: A disease in which your blood sugar levels are above normal.

douching: Rinsing or cleaning out the vagina, usually with a pre-packaged mix of fluids.

drug: A chemical compound or substance that can alter the structure and function of the body. Psychoactive drugs affect the function of the brain, and some of these may be illegal to use and possess.

dysmenorrhea: Painful menstrual periods that can also go along with nausea and vomiting and either constipation or diarrhea. Dysmenorrhea is common among teenagers.

eating disorder: An illness that involves serious problems with normal eating behaviors, such as feelings of distress and concern about body shape or weight, severe overeating, or starving oneself.

ejaculation: The release of semen (whitish fluid that contains sperm) from a man's penis.

endometriosis: A condition where tissue that normally lines the uterus grows in other areas of the body. This can cause pain, irregular menstrual bleeding, and infertility for some women.

fallopian tube: One of a pair of organs that connect the ovaries to the uterus.

genital area: The area around the vagina, penis, scrotum, anus, and thigh.

gland: A cell, group of cells, or organ that makes chemicals and releases them for use by other parts of the body or to be excreted.

gynecologist: A doctor who has special training in caring for a women's reproductive organs and system.

hazing: A humiliating or degrading act expected of someone joining a group. It may cause physical or emotional harm, even if the person wants to participate. Hazing occurs with sports teams, social groups, and fraternities or sororities.

hormone: A chemical substance formed in glands in the body and carried in the blood to organs and tissues, where it influences function, structure, and behavior.

immunization: A treatment that protects your body against infection from certain diseases, such as the measles, whooping cough, and chicken pox.

meningitis: A dangerous infection that affects the brain and spinal cord.

menstruation: The blood flow from the uterus that happens about every 28 days in women of childbearing age who are not pregnant. Commonly called a woman's period.

mental illness: A health condition that changes a person's thinking, feelings, or behavior (or all three) and that causes the person distress and difficulty in functioning.

nicotine: The addictive drug in tobacco. Nicotine activates a specific type of acetylcholine receptor.

obesity: Having too much body fat. Obesity is more extreme than being overweight, which means weighing too much. Obesity is measured using body mass index.

obsessive-compulsive disorder (OCD): An anxiety disorder in which a person experiences recurrent unwanted thoughts or rituals that the individual cannot control.

oppositional defiant disorder (ODD): A disruptive pattern of behavior of children and adolescents that is characterized by defiant, disobedient, and hostile behaviors directed toward adults in positions of authority.

oral sex: Sucking and/or licking a partner's sex organ.

ovary: One of a pair of the female reproductive organs on each side of the uterus that contain eggs and make female hormones. An ovary is about the size of an almond or grape.

ovulation: When an ovary releases an egg, about once each month, as part of the menstrual cycle.

panic disorder: An anxiety disorder in which people have feelings of terror, rapid heartbeat, and rapid breathing that strike suddenly and repeatedly with no warning.

pap test: A test done on a sample of cells collected from the cervix to look for cell changes that could be cancer or that could turn into cancer.

peer pressure: Social pressure on somebody to act or dress a certain way to be accepted as part of a group.

penis: A male sex organ.

phobia: An intense fear of something that poses little or no actual danger.

posttraumatic stress disorder (PTSD): Disorder in which a stressful experience is traumatic and produces severe, recurring symptoms.

psychotherapy: A treatment method for mental illness in which a mental health professional and a patient discuss problems and feelings to find solutions. Psychotherapy can help individuals change their thought or behavior patterns or understand how past experiences affect current behaviors.

puberty: The process of developing from a child to sexual maturity, when a person becomes capable of having children.

pubic area: On and around the genitals.

reproductive organ: A body part involved in producing a baby. In a female, they include the uterus, ovaries, fallopian tubes, and vagina. In a male, they include the testicles and penis.

schizophrenia: A chronic, severe, and disabling brain disease. People with schizophrenia often suffer terrifying symptoms such as hearing internal voices or believing that other people are reading their minds, controlling their thoughts, or plotting to harm them.

scoliosis: When the spine curves away from the middle of the body to the side.

semen: Whitish fluid containing sperm that comes out of the male's penis. Also known as cum.

sex hormones: Hormones that are found in higher quantities in one sex than in the other. Male sex hormones are the androgens, which include testosterone; and the female sex hormones are the estrogens and progesterone.

sexual assault: Any type of sexual activity that you do not agree to, including touching you, forcing you to touch someone, and forcing a body part into your vagina, rectum (bottom), or mouth. Another term for this can be molestation.

sexual contact: Any type of touching during sexual activity between two people, including sexual intercourse, oral sex, and skin-to-skin contact in the genital area (around the vagina, penis, scrotum, anus, and thigh).

sexual intercourse: When a man's penis is put into a woman's vagina.

sexually transmitted disease (STD): Infection that is spread from person to person through sexual contact. Also called sexually transmitted infection.

sperm: Cell found in semen that can unite with a female's egg after having sexual intercourse and lead to pregnancy.

syphilis: A sexually transmitted disease caused by bacteria that progresses in stages. Without treatment, the infection can cause damage throughout the body and even death.

testosterone: A male hormone that controls many of the changes males go through during puberty—deeper voice, body and facial hair, and the making of sperm.

tobacco: A plant widely cultivated for its leaves, which are used primarily for smoking.

uterus: A pear-shaped, hollow organ in a female's pelvis where a baby develops during pregnancy.

vagina: A muscular passage that leads down from the cervix to the outside of a female's body. During menstruation, menstrual blood flows from the uterus through the cervix and out of the body through the vagina. Also called the birth canal

virus: A kind of germ that can infect cells and cause disease.

vulva: The external female reproductive organ, which covers the entrance to the vagina.

Chapter 71

Directory of Adolescent Health Organizations for Parents and Teens

Government Agencies That Provide Information about Adolescent Health

Agency for Healthcare Research and Quality (AHRQ)
Office of Communications and Knowledge Transfer
5600 Fishers Ln.
Rockville, MD 20857
Phone: 301-427-1364
Fax: 301-427-1873
Website: www.ahrq.gov

Centers for Disease Control and Prevention (CDC)
1600 Clifton Rd.
Atlanta, GA 30333
Phone: 404-639-3311
Toll-Free: 800-CDC-INFO
(800-232-4636)
Toll-Free TTY: 888-232-6348
Website: www.cdc.gov
E-mail: cdcinfo@cdc.gov

Resources in this chapter were compiled from several sources deemed reliable; all contact information was verified and updated in November 2017.

*Child Welfare Information
Gateway*
Children's Bureau/ACYF
330 C St. S.W.
Washington, DC 20201
Toll-Free: 800-394-3366
Website: www.childwelfare.gov
E-mail: info@childwelfare.gov

Eunice Kennedy Shriver
*National Institute on
Child Health and Human
Development (NICHD)*
P.O. Box 3006
Rockville, MD 20847
Phone: 301-496-5133
Toll-Free Fax: 866-760-5947
Toll-Free: 800-370-2943
Toll-Free TTY: 888-320-6942
Website: www.nichd.nih.gov
E-mail:
nichdinformationresourcecenter@
mail.nih.gov

*Federal Interagency Forum
on Child and Family
Statistics*
Phone: 301-458-4082
Website: www.childstats.gov

*Federal Trade Commission
(FTC)*
600 Pennsylvania Ave. N.W.
Washington, DC 20580
Phone: 202-326-2222
Website: www.ftc.gov

*Health Resources and
Services Administration
(HRSA)*
5600 Fishers Ln.
Rockville, MD 20857
Phone: 301-443-3376
Toll-Free: 800-221-9393
Toll-Free TTY: 877-897-9910
Website: www.hrsa.gov

Healthfinder®
National Health Information
Center (NHIC)
P.O. Box 1133
Washington, DC 20013-1133
Phone: 301-565-4167
Fax: 301-984-4256
Toll-Free: 800-336-4797
Website: www.healthfinder.gov
E-mail: healthfinder@nhic.org

*National Cancer Institute
(NCI)*
NCI Office of Communications
and Education, Public Inquiries
Office
9609 Medical Center Dr.
Bethesda, MD 20892-9760
Phone: 240-276-6600
Toll-Free: 800-4-CANCER
(800-422-6237)
Toll-Free TTY: 800-332-8615
Website: www.cancer.gov
E-mail: cancergovstaff@mail.nih
.gov

National Diabetes Education Program (NDEP)
Toll-Free: 800-860-8747
Toll-Free TTY: 866-569-1162
Website: www.niddk.nih.
gov/health-information/
communication-programs/ndep
E-mail: healthinfo@niddk.nih.
gov

National Highway Traffic Safety Administration (NHTSA)
1200 New Jersey Ave. S.E.
Washington, DC 20590
Toll-Free: 888-327-4236
Toll-Free TTY: 800-424-9153
Website: www.nhtsa.gov

National Institute of Arthritis and Musculoskeletal and Skin Diseases (NIAMS)
Information Clearinghouse,
National Institutes of Health
(NIH)
1 AMS Cir.
Bethesda, MD 20892-3675
Phone: 301-495-4484
Fax: 301-718-6366
Toll-Free: 877-226-4267
TTY: 301-565-2966
Website: www.niams.nih.gov
E-mail: niamsinfo@mail.nih.gov

National Institute of Diabetes, Digestive and Kidney Diseases (NIDDK)
Office of Communications &
Public Liaison
31 Center Dr. MSC 2560
Bldg. 31 Rm. 9A06
Bethesda, MD 20892-2560
Phone: 301-496-3583
Toll-Free: 800-472-0424
Website: www.niddk.nih.gov
E-mail: niddkinquiries@nih.gov

National Institute of Neurological Disorders and Stroke (NINDS)
NIH Neurological Institute
P.O. Box 5801
Bethesda, MD 20824
Phone: 301-496-5751
Toll-Free: 800-352-9424
Website: www.ninds.nih.gov

National Institute on Alcohol Abuse and Alcoholism (NIAAA)
5635 Fishers Ln.
Rm. 2005 MSC 9304
Bethesda, MD 20892-9304
Phone: 301-443-2857
Toll-Free: 888-MY-NIAAA
(888-696-4222)
Website: www.niaaa.nih.gov
E-mail: niaaaweb-r@exchange
.nih.gov

National Institute on Deafness and Other Communication Disorders (NIDCD)
National Institutes of Health (NIH)
31 Center Dr. MSC 2320
Bethesda, MD 20892-2320
Website: www.nidcd.nih.gov
E-mail: nidcdinfo@nidcd.nih.gov

National Institute on Drug Abuse (NIDA)
6001 Executive Blvd.
Rm. 5213 MSC 9561
Bethesda, MD 20892
Phone: 301-443-1124
Website: www.drugabuse.gov

National Institute on Mental Health (NIMH)
Science Writing, Press, and Dissemination Branch
6001 Executive Blvd. MSC 9663
Rm. 6200
Bethesda, MD 20892-9663
Phone: 301-443-4513
Fax: 301-443-4279
Toll-Free: 866-615-6464
Toll-Free TTY: 866-415-8051
TTY: 301-443-8431
Website: www.nimh.nih.gov
E-mail: nimhinfo@nih.gov

National Institutes of Health (NIH)
9000 Rockville Pike
Bethesda, MD 20892
Phone: 301-496-4000
TTY: 301-402-9612
Website: www.nih.gov
E-mail: nihinfo@od.nih.gov

National Women's Health Information Center (NWHIC)
Office on Women's Health (OWH)
200 Independence Ave. S.W.
Washington, DC 20201
Toll-Free: 800-994-9662
Website: www.womenshealth.gov

National Youth Anti-Drug Media Campaign
White House, Office of National Drug Control Policy (ONDCP)
P.O. Box 6000
Rockville, MD 20849-6000
Fax: 301-519-5212
Website: www.whitehouse.gov/ondcp

Striving To Reduce Youth Violence Everywhere (STRYVE)
Centers for Disease Control and Prevention (CDC)
Website: www.cdc.gov/violenceprevention/stryve

Substance Abuse and Mental Health Services Administration (SAMHSA)
SAMHSA's Health Information Network
5600 Fishers Ln.
Rockville, MD 20857
Fax: 240-221-4292
Toll-Free: 877-726-4727
Toll-Free TTY: 800-487-4889
Website: www.samhsa.gov

U.S. Department of Education (ED)
400 Maryland Ave. S.W.
Washington, DC 20202
Phone: 202-401-2000
Toll-Free: 800-USA-LEARN
(800-872-5327)
Toll-Free TTY: 800-437-0833
Website: www.ed.gov

U.S. Department of Health and Human Services (HHS)
200 Independent Ave. S.W.
Washington, DC 20201
Toll-Free: 877-696-6775
Website: www.hhs.gov

U.S. Department of Labor (DOL)
200 Constitution Ave. N.W.
Washington, DC 20210
Toll-Free: 866-4-USA-DOL
(866-4487-2365)
Toll-Free TTY: 877-889-5627
Website: www.dol.gov

U.S. Food and Drug Administration (FDA)
10903 New Hampshire Ave.
Silver Spring, MD 20993
Toll-Free: 888-INFO-FDA
(888-463-6332)
Website: www.fda.gov

U.S. National Library of Medicine (NLM)
8600 Rockville Pike
Bethesda, MD 20894
Phone: 301-594-5983
Toll-Free: 888-FIND-NLM
(888-346-3656)
Website: www.nlm.nih.gov
E-mail: custserv@nlm.nih.gov

Private Agencies That Provide Information about Adolescent Health

AAA Foundation for Traffic Safety
607 14th St. N.W.
Ste. 201
Washington, DC 20005
Phone: 202-638-5944
Fax: 202-638-5943
Website: www.aaafoundation.org
E-mail: info@aaafoundation.org

American Academy of Child and Adolescent Psychiatry (AACAP)
3615 Wisconsin Ave. N.W.
Washington, DC 20016-3007
Phone: 202-966-7300
Fax: 202-464-0131
Website: www.aacap.org
E-mail: clinical@aacap.org

**American Academy of
Dermatology (AAD)**
930 E. Woodfield Rd.
Schaumburg, IL 60173
Phone: 847-330-0230
Fax: 847-240-1859
Toll-Free: 888-462-DERM
(888-462-3376)
Website: www.aad.org

**American Academy of Family
Physicians (AAFP)**
11400 Tomahawk Creek Pkwy
Leawood, KS 66211-2680
Phone: 913-906-6000
Fax: 913-906-6075
Toll-Free: 800-274-2237
Website: www.aafp.org

**American Academy of
Pediatrics (AAP)**
141 N.W. Pt. Blvd.
Elk Grove Village, IL
60007-1098
Fax: 847-434-8000
Toll-Free: 800-433-9016
Website: www.aap.org
E-mail: international@aap.org

**American Association of
Diabetes Educators (AADE)**
200 W. Madison St.
Ste. 800
Chicago, IL 60606
Toll-Free: 800-338-3633
Website: www.diabeteseducator.
org

**American Association of
Suicidology (AAS)**
5221 Wisconsin Ave. N.W.
Washington, DC 20015
Phone: 202-237-2280
Fax: 202-237-2282
Toll-Free: 800-273-8255
Website: www.suicidology.org

**American Childhood Cancer
Organization (ACCO)**
6868 Distribution Dr.
Beltsville, MD 20705
Phone: 301-962-3520
Fax: 301-962-3521
Toll-Free: 855-858-2226
Website: www.acco.org

**American College of
Obstetricians and
Gynecologists (ACOG)**
409 12th St. S.W.
Washington, DC 20024-2188
Phone: 202-638-5577
Toll-Free: 800-673-8444
Website: www.acog.org

**American College of Sports
Medicine (ACSM)**
401 W. Michigan St.
Indianapolis, IN 46202-3233
Phone: 317-637-9200
Fax: 317-634-7817
Website: www.acsm.org

American Diabetes Association
National Call Center
2451 Crystal Dr.
Ste. 900
Arlington, VA 22202
Toll-Free: 800-DIABETES
(800-342-2383)
Website: www.diabetes.org
E-mail: askada@diabetes.org

American Heart Association (AHA)
National Center
7272 Greenville Ave.
Dallas, TX 75231
Toll-Free: 800-AHA-USA-1
(800-242-8721)
Website: www.heart.org

American Medical Association (AMA)
AMA Plaza 330 N. Wabash Ave.
Ste. 39300
Chicago, IL 60611-5885
Toll-Free: 800-621-8335
Website: www.ama-assn.org

American Psychiatric Association (APA)
1000 Wilson Blvd.
Ste. 1825
Arlington, VA 22209-3901
Phone: 703-907-7300
Toll-Free: 888-357-7924
Website: www.psych.org
E-mail: apa@psych.org

American Psychological Association (APA)
750 First St. N.E.
Washington, DC 20002-4242
Phone: 202-336-5500
Toll-Free: 800-374-2721
TDD/TTY: 202-336-6123
Website: www.apa.org

American Sexual Health Association (ASHA)
P.O. Box 13827
Research Triangle Park, NC 27709
Phone: 919-361-8400
Fax: 919-361-8425
Websites: www.ashasexualhealth.org
E-mail: info@ashasexualhealth.org

Anxiety Disorders Association of America (ADAA)
8701 Georgia Ave.
Ste. 412
Silver Spring, MD 20910
Phone: 240-485-1001
Fax: 240-485-1035
Website: www.adaa.org
E-mail:information@adaa.org

Center for Young Women's Health (CYWH)
333 Longwood Ave.
Fifth Fl.
Boston, MA 02115
Phone: 617-355-2994
Fax: 617-730-0186
Website: www.youngwomenshealth.org

Child and Adolescent Bipolar Foundation (CABF)
Website: www.bpkids.org

Cincinnati Children's Hospital Medical Center
3333 Burnet Ave.
Cincinnati, OH 45229-3026
Phone: 513-636-4200
Toll-Free: 800-344-2462
TTY: 513-636-4900
Website: www.
cincinnatichildrens.org

Cleveland Clinic
9500 Euclid Ave.
Cleveland, OH 44195
Toll-Free: 800-223-2273
Website: www.
my.clevelandclinic.org

Crimes Against Children Research Center (CCRC)
University of New Hampshire
15 Academic Way
McConnell Hall Ste. 125
Durham, NH 03824
Phone: 603-862-1888
Fax: 603-862-1122
Website: www.unh.edu

Depression and Bipolar Support Alliance (DBSA)
55 E. Jackson Blvd.
Ste. 490
Chicago, Illinois 60604
Fax: 312-642-7243
Toll-Free: 800-826-3632
Website: www.dbsalliance.org

Guttmacher Institute
125 Maiden Ln.
Seventh Fl.
New York, NY 10038
Phone: 212-248-1111
Fax: 212-248-1951
Toll-Free: 800-355-0244
Website: www.guttmacher.org

The Hormone Foundation
2055 L St. N.W.
Ste. 600
Washington, DC 20036
Phone: 202-971-3636
Toll-Free: 888-363-6274
Website: www.hormone.org

Immunization Action Coalition (IAC)
2550 University Ave. W.
Ste. 415 N.
St. Paul, MN 55114
Phone: 651-647-9009
Fax: 651-647-9131
Website: www.immunize.org

International OCD (Obsessive-Compulsive Disorder) Foundation
P.O. Box 961029
Boston, MA 02196
Phone: 617-973-5801
Fax: 617-973-5803
Website: www.iocdf.org
E-mail: info@iocdf.org

Juvenile Arthritis Alliance
Arthritis Foundation
1355 Peachtree St. N.E.
Ste. 600
Atlanta, GA 30309
Phone: 404-872-7100
Toll-Free: 800-283-7800
Website: www.arthritis.org

Juvenile Diabetes Research Foundation (JDRF)
26 Bdwy.
14th Fl.
New York, NY 100004
Fax: 212-785-9595
Toll-Free: 800-533-CURE
(800-533-2873)
Website: www.jdrf.org
E-mail: info@jdrf.org

Kaiser Family Foundation
2400 Sand Hill Rd.
Menlo Park, CA 94025
Phone: 650-854-9400
Fax: 650-854-4800
Website: www.kff.org

Mayo Clinic
13400 E. Shea Blvd.
Scottsdale, AZ 85259
Phone: 480-301-8000
Website: www.mayoclinic.org

Mental Health America
500 Montgomery St.
Ste. 820
Alexandria, VA 22314
Phone: 703-684-7722
Fax: 703-684-5968
Toll-Free: 800-969-6642
Website: www.
mentalhealthamerica.net

National Adolescent Health Information Center (NAHIC)
P.O. Box 0503
LHTS Ste. 245
San Francisco, CA 94143-0503
Phone: 415-502-4856
Fax: 415-502-4858
Website: www.nahic.ucsf.edu

National Alliance on Mental Illness (NAMI)
3803 N. Fairfax Dr.
Ste. 100
Arlington, VA 22203
Phone: 703-524-7600
Fax: 703-524-9094
Toll-Free: 800-950-6264
Website: www.nami.org

National Campaign to Prevent Teen and Unplanned Pregnancy
1776 Massachusetts Ave. N.W.
Ste. 200
Washington, DC 20036
Phone: 202-478-8500
Fax: 202-478-8588
Website: www.
thenationalcampaign.org

National Center for Missing and Exploited Children (NCMEC)
Charles B. Wang International
Children's Bldg.
699 Prince St.
Alexandria, VA 22314-3175
Phone: 703-224-2150
Fax: 703-224-2122
Toll-Free: 800-843-5678
Website: www.missingkids.com

National Safety Council (NSC)
1121 Spring Lake Dr.
Itasca, IL 60143-3201
Phone: 630-285-1121
Fax: 630-285-1434
Toll-Free: 800-621-7615
Website: www.nsc.org
E-mail: customerservice@nsc.org

National Scoliosis Foundation (NSF)
5 Cabot Pl.
Stoughton, MA 02072
Fax: 781-341-8333
Toll-Free: 800-NSF-MYBACK
(800-673-6922)
Website: www.scoliosis.org
E-mail: nsf@scoliosis.org

National Youth Network
Website: www.nationalyouth.com

Nemours Foundation Center for Children's Health Media
Nemours/Alfred I. duPont
Hospital for Children
1600 Rockland Rd.
Wilmington, DE 19803
Phone: 302-651-4186
Website: www.nemours.org
E-mail: info@teenshealth.org

Palo Alto Medical Foundation (PAMF)
Phone: 650-321-4121
Toll-Free: 888-398-5677
Website: www.pamf.org

Parents, Families, and Friends of Lesbians and Gays (PFLAG)
1828 L St. N.W.
Ste. 660
Washington, DC 20036
Phone: 202-467-8180
Fax: 202-467-8194
Website: www.pflag.org
E-mail: info@pflagflagstaff.org

Partnership for Drug-Free Kids
352 Park Ave. S.
Ninth Fl.
New York, NY 10010
Phone: 212-922-1560
Fax: 212-922-1570
Website: www.drugfree.org

Pew Internet and American Life Project
The Pew Research Center
1615 L St. N.W.
Ste. 800
Washington, DC 20036
Phone: 202-419-4300
Fax: 202-419-4349
Website: www.pewinternet.org
E-mail: info@pewinternet.org

Planned Parenthood
Planned Parenthood Federation
of America
123 William St.
10th Fl.
New York, NY 10038
Phone: 212-541-7800
Toll-Free: 800-230-PLAN
(800-230-7526)
Website: www.plannedparenthood.org

SAFE Alternatives (Self-Abuse Finally Ends)
8000 Bonhomme
Ste. 211
St. Louis, MO 63105
Phone: 630-819-9505
Toll-Free Fax: 888-296-7988
Website: www.selfinjury.com

Sex, Etc.
Rutgers University
41 Gordon Rd.
Ste. C
Piscataway, NJ 08854
Website: www.sexetc.org
E-mail: sexetc@rci.rutgers.edu

Sexuality Information and Education Council of the United States (SIECUS)
1012 14th St. N.W.
Ste. 1108
Washington, DC 20005
Phone: 202-265-2405
Fax: 212-819-9776
Website: www.siecus.org
E-mail: info@siecus.org

Society for Adolescent Health and Medicine (SAHM)
1 Parkview Plaza
Ste. 800
Oakbrook Terrace, IL 60181
Phone: 847-686-2246
Fax: 847-686-2251
Website: www.adolescenthealth.org
E-mail: info@adolescenthealth.org

Students Against Destructive Decisions (SADD)
1440 G St.
Washington, DC 20005
Phone: 508-481-3568
Website: www.sadd.org

Suicide Awareness Voices of Education (SAVE)
8120 Penn Ave. S.
Ste. 470
Bloomington, MN 55431
Phone: 952-946-7998
Toll-Free: 800-273-8255
Website: www.save.org

TeenGrowth
11274 W. Hillsborough Ave.
Website: www.teengrowth.com

World Health Organization (WHO)
20 Ave. Appia
1211 Geneva 27
Switzerland
Website: www.who.int

Young Men's Health (YMH)
333 Longwood Ave.
Fifth Fl.
Boston, MA 02115
Phone: 617-355-2994
Website: www.youngmenshealthsite.org

Hotlines and Referral Services for Teens: General Help

Covenant House
461 Eighth Ave.
New York, NY 10001
Toll-Free: 800-388-3888
Website: www.covenanthouse.
org
E-mail: info@covenanthouse.org

Girls and Boys Town
National Hotline
Crawford St.
Boys Town, NE 68010
Phone: 310-855-4673
Toll-Free: 800-852-8336
Website: teenlineonline.org/yyp/
girls-boys-town-national-hotline

Hotlines and Referral Services for Teens: Assistance for Specific Concerns

Al-Anon Family Groups
1600 Corporate Landing Pkwy.
Virginia Beach, VA 23454-5617
Phone: 757-563-1600
Fax: 757-563-1656
Website: www.al-anon.org

American Pregnancy
Helpline
Toll-Free: 866-942-6466
Website: www.thehelpline.org
E-mail: aph@thehelpline.org

Centers for Disease Control
and Prevention (CDC)
Sexually Transmitted
Disease Hotline
1600 Clifton Rd.
Atlanta, GA 30333
Toll-Free: 800-CDC-INFO
(800-232-4636)
Toll-Free TTY: 888-232-6348
Website: www.cdc.gov/std

National Clearinghouse
for Alcohol and Drug
Information (NCADI)
5600 Fishers Ln.
Rockville, MD 20857
Fax: 240-221-4292
Toll-Free: 877-726-4727
Toll-Free TTY: 800-487-4889
Website: www.samhsa.gov/
find-help/national-helpline

National Domestic Violence
Hotline
PO Box 161810
Austin, TX 78716
Phone: 512-453-8117
Toll-Free: 800-799-7233
Toll-Free TTY: 800-787-3224
Website: www.ndvh.org
E-mail: hotline.requests@ndvh.
org

National Runaway Safeline (NRS)
3141B N. Lincoln
Chicago, IL 60657
Phone: 773-880-9860
Fax: 773-929-5150
Toll-Free: 800-RUNAWAY
(800-799-7233)
Website: www.1800runaway.org

National Suicide Hotline
Toll-Free: 800-786-2929
Website: www.hopeline.com

Planned Parenthood Federation of America
123 William St.
10th Fl.
New York, NY 10038
Toll-Free: 800-430-4907
Website: www.
plannedparenthood.org

Rape, Abuse & Incest National Network (RAINN)
Toll-Free: 800-656-4673
Website: www.rainn.org

SAFE Alternatives (Self-Abuse Finally Ends)
8000 Bonhomme
Ste. 211
St. Louis, MO 63105
Phone: 630-819-9505
Toll-Free Fax: 888-296-7988
Website: www.selfinjury.com

Index

Index

Page numbers followed by 'n' indicate a footnote. Page numbers in *italics* indicate a table or illustration.

A

AAA Foundation for Traffic Safety, contact 721
abortion, statistics 178
absent menstrual periods, described 237
abstinence
  defined 711
  overview 293–5
  sexually transmitted diseases 264
  unplanned pregnancy 264
"Abstinence" (HHS) 293n
abuse-deterrent formulations (ADF), opioid medications 557
abusive relationship
  overview 679–82
  stalking 674
academic performance
  attention deficit hyperactivity disorder 11
  cognitive enhancers 555
  sleep deprivation 166
  substance use disorder 569
  youth violence 662

acne
  cosmetic surgery 162
  defined 711
  hormonal birth control 309
  overview 333–7
  puberty 185
"Acne" (NIAMS) 333n
acromegaly, described 363
actinic keratoses, described 620
addiction
  adolescent brain 503
  benzodiazepines 552
  central nervous system (CNS) depressants 560
  cognitive enhancers 555
  defined 711
  drug abuse 509
  inhalants 568
  marijuana use 540
  methadone 559
  nicotine 516
  opioids 550
  prescription drug addiction 558
  stimulants 554
ADHD *see* attention deficit hyperactivity disorder
adolescence
  alcohol use 49
  brain development overview 25

adolescence, *continued*
defined 711
"Adolescent and School Health—
Positive Parenting Practices"
(CDC) 425n
"Adolescent and School Health—
School Connectedness" (CDC) 412n
adolescent depression, adolescent well
being 55 ·
"Adolescent Development E-Learning
Module" (OAH) 25n
"Adolescent Development—Mental
Health in Adolescents" (OAH) 431n
"Adolescent Health" (ODPHP) 15n
adolescent population, depicted *4*
adrenaline
nicotine addictive 518
test anxiety 405
adult-onset diabetes, defined 356
adverse childhood experiences (ACEs),
trauma 18
aerobic activity, adolescent fitness 139
aerosols
cosmetics 610
inhalants 563
Affordable Care Act (ACA)
low-cost birth control 311
sexually transmitted diseases 277
substance abuse treatment
services 573
age factor
delayed puberty 257
growing pains 360
HPV vaccine 100
menstrual cycle 222
suicide statistics 497
testicular cancer 200
youth gangs 694
Agency for Healthcare Research and
Quality (AHRQ), contact 717
aggression, defined 711
aggressive behavior, amygdala and
frontal cortex 30
Al-Anon Family Groups, contact 728
alcohol abuse
parental involvement 537
gangs 698
genetic traits 536
self-harm 494

alcoholic, defined 711
alcoholism, defined 711
allergies
defined 711
overview 339–41
"Allergies" (CDC) 339n
"Allergy" (NIH) 339n
amenorrhea
defined 712
described 238
American Academy of Child and
Adolescent Psychiatry (AACAP),
contact 721
American Academy of Dermatology
(AAD), contact 722
American Academy of Family
Physicians (AAFP), contact 722
American Academy of Pediatrics
(AAP), contact 722
American Association of Diabetes
Educators (AADE). contact 722
American Association of Suicidology
(AAS), contact 722
American Childhood Cancer
Organization (ACCO), contact 722
American College of Obstetricians and
Gynecologists (ACOG), contact 722
American College of Sports Medicine
(ACSM), contact 722
American Diabetes Association,
contact 723
American Heart Association (AHA),
contact 723
American Medical Association (AMA),
contact 723
American Pregnancy Helpline,
contact 728
American Psychiatric Association
(APA), contact 723
American Psychological Association
(APA), contact 723
American Sexual Health Association
(ASHA), contact 723
"America's Children in Brief: Key
National Indicators of Well Being"
(ChildStats.gov) 33n
amotivational syndrome,
marijuana 543
amphetamine, inhalants 568

anal sex, defined 712
androgens, erectile dysfunction 190
anemia
  anorexia nervosa 479
  defined 712
anorexia nervosa
  defined 712
  described 479
  psychotherapies 482
"Antidepressant Medications
  for Children and Adolescents:
  Information for Parents and
  Caregivers" (NIMH) 446n
antidepressants
  childhood mental disorders 438
  eating disorders 482
  erectile dysfunction 190
  overview 446–9
  premenstrual syndrome 235
  repetitive stress injuries 650
antigang policies, gang crime 694
anxiety disorders
  defined 712
  overview 452–7
  premenstrual syndrome 234
"Anxiety Disorders" (NIMH) 452n
Anxiety Disorders Association of
  America (ADAA), contact 723
apex, depicted *645*
"Are You a Working Teen?"
  (CDC) 633n
arthritis, described 365
asthma
  defined 712
  obesity 147
  overview 343–5
  smoking 528
  statistics 57
  stimulants 554
"Asthma" (NHLBI) 343n
"Asthma in Schools" (CDC) 343n
asthma triggers, defined 343
athlete's foot, described 630
attention deficit hyperactivity
  disorder (ADHD)
  defined 712
  overview 457–64
"Attention Deficit Hyperactivity
  Disorder" (NIMH) 457n

B

"BAM! Body and Mind—Body
  Smarts—Questions Answered"
  (CDC) 181n
barrier methods, contraception 298
behavioral therapy, defined 712
binge eating disorder (BED)
  defined 712
  described 480
bipolar disorder
  defined 712
  overview 467–72
"Bipolar Disorder in Children and
  Teens" (NIMH) 467n
birth control methods *see*
  contraception
"Birth Control Methods" (OWH) 297n
birth control pills, defined 712
blood alcohol concentration (BAC),
  driving 590
blood pressure, fats 106
BMI *see* body mass index
BMI percentile, described 144
"Body" (OWH) 211n
body dysmorphic disorder, defined 160
"Body—Getting Enough Sleep"
  (OWH) 169n
body hair
  gynecomastia 207
  puberty 216
body image, overview 158–62
body mass index (BMI)
  defined 712
  overview 144–8
body odor, puberty 184
boils, staphylococcal infections 381
bone strengthening, physical
  activity 136
borderline personality disorder,
  overview 472–8
"Borderline Personality Disorder"
  (NIMH) 472n
braces, malocclusion 389
brain
  adolescents 25
  alcohol use 533
  bipolar disorder 467
  caffeine 130

brain, *continued*
  depression 442
  described 503
  inhalants 563
  marijuana use 540
  meningococcal infection 375
  precocious puberty 253
  stimulants 461
brain circuits, medication-assisted
  treatment 559
brain development, overview 25–31
brain stem, defined 503
brain tumor, central precocious
  puberty 254
brain's plasticity, brain
  development 28
breast enlargement, male *see*
  gynecomastia
bulimia nervosa
  defined 712
  described 480
bullying
  lesbian, gay, bisexual, and
    transgender (LGBT) youth 324
  statistics 13
  youth violence 656
bupropion, smoking cessation 528
bursitis, defined 650
"The Buzz on Caffeine"
  (NIDA) 130n

C

caffeine use, overview 128–32
calcium
  bulimia nervosa 480
  intake recommendations 114
  premenstrual syndrome
    symptoms 236
"Calcium" (ODS) 114n
cancer
  pap test 230
  physical activity 137
  smokeless tobacco 521
  tanning beds 122
"Cancer in Children and Adolescents"
  (NCI) 347n
cannabis, defined 539
carcinogens, defined 521

cardiovascular disease
  calcium 118
  obesity 9
  sleep 169
carpal tunnel syndrome, defined 650
cataracts, tanning 621
CDC *see* Centers for Disease Control
  and Prevention
"CDC Releases Youth Risk Behaviors
  Survey Results" (CDC) 579n
Celexa (citalopram), depression 44
cellulitis, staphylococcal infections 381
Center for Young Women's Health
  (CYWH), contact 723
Centers for Disease Control and
  Prevention (CDC)
  contact 717
  publications
    allergies 339n
    asthma in schools 343n
    children's mental health 464n
    college health and safety 170n
    concussion 640n
    educating teenagers about
      sex 266n
    electronic aggression 598n
    energy drinks 129n
    epididymitis 198n
    HIV testing among
      adolescents 279n
    hookahs 523n
    HPV vaccination for young
      women 281n
    hygiene-related diseases 625n
    influenza (flu) 370n
    LGBT youth 323n
    meningococcal 375n
    monitoring teen's
      activities 425n
    mononucleosis 386n
    MRSA 380n
    physical activity 135n
    positive parenting 21n, 425n
    prevent sexually transmitted
      diseases 263n
    preventing flu 370n
    puberty 181n
    reproductive health 314n
    ringworm 625n

Centers for Disease Control and
Prevention (CDC)
publications, *continued*
school connectedness 412n
sexual activity
statistics 175n
sexual risk behaviors 175n
sleep deprivation 166n
smokeless tobacco 520n
STDs in adolescents 175n
suicide 497n
teen BMI 145n
teen dating violence 679n
teen drivers 584n
teen drivers safety 591n
teen monitoring 81n
teen pregnancy 175n
teen sleep habits 167n
Tourette syndrome 490n
underage drinking 532n
vaccines for children 101n
VISA/VRSA 380n
working teen 633n
young worker safety and
health 633n
Youth Risk Behavior
Surveillance System
(YRBSS) 579n
youth risk behaviors survey
results 579n
youth violence 656n
youth violence risks 661n
Centers for Disease Control and
Prevention (CDC) Sexually
Transmitted Disease Hotline,
contact 728
cerebral cortex, described 504
cervical cancer, pap test 230
cervix, described 212
Chantix (varenicline), smoking
cessation 528
"Characteristics of Healthy and
Unhealthy Relationships" (Youth.
gov) 418n
cheating, overview 409–11
"Cheating" (Omnigraphics) 409n
chewing tobacco, defined 520
Child and Adolescent Bipolar
Foundation (CABF), contact 724

"Child Development—Positive
Parenting Tips" (CDC) 21n
child maltreatment, youth
gang 696
child poverty, statistic 36
Child Welfare Information Gateway,
contact 718
childbearing in adolescents,
statistics 178
"Children's Mental Health—Behavior
or Conduct Problems" (CDC) 464n
children's oncology group (COG),
cancer treatment 351
chlamydia, statistics 177
"Chronic Diseases" (NIH) 329n
chronic illness, described 329
"Cigarette Smoking: Health Risks
and How to Quit (PDQ®)—Patient
Version" (NCI) 526n
Cincinnati Children's Hospital
Medical Center, contact 724
citalopram, depression 448
Cleveland Clinic, contact 724
clitoris
defined 713
depicted *212*
described 213
cocaine
brain 505
marijuana 542
cochlea, depicted *645*
cognitive behavioral therapy, mental
health problems 436
cognitive enhancers, described 554
college education, statistics 53
"College Health and Safety"
(CDC) 169n
communication, overview 63–7
concussion, overview 640–3
"Concussion Information Sheet"
(CDC) 640n
condoms
birth control 298
defined 713
human papillomavirus 286
safer sex 288
sexually transmitted
diseases 77
yeast infection 241

conduct disorder
  defined 713
  described 465
constitutional delay, described 257
"Consumer Updates—Think before
  You Ink: Are Tattoos Safe?"
  (FDA) 622n
contraception, overview 297–311
"Conversation Tools" (OAH) 63n
"Coping with Chronic Illness"
  (NIH) 329n
cosmetic surgery, described 162
"Cosmetic Surgery" (OWH) 162n
cosmetics, overview 610–4
"Cosmetics Safety Q&A: Shelf Life"
  (FDA) 610n
"Cosmetics: Tips for Women"
  (FDA) 610n
"Could I Get Pregnant If...?"
  (OWH) 316n
Covenant House, contact 728
Cowper's glands, defined 183
crash risk, teen drivers 584
Crimes Against Children Research
  Center (CCRC), contact 724
cryptorchidism, testicular self-
  examination 205
cutting, overview 493–5
"Cutting and Self-Harm" (OWH) 493n
cyberbullying, described 666
cysts
  defined 335
  hormonal birth control 309

D

dairy, bones 105
date rape, defined 713
dating violence, overview 679–82
"Dating Violence" (OWH) 679n
"Dealing with Drug Problems"
  (NIH) 509n
"Deciding about Sex" (OWH) 262n
decision making, drugs 570
dehydration, energy drinks 129
delayed puberty, described 257–9
dental dams, usage tips 288
dental X-rays, malocclusion 391
depilatories, described 615

depression
  bullied 667
  defined 713
  overview 442–6
  social anxiety disorder 453
Depression and Bipolar Support
  Alliance (DBSA), contact 724
detoxification, drug abuse 511
developmental milestones, physical
  and emotional changes 22
diabetes, defined 713
"Diabetes in Children and Teens"
  (NIH) 355n
diaphragm, yeast infections 242
diet and nutrition, weight
  management 104
dietary supplement
  calcium 115
  premenstrual syndrome 236
  vitamin D 122
diphtheria, Tdap vaccine 101
disinfecting, flu 372
disruptive behavior disorder,
  described 465
distracted driving, teen crashes 586
diuretics, calcium dietary
  supplements 120
dopamine
  drugs 505
  exercise 402
  inhalants 568
  marijuana 541
  stimulants 461
douching, defined 713
"Douching" (OWH) 245n
Down syndrome, cancer 349
driving safety, overview 584–95
drug, defined 713
drug abuse
  communication tips 69
  defined 509
drug paraphernalia, preventing
  substance abuse 510
"Drugs, Brains, and Behavior: The
  Science of Addiction" (NIDA) 503n
drunk driving and drugs, driving
  safety 588
dysmenorrhea, defined 713
dysthymic disorders, defined 433

E

ear canal, depicted *645*
eating disorders
    defined 713
    overview 478–82
"Eating Disorders" (NIMH) 478n
e-cigarettes, tobacco and nicotine
    products 529
economic circumstances, adolescent
    well-being 36
"Educating Teenagers about Sex in
    the United States" (CDC) 266n
Effexor (venlafaxine), antidepressant
    medications 448
egg (ovum), described 212
ejaculation, defined 713
electronic aggression, overview
    598–600
emergency contraception
    described 306
    sexual assault 689
emergency department, drug
    abuse 560
emotional bonds, positive
    parenting 60
emotional problems
    puberty 185
    talking to parents 85
endocannabinoids, defined 540
"Endocrine Diseases" (NIH) 363n
endometriosis, defined 713
endometrium, described 212
energy drinks, described 128
"Energy Drinks" (NCCIH) 128n
enlarged spleen, mononucleosis 386
environmental factors
    anxiety disorders 454
    cancer 349
    schizophrenia 488
epididymis, defined 181
epididymitis, described 197
"Epididymitis" (CDC) 197n
"Epstein-Barr—Mononucleosis"
    (CDC) 386n
Epstein-Barr virus,
    mononucleosis 386
erectile dysfunction (ED),
    overview 188–96

"Erectile Dysfunction (ED)"
    (NIDDK) 188n
escitalopram, depression 448
estrogen, menstrual cycle 219
Eunice Kennedy Shriver National
    Institute of Child Health and
    Human Development (NICHD)
    contact 718
    publications
        bullying 666n
        menstrual irregularities 237n
        precocious puberty 252n
        prenatal care 318n
        puberty 257n
euphoria, marijuana 541
excessive drinking, statistics 532
extraction, malocclusion 391
eye damage, tanning safety 621

F

facial disfigurement, malocclusion 390
"Fact Sheets—Underage Drinking"
    (CDC) 532n
"Facts about Bullying" (HHS) 671n
"Facts about Tourette Syndrome"
    (CDC) 490n
fallopian tubes
    defined 713
    described 212
"Family Checkup: Positive Parenting
    Prevents Drug Abuse" (NIDA) 67n
"Family Relationships—Parents,
    Stepparents, Grandparents, and
    Guardians" (OWH) 83n
fats, described 105
FDA *see* U.S. Food and Drug
    Administration
Federal Bureau of Investigation (FBI)
    publication
        sextortion 600n
Federal Interagency Forum on Child
    and Family Statistics
    contact 718
    publication
        adolescent well-being
            indicators 33n
Federal Trade Commission (FTC),
    contact 718

female condom, described 290
fiber, benefits 106
fibroids *see* uterine fibroids
fight-or-flight, test anxiety 405
flu *see* influenza
fluoxetine
    depression 447
    obsessive-compulsive disorder 485
fluvoxamine, depression 448
fruits and vegetables, weight
    control 104
FTC *see* Federal Trade Commission
"Fungal Diseases—Ringworm"
    (CDC) 625n

G

gamma-aminobutyric acid, CNS
    depressants 553
gang crime, youth gangs and
    violence 694
"Gang Involvement Prevention—
    Girls, Juvenile Delinquency, and
    Gangs" (Youth.gov) 693n
gang member, youth gangs and
    violence 694
"Gangs and Gang Crime—What Is a
    Gang?" (NIJ) 693n
"General Supports for Youth with
    Chronic Conditions and Disabilities
    and Their Families" (OAH) 329n
"General Information about MRSA in
    the Community" (CDC) 380n
"General Information about VISA/
    VRSA" (CDC) 380n
generalized anxiety disorder
    antianxiety medications 456
    described 452
    mental health disorders in
        adolescence 432
genes
    alcohol use 536
    allergies 339
    attention deficit hyperactivity
        disorder (ADHD) 460
    bipolar disorder 468
    calories 104
    puberty 184
    schizophrenia 488
    weight loss 153

Genetic and Rare Diseases
    Information Center (GARD)
    publication
        growth hormone
            deficiency 363n
genetic mutation, cancer in
    children 349
genital area
    defined 713
    gynecologist 230
    hair removal 615
    HPV vaccine 282
    jock itch 631
    sexually transmitted diseases
        (STDs) 276
    yeast infection 244
gigantism, growth disorders 363
Girls and Boys Town National
    Hotline, contact 728
glands
    acne 333
    defined 714
    delayed puberty 257
    endocrine diseases 364
    male reproductive system 181
    precocious puberty 253
    testicular cancer 201
glutamate
    addiction and adolescent
        brain 506
    schizophrenia 488
gonorrhea
    menstrual irregularities 239
    sexually transmitted
        diseases 177
graduated driver licensing programs
    (GDL), driving safety for teens 587
grains
    child's eating habits 150
    lose weight 154
    nutrition recommendations 104
growing pains, overview 360–2
"Growing Pains" (Omnigraphics) 360n
growth disorders, overview 363–4
"Growth Disorders" (NIH) 363n
growth hormone deficiency (GHD),
    described 363
"Growth Hormone Deficiency"
    (GARD) 363n

growth spurt
  adolescent brain development 27
  puberty 184
  repetitive stress injuries 651
guilt
  depression 443
  eating disorders 481
  peer pressure 421
  sexual coercion 686
Guttmacher Institute, contact 724
gynecologist
  defined 714
  overview 228–31
  sexually transmitted diseases
    (STDs) 278
gynecomastia, overview 206–9
"Gynecomastia (Male Breast
  Development)" (Omnigraphics) 206n

H

hair removal
  overview 614–6
  pubic hair 216
"Having Body Image Issues"
  (OWH) 158n
hazing
  defined 714
  overview 677–8
"Hazing vs. Bullying"
  (OWH) 677n
health
  adolescent brain development 26
  drinking levels among youth 532
  food choices for teens 109
  nutrition recommendations for
    teens 103
  physical activity 134
  weight management 144
health insurance
  adolescent health 16
  cosmetic surgery 163
  healthcare 39
  paying for vaccines 101, 285
  secure parental employment 38
  sexually transmitted diseases
    (STDs) 277
  socioeconomic status 7
  see also insurance coverage

health problems
  adolescent health 9, 16
  birth control pills 307
  body image 161
  calcium 117
  chronic illness 329
  diabetes 355
  physical activity and obesity 137
  self-harm 493
  sexually transmitted diseases
    (STDs) 264
  suicide 497
  weight control 104, 149
Health Resources and Services
  Administration (HRSA), contact 718
Healthfinder®, contact 718
healthy choices
  adolescent brain development 31
  weight control 150
healthy eating
  erectile dysfunction 195
  nutrition recommendations for
    teens 104, 109
  physical activity and obesity 137
  weight management 149
"Healthy Friendships in Developing
  Adolescents" (HHS) 418n
healthy relationships
  parental monitoring 427
  positive parenting 60
  versus Unhealthy Relationships 420
"Healthy Schools—The Buzz on
  Energy Drinks" (CDC) 128n
"Healthy Schools—Physical Activity
  Facts" (CDC) 134n
healthy sexual decisions
  overview 262–6
  sexually transmitted diseases
    (STDs) 76
healthy snack, weight management in
  teens 151
healthy weight
  body mass index 144
  diabetes 357
  eating disorders 479
  erectile dysfunction 196
  medical care and your teen 92
  nutrition recommendations for
    teens 103

healthy weight, *continued*
  overweight 148, 153
  physical activity and obesity 137
  prenatal care 318
"Healthy Weight—About Child and
  Teen BMI" (CDC) 144n
hearing damage, noise induced
  hearing loss 643
heart disease
  calcium 119
  diabetes 357
  hookahs 524
  physical activity and obesity 56,
    104, 137
  stress 401
heavy menstrual periods, menstrual
  irregularities 238
"Helping Children and Adolescents
  Cope with Violence and Disasters:
  What Parents Can Do" (NIMH) 701n
"Helping Your Child Feel Connected
  to School" (CDC) 412n
hepatitis B, vaccine 265, 275
heredity
  adolescent brain
    development 25
  precocious puberty 253
  see also genes
heroin
  addiction and adolescent brain 505
  gynecomastia 207
  prescription drugs 550
  preventing and treating substance
    abuse 511
HHS *see* U.S. Department of Health
  and Human Services
high school smokers, nicotine
  addiction 519
"HIV/AIDS—Tips for Using Condoms
  and Dental Dams" (VA) 287n
"HIV/AIDS—What Is 'Safer Sex'?"
  (VA) 287n
HIV counseling, sexually transmitted
  diseases (STDs) and their
  prevention 281
HIV testing
  overview 279–81
  Youth Risk Behavior Surveillance
    System (YRBSS) 581

"HIV Testing among Adolescents"
  (CDC) 279n
homicide
  school-associated violent deaths 660
  underage drinking 533
  youth violence 656
homophobia, LGBT youth 325
hookahs
  overview 523–25
  tobacco and nicotine products 529
  see also water pipes
hormonal birth control
  birth control pills 307
  menstrual irregularities 239
  premenstrual syndrome (PMS) 235
The Hormone Foundation, contact 724
hormones
  birth control pills 307
  calcium 114
  defined 714
  delayed puberty 257
  developmental milestones 22
  endocrine diseases 364
  female reproductive system 211
  gynecomastia 206
  precocious puberty 255
  puberty 183
  stress 401
  tabulated *301*
  testicles 182
"How to Clean and Disinfect Schools
  to Help Slow the Spread of Flu"
  (CDC) 370n
"How the Female Reproductive
  System Works" (OWH) 211n
HPV *see* human papillomavirus
"HPV Vaccine Information for Young
  Women" (CDC) 281n
human immunodeficiency virus (HIV)
  abstinence 294
  practicing safer sex 287
  sexual health trends 176
  testing among adolescents 279
  vaginal yeast infections 240
human papillomavirus (HPV),
  vaccine 281
hydrocele, described 198
"Hydrocele" (Omnigraphics) 197n
hymen, described 212

hyperactivity
  attention deficit hyperactivity
    disorder (ADHD) 457
  youth violence 661
hypoallergenic cosmetics,
  described 612
hypogonadism
  delayed puberty 257
  erectile dysfunction 194
  gynecomastia 207

I

"If You Need to Lose Weight"
  (OWH) 153n
illicit drugs
  addiction 47
  borderline personality disorder 478
  mental health and substance use
    disorder 433
  prescription drug misuse 548
  stress management techniques 455
immune system
  allergies 339
  diabetes 356
  flu 371
  juvenile arthritis 366
  skin cancer 619
  tabulated *566*
  tanning 616
  vaginal yeast infections 240
  vitamin D 121
Immunization Action Coalition (IAC),
  contact 724
immunizations
  defined 714
  meningococcal infection 379
  prenatal care 318
  see also vaccines
impetigo, staphylococcal
  infections 381
Implanon, tabulated *300*
"Importance of Physical Activity"
  (HHS) 136n
income levels, teen pregnancy 315
incus, depicted *645*
infant mortality
  adolescent births 35
  statistics 55

infectious mononucleosis *see*
  mononucleosis
influenza (flu), overview 370–4
"Information and Advice about MRSA
  for School and Daycare Officials"
  (CDC) 380n
infrequent menstrual periods,
  menstrual irregularities 238
inguinal hernia, described 199
"Inguinal Hernia" (NIDDK) 197n
inguinal orchiectomy, testicular
  cancer 203
inhalants, overview 563–8
"Inhalants" (NIDA for Teens) 563n
insomnia
  energy drinks 129
  opioid misuse 551
insurance coverage *see* health
  insurance
intermenstrual bleeding, menstrual
  irregularities 238
International OCD (Obsessive-
  Compulsive Disorder) Foundation,
  contact 724
intimate partner violence
  dating violence 679
  healthy relationships 13
intrauterine devices (IUD)
  menstrual irregularities 239
  tabulated *300*
  types of birth control 298, 307
iron
  calcium 119
  hormonal birth control 309
  nutrition recommendations for
    teens 106
"Irregularities" (NICHD) 237n
IUD *see* intrauterine devices

J

jaw surgery, defined 392
jock itch, described 631
"Jock Itch" (Omnigraphics) 625n
juvenile arthritis,
  overview 365–7
"Juvenile Arthritis" (NIAMS) 365n
Juvenile Arthritis Alliance,
  contact 725

juvenile delinquency
  child maltreatment 36
  youth gangs 695
Juvenile Diabetes Research
  Foundation (JDRF), contact 725

K

Kaiser Family Foundation,
  contact 725
"Key Facts about Influenza (Flu)"
  (CDC) 370n
kidney disease
  diabetes 357
  erectile dysfunction 190
kidney stones, defined 119
kissing disease *see* mononucleosis
Klinefelter syndrome, delayed
  puberty 258

L

labia
  defined 213
  depicted *212*
lactose intolerance, calcium 116
lesbian, gay, bisexual, and
  transgender (LGBT) youth,
  overview 323–6
"Lesbian, Gay, Bisexual, and
  Transgender Health—LGBT Youth"
  (CDC) 323n
leukemia, statistics 348
Lexapro (escitalopram),
  depression 448
limbic system, described 504
low-cost birth control, described 311
luteinizing hormone (LH),
  defined 221
Luvox (fluvoxamine), depression 448

M

magic foods, healthy food
  choices 111
magnetic resonance imaging (MRI)
  brain development 27
  gynecomastia 207
  puberty 255
  skin safety 624

major depressive disorder
  depression 446
  mood disorders 433
"Make the Most of Your Child's
  Visit to the Doctor (Ages 11 to 14)"
  (ODPHP) 90n
"Make the Most of Your Child's
  Visit to the Doctor (Ages 15 to 17)"
  (ODPHP) 95n
male breast development *see*
  gynecomastia
male breast enlargement *see*
  gynecomastia
"The Male Reproductive System"
  (Omnigraphics) 181n
malleus, depicted *645*
malocclusion, overview 389–92
"Malocclusion" (Omnigraphics) 389n
manic episode, bipolar disorder 467
marijuana
  adolescent brain 505
  overview 539–46
  sleep habits 168
  substance abuse 67
"Marijuana: Facts Parents Need to
  Know" (NIDA) 539n
Mayo Clinic, contact 725
medication-assisted treatment (MAT),
  described 559
medications
  asthma 343
  athlete's foot 630
  attention deficit hyperactivity
    disorder 461
  bipolar disorder 470
  central nervous system
    depressants 552
  depression 449
  gynecomastia 208
  immune suppression system 622
  marijuana 543
  meningococcal disease 375
  menstrual irregularities 238
  mental disorders 435
  obsessive-compulsive disorder 485
  precocious puberty 256
  prenatal care 320
  repetitive stress injuries 650
  social anxiety disorder 453
  stress management 456

melanoma
  skin cancer 619
  sunburn 617
memory impairment, marijuana 541
meningitis
  defined 714
  meningococcal disease 376
  vaccines 100
"Meningococcal" (CDC) 375n
meningococcal disease, overview
  375–80
menopause
  premenstrual syndrome (PMS) 231
  puberty 219
  vaginal yeast infections 240
menstrual cycle
  menstrual irregularities 237
  pregnancy 317
"Menstrual Cycle" (OWH) 219n
menstruation
  defined 714
  overview 219–25
Mental Health America, contact 725
mental health issues, suicide
  risks 498
mental illness
  bipolar disorder 467
  co-occurring disorders 433
  defined 714
  trauma stress 706
mentoring, described 700
methadone
  gynecomastia 207
  medication-assisted
    treatment 559
methicillin-resistant Staphylococcus
  aureus (MRSA), described 381
Microsporum canis, ultraviolet
  light 628
"Misuse of Prescription Drugs"
  (NIDA) 547n
"Monitoring Your Teen's Activities:
  What Parents and Families Should
  Know" (CDC) 80n, 425n
mononucleosis, overview 386–8
mood disorders
  borderline personality disorder 472
  described 433
mood episodes, bipolar disorder 468

"Most U.S. Middle and High Schools
  Start the School Day Too Early"
  (CDC) 166n
motor vehicle related (MVR) injury,
  adolescents 46
MRSA *see* methicillin-resistant
  Staphylococcus aureus
muscle strengthening, physical
  activity 135
mutual monogamy,
  described 266
myelin, adolescent brain
  development 27

N

naltrexone, substance abuse 559
National Adolescent Health
  Information Center (NAHIC),
  contact 725
National Alliance on Mental Illness
  (NAMI), contact 725
National Campaign to Prevent
  Teen and Unplanned Pregnancy,
  contact 725
National Cancer Institute (NCI)
  contact 718
  publications
    cancer 347n
    testicular cancer 200n
National Center for Missing and
  Exploited Children (NCMEC),
  contact 725
National Clearinghouse for Alcohol
  and Drug Information (NCADI),
  contact 728
National Diabetes Education Program
  (NDEP), contact 719
National Domestic Violence Hotline,
  contact 728
National Heart, Lung, and Blood
  Institute (NHLBI)
  publication
    asthma 343n
National Highway Traffic Safety
  Administration (NHTSA)
  contact 719
  publication
    teen driving 587n

National Institute of Arthritis and
Musculoskeletal and Skin Diseases
(NIAMS)
  publications
    acne 333n
    juvenile arthritis 365n
    scoliosis 393n
National Institute of Diabetes and
Digestive and Kidney Diseases
(NIDDK)
  contact 719
  publications
    diabetes 355n
    erectile dysfunction 188n
    inguinal hernia 197n
    perineal injury in males 197n
    teen health guide 103n
    weight management 148n
National Institute of Justice (NIJ)
  publication
    gang violence 693n
National Institute of Mental Health
(NIMH)
  contact 720
  publications
    antidepressant
      medications 446n
    anxiety disorders 452n
    attention deficit hyperactivity
      disorder 457n
    bipolar disorder 467n
    borderline personality
      disorder 472n
    children with mental
      illness 435n
    coping with
      disaster 701n
    eating disorders 478n
    obsessive-compulsive
      disorder 482n
    schizophrenia 486n
    teen depression 442n
National Institute of Neurological
Disorders and Stroke (NINDS),
  contact 719
National Institutes of Health (NIH)
  contact 720
  publications
    allergy 339n

National Institutes of Health (NIH)
  publications, *continued*
    chronic illness/diseases 329n
    diabetes 355n
    drug problems 509n
    endocrine diseases 363n
    growth disorders 363n
    positive parenting 60n
    scoliosis 393n
    staphylococcal infections 380n
    teen development 21n
National Institute on Alcohol Abuse
and Alcoholism (NIAAA)
  contact 719
  publications
    peer pressure 421n
    preventing childhood alcohol
      use 534n
National Institute on Deafness and
Other Communication Disorders
(NIDCD)
  contact 720
  publication
    noise-induced hearing
      loss 643n
National Institute on Drug Abuse
(NIDA)
  contact 720
  publications
    addiction and adolescent
      brain 503n
    caffeine 130n
    helping your teen with drug
      problem 569n
    marijuana 539n
    prescription drugs misuse 547n
    substance abuse 67n
National Institute on Drug Abuse
(NIDA) for Teens
  publications
    coping up with stress 399n
    inhalants 563n
National Runaway Safeline (NRS),
  contact 729
National Safety Council (NSC),
  contact 726
National Scoliosis Foundation (NSF),
  contact 726
National Suicide Hotline, contact 729

National Women's Health Information Center (NWHIC), contact 720
National Youth Anti-Drug Media Campaign, contact 720
National Youth Network, contact 726
natural rhythm methods, birth control 307
NCI *see* National Cancer Institute
NDEP *see* National Diabetes Education Program
needle epilators, hair removal 614
neighborhood
    communication 64
    safety 13
    youth violence 662
neisseria meningitidis, meningococcal disease 375
Nemours Foundation Center for Children's Health Media, contact 726
neonatal abstinence syndrome (NAS), prescription drug abuse 555
neurons
    addiction 504
    brain development 25
neurotransmitters
    defined 504
    schizophrenia 488
NIAAA *see* National Institute on Alcohol Abuse and Alcoholism
NIAMS *see* National Institute of Arthritis and Musculoskeletal and Skin Diseases
NICHD *see Eunice Kennedy Shriver* National Institute of Child Health and Human Development
nicotine
    defined 714
    drug abuse 509
    drug treatment 527
    smokeless tobacco 521
nicotine addiction, overview 516–9
"Nicotine Addiction and Your Health" (HHS) 516n
"Nicotine and Addiction" (HHS) 516n
nicotine replacement products, drug treatment 528

NIDCD *see* National Institute on Deafness and Other Communication Disorders
NIDDK *see* National Institute of Diabetes and Digestive and Kidney Diseases
NIMH *see* National Institute of Mental Health
"Nine Tips to Help You Cope with Stress" (NIDA for Teens) 399n
nitrites, described 564
nocturnal erection test, erectile dysfunction 193
nodules, acne 335
noise damage, described 645
"Noise Induced Hearing Loss" (NIDCD) 643n
noise induced hearing loss (NIHL), described 643
nonconscious memory system, drug addiction 506
nonfatal injuries
    work safety 633
    youth violence 659
nontobacco products, nicotine use 525
nutrition *see* diet and nutrition
nutrition facts label
    calories 112
    eating habits 151
    fats 106

O

obesity
    body image 158
    defined 714
    depression 55
    diabetes 356
    male reproductive concerns 207
    physical activity 134
    sleep 169
    statistics 9
    stimulants 554
    stress 401
obsessive-compulsive disorder (OCD)
    defined 714
    overview 482–6
"Obsessive-Compulsive Disorder" (NIMH) 482n

OCD *see* obsessive-compulsive
disorder
Office of Adolescent Health (OAH)
publications
adolescent brain
development 25n
chronic health problems 329n
communicating with your
child 63n
mental health in
adolescents 431n
trends in teen pregnancy and
childbearing 175n
Office of Dietary
Supplements (ODS)
publications
calcium 114n
vitamin D 121n
Office of Disease Prevention and
Health Promotion (ODPHP)
publications
adolescent health 15n
tobacco, alcohol, and drugs 67n
healthy relationships 72n
sex 75n
visiting the doctor (ages 11
to 14) 90n
visiting the doctor (ages 15
to 17) 95n
physical activity guidelines for
adolescents 138n
Office on Women's Health (OWH)
publications
birth control methods 297n
body image 158n
cosmetic surgery 162n
cutting and self-harm 493n
dating violence 679n
deciding about sex 262n, 293n
douching 245n
emotional problems 83n
family relationships 83n
female reproductive
system 211n
gynecologist 228n
hazing versus bullying 677n
lose weight 153n
menstrual cycle 219n
pregnancy 316n

Office on Women's Health (OWH)
publications, *continued*
premenstrual syndrome
(PMS) 231n
puberty 211n
self-esteem and self-
confidence 158n
sleep 169n
stalking 673n
STDs and STIs 274n
stress 399n
vaginal yeast infections 240n
oligomenorrhea, menstrual
irregularities 238
Omnigraphics
publications
cheating 409n
growing pains 360n
gynecomastia (male breast
development) 206n
hydrocele 197n
jock itch 625n
male reproductive
system 181n
malocclusion 389n
repetitive stress injuries in
teens 648n
spermatocele 197n
test anxiety 404n
testicular self-
examination 200n
opioid overdose, naloxone 560
opioids
central nervous system
depressants 561
described 550
marijuana 542
substance use disorder 511
oppositional defiant
disorder (ODD)
defined 714
described 464
oral contraceptives, birth control 306
oral health, described 41
oral sex
abstinence 264
defined 714
sexually transmitted
diseases 290

osteoporosis
  calcium 117
  eating disorders 479
  physical activity 134
ovaries
  birth control 307
  defined 715
  delayed puberty 257
  douche 246
  female reproductive system 211
  pelvic exam 230
overweight
  body mass index 145
  physical inactivity 134
  precocious puberty 253
  statistics 9
  type 2 diabetes 357
  weight management 149
ovulation
  defined 715
  described 220
ovum, female reproductive system 212

P

pads/tampons, menstrual cycle 222
painful periods, dysmenorrhea 238
Palo Alto Medical Foundation
  (PAMF), contact 726
panic disorder
  defined 715
  described 453
pap test
  cervical cancer 285
  defined 715
  described 230
papules, acne 334
parent management training (PMT),
  psychosocial therapies 436
parent-teen driving agreement, safe
  driving 591
"Parents Are the Key to Safe Teen
  Drivers" (CDC) 591n
Parents, Families, and Friends
  of Lesbians and Gays (PFLAG),
  contact 726
parental monitoring
  described 80
  overview 425–30

parenting
  alcohol use 535
  monitoring 425
  positive 62
  pregnancy 321
"Parenting to Prevent Childhood
  Alcohol Use" (NIAAA) 534n
paroxetine, antidepressant
  medications 447
Partnership for Drug-Free Kids,
  contact 726
Paxil (paroxetine), antidepressant
  medications 447
PCOS *see* polycystic ovary syndrome
peer pressure
  dating relationships 418
  defined 715
  overview 421–4
"Peer Pressure" (NIAAA) 421n
pelvic exam, described 230
pelvic inflammatory disease (PID)
  described 278
  hormonal birth control 309
penis
  defined 715
  described 181
  erectile dysfunction 191
  human papillomavirus vaccines 282
  testicular cancer 205
perineal injury, described 199
"Perineal Injury in Males"
  (NIDDK) 197n
period *see* menstrual cycle
pertussis (whooping cough),
  vaccine 101
Pew Internet and American Life
  Project, contact 726
phobia, defined 715
photokeratitis, described 621
physical activity
  behavior disorder 466
  calcium 117
  erectile dysfuntion 193
  nutrition recommendation 103
  obesity 56
  overview 134–41
  premenstrual syndrome 234
  sleep habits 167
  statistics 9

physical changes, puberty 217

physical environment, adolescent well-being 42

physical examination
  growing pain 361
  skin safety 631

physical therapy, recurrent stress injuries 650

pilosebaceous units, acne 333

pimples *see* acne

pinna, depicted *645*

pituitary gland
  growth disorders 363
  hypogonadism 258
  menstrual irregularities 238

Planned Parenthood. contact 726

Planned Parenthood Federation of America, contact 729

plastic surgery, cosmetic surgery 163

PMDD *see* premenstrual dysphoric disorder

PMS *see* premenstrual syndrome

pneumonia, methicillin-resistant Staphylococcus aureus 381

polycystic ovary syndrome (PCOS), menstrual cycle 221

pornography, Internet safety 602

positive parenting, overview 60–2

"Positive Parenting—Building Healthy Relationships with Your Kids" (NIH) 60n

positive youth development (PYD), described 19

posttraumatic stress disorder (PTSD)
  defined 715
  stress 706

potency, marijuana 541

poverty levels *see* income levels

PPFA *see* Planned Parenthood Federation of America

precocious puberty, overview 252–6

preconception care, prenatal care 318

preeclampsia, defined 118

pregnancy
  abstinence 265
  menstrual cycle 219
  menstrual irregularities 238

pregnancy, *continued*
  parental monitoring 425

sexual assault 688

sexually transmitted infections 306

statistics 176

vaccine 283

premature aging, described 618

premenstrual dysphoric disorder (PMDD), premenstrual syndrome 232

premenstrual syndrome (PMS), overview 231–7

"Premenstrual Syndrome (PMS)" (OWH) 231n

prenatal care, described 319

"Prenatal Care" (NICHD) 318n

prescription drug abuse, described 548

prescription medicine abuse, overview 547–61

"Preventing Tobacco Use among Youth and Young Adults Fact Sheet" (HHS) 516n

prolonged menstrual bleeding, menstrual irregularities 239

prostate gland, male reproductive system 181

psychotherapy
  bipolar disorder 470
  defined 715
  described 454
  eating disorder 481
  mental health disorder 435

psychotropic medications, described 436

PTSD *see* posttraumatic stress disorder

puberty
  defined 715
  described 183
  female sexual development 213
  schizophrenia 488
  see also delayed puberty; precocious puberty

"Puberty and Precocious Puberty: Overview" (NICHD) 252n

"Puberty and Precocious Puberty: Condition Information" (NICHD) 257n

pubic area, defined 715

pubic hair, precocious puberty 253

Q

QuitGuide, described 530
quitSTART, described 530

R

race and ethnicity,
statistics 6
rape
date rape drugs 682
defined 683
juvenile arrests 660
Rape, Abuse & Incest National
Network (RAINN), contact 729
receptors, described 504
reflex, conditioning 507
"Removing Hair Safely" (FDA) 614n
repetitive stress injuries,
overview 648–52
"Repetitive Stress Injuries in Teens"
(Omnigraphics) 648n
"Reproductive Health—Teen
Pregnancy" (CDC) 314n
reproductive organ, defined 715
reproductive system
female 211
male 181
rhythm method, birth control 307
ringworm, described 625
"Risk and Protective Factors—Youth
Violence" (CDC) 661n
risk factors
anxiety disorder 454
bullying 668
growing pains 361
gynecomastia 206
meningococcal
disease 375
schizophrenia 487
suicide 497
testicular cancer 201
Tourette syndrome 492
youth violence 661
risk-taking, driving 587
"The Risks of Tanning"
(FDA) 616n
risperidone, antipsychotic
medication 485

S

SAFE Alternatives (Self- Abuse
Finally Ends), contact 727, 729
safer sex, overview 287–92
salicylic acid, acne treatment 335
saliva, meningococcal disease 376
SAMHSA *see* Substance Abuse
and Mental Health Services
Administration
saturated fat, healthy eating 105
schizophrenia
defined 715
overview 486–9
"Schizophrenia" (NIMH) 486n
school, attention deficit hyperactivity
disorder 459
school violence, statistics 659
scoliosis
defined 715
overview 393–5
"Scoliosis" (NIH) 393n
"Scoliosis in Children and
Adolescents" (NIAMS) 393n
scrotum, described 182
sebaceous gland, depicted *334*
sebum, described 333
secondhand smoke, health risks 43
secure parental employment,
adolescent well being 38
selective serotonin reuptake inhibitors
(SSRIs), described 485
self-esteem
distorted body image 479
overview 158–62
"Self-Esteem and Self-Confidence"
(OWH) 158n
self-injury, overview 493–5
semen
defined 715
pregnancy risk 265
semicircular canals, depicted *645*
seminal vesicles, male reproductive
system 181
septicemia, meningococcal disease 375
sertraline, antidepressant
medications 447
sex education, overview 266–71
Sex, Etc., contact 727

sex hormones, defined 716
"Sextortion Affecting Thousands of
   U.S. Children" (FBI) 600n
sexual activity
   abstinence 293
   safer sex 94
   sexual coercion 685
   statistics 175
   teen pregnancy 314
"Sexual Activity, Contraceptive Use,
   and Childbearing of Teenagers
   Aged 15–19 in the United States"
   (CDC) 175n
sexual assault
   defined 716
   overview 683–92
"Sexual Assault" (HHS) 683n
sexual coercion, described 685
sexual contact, defined 716
sexual exploitation, sextortion 600
sexual health trends, overview 175–9
sexual intercourse, defined 716
"Sexual Risk Behaviors: HIV, STD,
   and Teen Pregnancy Prevention"
   (CDC) 175n
Sexuality Information and Education
   Council of the United States
   (SIECUS), contact 727
sexually transmitted diseases (STDs)
   abstinence 264
   defined 716
   overview 274–9
   safer sex 287
   statistics 176
"Sexually Transmitted Diseases
   (STDs)—How You Can Prevent
   Sexually Transmitted Diseases"
   (CDC) 262n
sildenafil (Viagra), erectile
   dysfunction medication 194
skin problems, acne 333
sleep deprivation, overview 166–9
smokefree app, described 529
"Smokefree Apps" (HHS) 526n
smokeless tobacco, overview 520–2
"Smokeless Tobacco (Dip, Chew,
   Snuff)" (CDC) 520n
"Smokeless Tobacco: Get the Facts"
   (HHS) 520n

smoking, health risks 48
"Smoking and Tobacco Use—
   Hookahs" (CDC) 523n
snuff, smokeless tobacco 520
social-development strategies, youth
   violence prevention 657
social media
   cyberbullying 666
   cyberstalking 674
   safety tips 603
   statistics 604
social networking, overview 603–7
social phobia, described 453
Society for Adolescent Health and
   Medicine (SAHM), contact 727
solar keratoses, described 620
speculum, pelvic exam 230
sperm
   defined 716
   pregnancy 316
spermatocele, described 199
"Spermatocele" (Omnigraphics) 197n
spermicides, described 308
spice, described 543
stalking, overview 673–6
"Stalking" (OWH) 673n
stapes, depicted *645*
staphylococcal infections,
   overview 380–5
"Staphylococcal Infections"
   (NIH) 380n
Staphylococcus aureus, staph
   infections 380
statistics
   adolescent health 3
   adolescent well-being 33
   adolescent workers 633
   bullying 660
   childhood cancers 348
   inhalants use 564
   marijuana use 540
   meningococcal disease 379
   sex education 266
   sexual health trends 175
   suicide 497
   teen pregnancy 314
   tobacco use 522
   underage drinking 532
   youth violence 658

STD *see* sexually transmitted diseases
"STDs in Adolescents and Young
Adults" (CDC) 175n
sterilization, birth control method 298
steroid injections, repetitive stress
injuries treatment 650
stimulants, energy drinks 128
stress, overview 399–402
"Stress and Your Health" (OWH) 399n
stress fractures, defined 649
Striving To Reduce Youth Violence
Everywhere (STRYVE), contact 720
Students Against Destructive
Decisions (SADD), contact 727
"Students—Teens" (USDA) 109n
substance abuse, communication tips 67
Substance Abuse and Mental Health
Services Administration (SAMHSA),
contact 720
suicide, overview 497–9
"Suicide among Youth" (CDC) 497n
Suicide Awareness Voices of
Education (SAVE), contact 727
"Suicide Prevention" (Youth.gov) 497n
sunburn, described 616
sweat glands, puberty 184
syphilis, defined 716

T

"Take Charge of Your Health: A Guide
for Teenagers" (NIDDK) 103n
"Talk to Your Kids about Sex"
(ODPHP) 75n
"Talk to Your Kids about Tobacco,
Alcohol, and Drugs" (ODPHP) 67n
"Talk with Your Teen about Healthy
Relationships" (ODPHP) 72n
"Talking with Teens about Peer
Relationships: How You Make a
Difference" (HHS) 425n
tattoos
gangs 695
overview 622–5
taurine, energy drinks 128
technology
Internet safety 599
online dating 681
stalking 673

"Technology and Youth: Protecting
Your Child from Electronic
Aggression" (CDC) 598n
"Teen Depression" (NIMH) 442n
"Teen Development" (NIH) 21n
teen drivers, overview 584–7
"Teen Driving" (NHTSA) 587n
"Teen Drivers: Get the Facts"
(CDC) 584n
teen pregnancies
overview 314–21
statistics 179
unplanned 263
"Teen Pregnancy—About Teen
Pregnancy" (CDC) 175n
"Teen Sleep Habits—What Should
You Do?" (CDC) 166n
TeenGrowth, contact 727
"Teens' Social Media Use: How They
Connect and What It Means for
Health" (HHS) 603n
tendonitis, recurrent stress
injuries 650
test anxiety, overview 404–9
"Test Anxiety" (Omnigraphics) 404n
testicles
common disorders 197
peripheral precocious puberty 254
testicular cancer, overview 200–5
"Testicular Cancer Treatment
(PDQ®)—Patient Version"
(NCI) 200n
testicular self-examination (TSE),
described 204
"Testicular Self-Examination"
(Omnigraphics) 200n
testosterone, defined 716
tests
bipolar disorder 470
flu 372
precocious puberty 255
sexually transmitted diseases 277
test anxiety 405
tetanus, vaccine 101
THC (delta-9-tetrahydrocannabinol),
marijuana 540
threading, skin safety 615
tinea infections, overview 625–31
tinea pedis, ringworm 626

"Tip Sheets for Parents and
Caregivers" (HHS) 320n
tobacco, defined 716
tobacco use, described 11
tolerance, prescription medicine
abuse 551
topical medicines, acne 335
Tourette syndrome,
overview 490–2
toxic shock syndrome (TSS), female
hygiene 224
transporters, brain 504
trauma, described 701
"Treatment of Children with Mental
Illness" (NIMH) 435n
"Trends in Teen Pregnancy and
Childbearing" (OAH) 175n
TSE *see* testicular self-examination
TSS *see* toxic shock syndrome
tumor markers, testicular cancer 202
"2008 Physical Activity Guidelines for
Americans" (ODPHP) 138n

U

underage drinking
drunk driving 588
overview 532–4
"Understanding Teen Dating
Violence" (CDC) 679n
"Understanding the Effects
of Maltreatment on Brain
Development" (HHS) 25n
"Understanding Youth Violence"
(CDC) 656n
undescended testicle, testicular
cancer 201
unintentional overdose deaths,
prescription medicine abuse 547
unplanned pregnancy
abstinence 294
healthy sexual
decisions 262
unsafe behaviors, parental
monitoring 81
urethra
described 182
erectile dysfunction 195
male reproductive system 181

U.S. Department of Agriculture
(USDA)
publication
healthy food choices for
teens 109n
U.S. Department of Education (ED),
contact 721
U.S. Department of Health and
Human Services (HHS)
contact 721
publications
abstinence 293n
brain development 25n
bullying 671n
healthy relationship 418n
nicotine addiction 516n
parental tips 320n
peer relationships 425n
physical activity 136n
sexual assault 683n
smokefree 526n
smokeless tobacco 520n
social media use 603n
statistics on adolescent 3n
tobacco use prevention 516n
vaccines 100n
U.S. Department of Labor (DOL),
contact 721
U.S. Department of Veterans Affairs
(VA)
publications
safe sex 287n
tips for using condoms and
dental dams 287n
U.S. Food and Drug Administration
(FDA)
contact 721
publications
cosmetics 610n
hair removal 614n
tanning risks 616n
tattoo safety 622n
U.S. National Library of Medicine
(NLM), contact 721
uterine fibroids, menstrual
irregularities 239
uterus
birth control 307
defined 716